Counseling and Psychotherapy

Counseling and Psychotherapy: Theoretical Analyses and Skills Applications

Leroy G. Baruth
University of South Carolina

Charles H. Huber
Child Guidance Clinic of Jacksonville, Florida

Macmillan Publishing Company
866 Third Avenue New York, New York   10022

Maxwell Macmillan Canada, Inc.
1200 Eglinton Avenue East, Suite 200
Don Mills, Ontario M3C 3N1

Library of Congress Cataloging-in-Publication Data

Library of Congress Catalog Card Number: 84-61382
International Standard Book Number: 0-675-20229-X
Printed in the United States of America

Print   4 5 6 7 8   Year 2 3 4 5 6 7

This book was set in Frutiger
Production Editor: Mary Henkener
Cover Design Coordination: Cathy Watterson
Text Designer: Cynthia Brunk

Photo credits:
pp. xiv, 10, 134, Ginny Halloran; p. 21, Alan Cliburn; p. 148, Randall D. Williams, photo reproduced by permission of the Licking County Board of Mental Retardation; pp. 155, 288, 329, Jean Greenwald; p. 26 courtesy of Rollo May; p. 48 © 1970 Real People Press/Deke Siman, photographer; pp. 59, 62, 78, 161, 204, 240, 311, 316, 327, Strix Pix; p. 95 courtesy of the Institute for Rational-Emotive Therapy; p. 101 C. Quinlan; p. 117, Nationwide Insurance Company; p.176, Nozizwe S. p. 246 © Jack Hamilton; p. 310, Robert Maust.

Preface

Theoretical models of counseling and psychotherapy have many important purposes. Conceptually, they serve as catalysts of new hypotheses, thus refining current ideas and stimulating theory development. These models also serve three functions essential to successful intervention.

First, theoretical models enable therapists to organize the immense amount of information they face so that hypotheses can be proposed to guide the course of therapy.

Second, theoretical models help therapists understand adaptive and maladaptive human functioning. Although appropriate modes of functioning are primarily defined by prevailing societal values and norms, theory underscores and explains how and why humans feel, think, and act the way they do.

Finally, theoretical models provide a conceptual foundation for developing and determining appropriate therapeutic strategies. In doing so, they suggest a plan for therapists to pursue in helping clients.

Theoretical approaches, however, are not sets of techniques. They are *theories* of human functioning; ways of understanding people that can be used to help them change. Using a particular theoretical basis in counseling and psychotherapy simply means working with clients according to its principles: its view of human nature, its goals for therapy, its ideal therapeutic process. Therapists, however, need means to apply theory: techniques, or *skills*.

The skills used in counseling and psychotherapy for some time were viewed as almost mystical—immune to systematic study and definition. Research of the past decade and a half, however, has clearly shown that certain key dimensions of how clients are interviewed underly all counseling and therapeutic approaches. The extensive and rigorous research of Carkhuff and his associates (Carkhuff, 1969, 1971, 1972, 1973; Carkhuff & Berenson, 1967; Truax & Carkhuff, 1967) has resulted in a scientific model made up of phases that spell out specific techniques used in effective therapy. Not only does this model provide the required therapist tasks for each of its phases, but it also delineates the skills needed to complete these tasks.

Using Carkhuff's work, and independently, others have similarly categorized essential therapist skills within their own *systematic skills* models (Cormier & Cormier, 1979; Egan, 1975,

1982; Hackney & Nye, 1973; Ivey, 1971; Ivey & Authier, 1978; Ivey & Simek-Downing, 1980; Okun, 1982). All of these writers strongly believe that a systematic set of therapist skills is vital in effective counseling and psychotherapy.

We share this belief. Theory offers goals to pursue and a systematic skills model provides an organized means of achieving them. Combining theoretical knowledge with skills expertise results in effective and efficient counseling and psychotherapeutic efforts.

The major concern of the faculty and students of any counseling and psychotherapy training program is integrating theory (forming a conceptual knowledge base) with techniques and procedures (a specific skill repertoire). Field experiences all too soon follow classroom coursework. If students lack both an understanding of theory and technique and the ability to effectively integrate them, these field placements become an anxiety-producing and disappointing learning endeavor in which clients can be more harmed then helped. Students often remark on the need to combine theory and technique in a more understandable, let alone pragmatic, manner.

We recall our own fears as beginning clinicians when we first tried to integrate the theory and technique we learned and experimented with in class. Although our textbooks explained both theory and techniques quite well, these resources rarely suggested the specific skills best suited for implementing specific theoretical concepts. This knowledge came later through trial and error (unfortunately so for our clients) and clinical supervision. Supervisors, knowledgeable and skilled from hours of contacts with clients, taught us how to augment and integrate conceptualizations with specific skills to best help our clients.

As both practicing clinicians and educators, we have codified the aforementioned "oral supervisory teachings" to combine theory and

skills in a concrete, structured, and *integrated* way. Should you choose to use rational-emotive, person-centered, or any of the other intervention theories we discuss, you will be able to understand how best to implement their specific concepts by using effective skills. Further, we suggest that you try to become equally competent at using specific skills in and of themselves.

The book is divided into four major Parts. Part I sets the stage for the theoretical analyses and skills applications to come. Chapter 1 describes a framework for learning specific theoretical approaches, skills with which to implement them, and how to apply these skills. Part II explains the major theoretical approaches to counseling and psychotherapy. Part III provides the means of putting theory into practice: skills. As well as explaining skills, these chapters in this Part discuss how the particular skills can be used to implement each of the major theories in Part II. Finally, Part IV discusses how clinical accountability can help both clients and counselors in making therapy more effective. Chapters 11 and 12 consider two primary points: (a) the belief that therapy has inherent obstacles that must be dealt with if it is to be successful, and (b) that as professionals, therapists must adhere to recognized standards of competence and certification, practice according to stated ethical standards, and constantly strive to improve the services they offer by acting as therapist/researchers and research consumers.

We have provided clinical examples and case illustrations throughout all four Parts to help you to internalize and understand the concepts and skills we present. We recommend that you always remember that clients are complex human beings. The models of human functioning we present are simplified for convenience. Much literature has been devoted to *each* of the theories we present, and we urge you to explore it. At the end of each chapter we list recommended resources to guide you to additional information.

Finally, any form of counseling or psychotherapy is more than just using theory or applying techniques. It is the personality of the therapist and the attitude he or she has toward clients, the world, and self. Continuing self-exploration and growth should always be a goal concurrent with one's professional training and career.

We would like to thank a number of reviewers for their constructive suggestions during manuscript development. They include Ursula Delworth, University of Iowa; Beverly Celotta, Celotta & Jacobs Associates; James Fruehling, Northeastern Illinois University; and Gail Hackett, Ohio State University.

We are especially grateful to the individuals who worked with us on the audio tape that accompanies this book: Walter Bailey, Seana Baruth, Bob Bowman, Margaret Burggraf, Maurice Campbell, Patricia Lambert, Courtney Neale, and Al Turner. We are particularly indebted to Vicki Knight, administrative editor, and Mary Henkener, production editor, both with Charles E. Merrill Publishing Company.

Contents

3

Behaviorally-Oriented Approaches 57

4

Cognitively-Oriented Approaches 93

5

Comparing and Contrasting: Clarifying a Pragmatic Therapeutic Position 129

**PART THREE
PUTTING THEORY INTO PRACTICE:
A SKILLS APPROACH**

6

The Course of Counseling and Psychotherapy 153

7

Phase One: Creating a Therapeutic Climate   171

8

Phase Two: Discriminating and Defining Client Problems   199

9

Phase Three: Goal Setting   224

10

Phase Four: Proactive Problem Intervention   259

PART FOUR
CLINICAL ACCOUNTABILITY

11

12

Part One

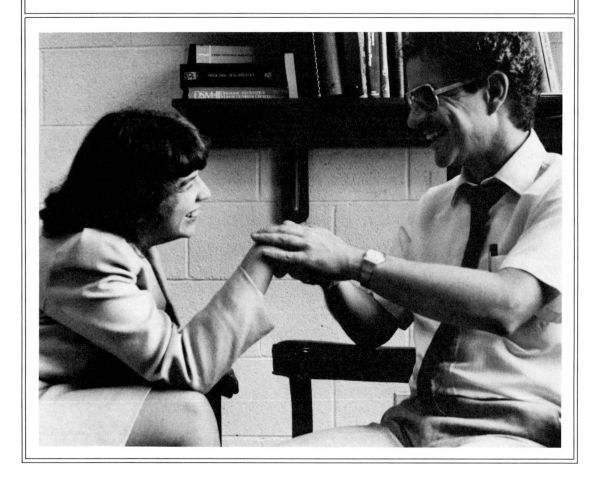

A Framework for Change: Establishing a Theoretical Base

Sure, I'm only 20 and already divorced! I realize I made a stupid mistake getting married at 17. Neither of us was ready to make such a commitment. But it seems like no one is willing to let me forget. I can't find a decent job; and my parents, well, the heck with them. Is something I did at 17 going to count against me the rest of my life?

Imagine a young man coming to you for therapy and telling you this story. What aspect about this situation do you consider most important from a therapeutic standpoint? On what might you first begin to focus? Most likely, you do have some thoughts on how to proceed and suggestions for the client. Your prescriptions come from your personal philosophy of helping—the philosophy you have developed from your experiences of the nature of human beings, your perceptions of the "good life," and your views on what constitutes a mature, well-functioning person.

Aspiring counselors and psychotherapists enter training to acquire the theory and accompanying skills to assist clients. To their study, they bring their own personalities as life has molded them. Most people can and do assist others by sharing their own methods of coping, how they help themselves, their friends, and their family to live more satisfying lives. A helper's effectiveness, however, must be judged in terms of degree.

"Helping" is not a neutral process; it is *for better or for worse* (Carkhuff & Anthony, 1979; Carkhuff & Berenson, 1976). If a distressed person finds a "high-level" helper, he or she is likely to psychologically improve, to begin to live more effectively according to a variety of outcome criteria. However, if he or she becomes involved with a "low-level" helper, it is quite likely that the client will get worse (Egan, 1975).

We hope to expand your personal philosophy of helping to ensure that you will function as an effective therapist. We begin, in chapter 1, by considering the importance of establishing a therapeutic base, the available theories, and a framework from which to work effectively with clients.

1

Developing a Pragmatic Therapeutic Position

Practicing counseling without an explicit theoretical rationale
is somewhat like flying a plane without a map and without
instruments.

(Corey, Corey, & Callanan, 1984, p. 102)

At the opening of his address "A House Divided," Abraham Lincoln conveyed a concern especially relevant to this chapter: "If we could first know where we are, and whither we are tending, we could better judge what to do, and how to do it."

Early, accurate assessment of clients' problems and specific therapeutic goals are the essence of initial therapy efforts. As the process continues therapists should know *what* they plan to do in their sessions with clients and *why* they will do it. This is the basic function of a therapeutic position—to make sense of clients' concerns and provide therapeutic direction.

ELEMENTS OF AN EFFECTIVE THERAPEUTIC POSITION

Theory applied to counseling and psychotherapy has been defined as a statement of general principles, verified by data, that explain certain phenomena (Shertzer & Stone, 1974). As such, theory deals with principles rather than practice; however, theory should not be viewed as removed from practice. Theory is not simply impractical ideas unrelated to day-to-day reality. Rather, theory is an essential underpinning of effective practice. George and Christiana (1981) further illustrate this point:

> When a counselor is baffled by a problem, he turns to theory to enlarge his perspective about the various alternatives. Since a theory's ability to explain what we are doing suggests the value of that theory, it follows that a theory would also suggest what needs to be done when we are faced with a problem. (p. 126)

Hansen, Stevic, and Warner (1982) have delineated five requirements of a good theory. These requirements can also be used to identify basic elements of an effective therapeutic position:

1. It must be clear, easily understood, and communicable. Its assumptions must form a coherent pattern and not be contradictory.
2. It is comprehensive. It supplies plausible explanations for a variety of phenomena in a variety of situations.
3. It is explicit enough to generate research. It is designed so that it can be subjected to the rigors of scientific inquiry.
4. It relates means to desired outcomes, stating specific procedures for achieving an end product. Defining outcomes without stating how to achieve them is not a formulation of theory but a mere statement of objectives (Williamson, 1965).

5. An effective therapeutic position is useful to its intended practition-ers. It provides the researcher with principles that can be subjected to experimental testing. It gives the therapist guidelines for using specific procedures with specific clients.

These elements form the *external* aspects of a therapeutic position; i.e., its guidelines for practice derived from a clearly formulated set of assumptions. These assumptions emanate from the established theoretical structure of the approach.

A second means of judging a theory is to examine how closely it matches your personal philosophy of helping, which comprises your ex-periences, your personality, your likes and dislikes, and your informal as-sumptions about people and what makes them tick. It's foolish to expect future counselors and psychotherapists to accept, let alone internalize, what might be foreign to their makeup. Shertzer and Stone (1974) likened this important compatibility to a counselor's wearing a suit of clothes:

> He cannot operate maturely and professionally in borrowed clothes. Preferably, his suit is tailor-made with the cloth and style selected upon the basis of his individual taste. (p. 250)

Personal values and experiences are a large part of the therapeutic position that counselors and psychotherapists develop. These variables likewise heavily influence a therapist's potential effectiveness. Williamson (1962) in this regard spoke of the "counselor as technique":

> I refer to the counselor himself as a technique of counseling; not only what he does or says in the interview, but how he conducts himself and the manner of often unverbalized communication. I suggest that the style of living of the counselor himself is an extremely important and effective technique in counseling. (p. 214)

It is essential that you explore your basic attitudes and beliefs and work to understand them better. As you proceed through this book, we encourage you to examine carefully what the various ideas presented mean to you. These personal associations will make up the *internal* ele-ments of your therapeutic position. How compatible are the various the-oretical concepts with your already internalized personal philosophy of helping?

An effective therapeutic position requires a person to understand, advance, and employ a conceptual framework of both external and inter-nal elements. From this position, your actual therapeutic practice can evolve. Strickland (1969) illustrates these elements and their relationship

FIGURE 1-1
The philosophy–theory–practice continuum. Adapted from "The philosophy–theory–practice continuum" by B. Strickland, 1969, *Counselor Education and Supervision, 8,* p. 165-75. Reprinted by permission.

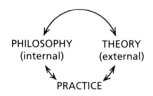

PHILOSOPHY   THEORY
(internal)   (external)

PRACTICE

to therapeutic practice in a "philosophy–theory–practice continuum." This continuum, pictured in Figure 1-1, illustrates how philosophy (internal elements), theory (external elements), and actual practice are interrelated.

Strickland depicts this relationship as continuous and cyclical. One can begin at any point on the continuum. Theory, for example, can develop from one's personal philosophy. Practice then emanates from the theoretical foundation, and is then reevaluated by using philosophical guidelines. In this way the three aspects of this philosophy–theory–practice continuum check and balance one another. The therapeutic practice is thus constantly redefined and improved. Strickland's tripart continuum is a graphic model for visualizing how the external and internal elements of an effective therapeutic position and actual counseling and psychotherapy practice are related.

THE GOAL-DIRECTED NATURE OF COUNSELING AND PSYCHOTHERAPY

The primary goal of counseling and psychotherapy is to help clients function better. Individuals who seek therapy are dissatisfied with their lives, either what they are doing or what they are failing to do. This dissatisfaction may stem from things public or private, internal or external, but in all cases clients are unhappy about their lives. Thus, positive *change* is always the goal of meaningful therapy.

Human beings *feel, act,* and *think*. How people function, both internally and with others, can be viewed as falling into three interrelated domains: the *affective,* the *behavioral,* and the *cognitive.* When people are distressed, their emotions (affect), their behavior, and their thoughts are all involved. One domain can dominate in creating or maintaining psychological distress. For example, how persons feel and act can be adversely influenced by what they are thinking ("life is terrible" = depressed feelings and slow, lethargic movement). Similarly, significantly changing any facet of how one acts can alter how one feels and thinks (working hard and succeeding at a project = good feelings of pride and accomplishment and thoughts such as "It's great to succeed!"). A change in one sphere of individuals' being or functioning will affect the other two spheres.

Most therapists frequently hear similar problems. How they receive clients' information and then investigate, analyze, assess, and ultimately deal with it can vary greatly from practitioner to practitioner. This variability is not surprising: more than 250 therapeutic approaches were reported in use at the beginning of this decade (Herink, 1980).

This book's organization reflects our belief that the major goal of each of the approaches to counseling and psychotherapy is positive change in primarily one domain of human functioning. While each approach does account for all three domains, one is primary. The three domains are: (1) affective—changing how a person *feels,* (2) behavioral—changing how a person *acts,* and (3) cognitive—changing how a person *thinks.* We reiterate that while our *primary* focus is on one domain, the other two are not ignored. Cognitive approaches, for example, emphasize changing clients' thoughts with a belief that affective and behavioral change will result.

To illustrate, we gave three colleagues the account of the young divorced client introduced at the beginning of Part One. We chose these three individuals because each claims a different therapeutic position emphasizing one of the three domains of human functioning. We asked each for their main hypotheses about the young man's difficulties and a potential course for therapy. Here are their replies.

1. **Affectively-Oriented Therapist.** My perceptions of this individual's difficulties are best explained by my view of the therapeutic process in general. Clients seek therapeutic assistance because there is a discrepancy between the way they feel about themselves and the way they would like to feel. They have a basic mistrust in themselves and are therefore, in a sense, out of touch with their true feelings. This mistrust creates an inability to express feelings and a tendency to externalize one's problem. If I were to work with this client, sessions would be focused on him, and he would be the one to decide the direction we would take. I would attempt to accept him and empathize with him and, while always being myself and offering genuine feelings, communicate this acceptance and empathic understanding to him. As therapy progressed, I would hope he would be able to express any fears, anxiety, guilt, shame, anger, or other feelings that he has deemed too negative to incorporate into his self-structure. Eventually, he might be able to trust himself more, become comfortable with those feelings that were previously unconscious, and become more internally evaluative as well as open to all of his experience.

2. **Behaviorally-Oriented Therapist.** Your client appears to lack assertive social skills, resulting in a learned helplessness and a loss of positive reinforcement. He also seems to be hypersensitive to criticism and rejection. Before beginning any therapeutic intervention, however, I would first want to more carefully assess his strengths and

weaknesses and clarify the behavior he wants to increase or decrease in frequency. In treatment we would begin by establishing baseline data (the present frequency of a specific behavior) for those behaviors he wants to change. This information would help us to determine where he is now, the amount of change desired, and how realistic that change might be. This procedure will further provide a basis for evaluating therapeutic progress. We would then make precise treatment goals and develop a plan with techniques that are designed to meet them. Throughout therapy, however, we want him to learn new skills that he can use to solve his problems and live more effectively.

3. **Cognitively-Oriented Therapist.** The client apparently tears himself down and is self-pitying and depressed; he has adopted these attitudes by thinking and believing thoughts such as "I must do well and be approved by significant others; isn't it awful that I'm not; and what a rotten person I am for not doing as well as I *must!*" or "The conditions under which I live should be easier and more enjoyable; isn't it horrible when they aren't; what a terrible world this is for not being as good as it *must!*" In working with this client, I would stress the value of applying logical as well as functional analysis in evaluating the irrational beliefs he appears to hold. For example, I would ask "Why *must* anything be as you *want* it to be?" In doing so, I would help him to change his thinking by replacing self-defeating, dysfunctional ideas with a more logical, rational philosophy of life.

Each of these therapists clearly advocate working with the client by emphasizing that domain of human functioning particular to his or her own therapeutic position. Numerous theoreticians and practitioners have written extensively about counseling and psychotherapy from similar specific points of view. Each point of view—the affective, behavioral, and cognitive—has strong advocates in both theory and practice who hasten to provide evidence supporting their views.

Rigid adherents to a particular therapeutic position, however, are receding into a minority, replaced by practitioners who use a diverse range of methods and concepts (Lazarus, 1981). We don't suggest that "one domain–focused" therapeutic approaches are inappropriate or ineffective. Rather, each has its limitations, and practitioners who recognize these deficits are placing the practical concerns of their clients' problems ahead of the theoretical constraints of a specific therapeutic approach. But in doing so many have embraced "a mish-mash of theories, a hugger-mugger of procedures, a galimarifry of therapies, and a charivaria of activities having not proper rationale, and incapable of being tested or evaluated" (Eysenck, 1970, p. 140). These therapists chose their therapeutic concepts and techniques largely by subjective appeal. "I use whatever makes sense to me and whatever I feel comfortable with" is often heard from these practitioners. This type of anti-theoretical and unsystematic therapeutic intervention can only breed confusion and ineffective therapy (Lazarus, 1981).

We respond to this dilemma by recommending that counselors and psychotherapists in training go through two stages to expand their present personal philosophy of helping and become more effective helpers: (1) choose and develop expertise in one basic therapeutic position that has been written about and tested, *then* (2) pursue a *systematic synthesis* of therapeutic concepts emanating from this position.

In undergoing this process, you must first become familiar with the major approaches to counseling and psychotherapy. You can then select one approach in which to firmly ground yourself. From this foundation you can judiciously select more diverse theoretical concepts and intervention strategies and synthesize them into a systematic and pragmatic therapeutic position.

WHY A PRAGMATIC THERAPEUTIC POSITION?

Choosing an established approach to counseling and psychotherapy has the advantage of offering a ready-made set of assumptions and counseling techniques. There is constancy of theory and method. Further, clinical experience and research based on an established approach frequently is backed by extensive data that validates its basic tenets. Allegiance to one basic approach also can provide a solid professional identity and often substantial status. (Brammer & Shostrom, 1982).

Evidence suggests, however, that no particular approach is totally effective for all persons and situations. In fact, the more effective practitioner tries to carefully screen clients for the characteristics that the practitioner can work with most effectively. Many therapists thus frequently seek clients who fit readily into the particular pattern with which the therapist feels most comfortable (Carkhuff & Berenson, 1977). However, many other therapists neither desire nor have the luxury of choosing clients they prefer. For these practitioners, a systematic synthesis of concepts built upon their basic therapeutic position is a more appropriate approach to take.

It is this latter approach we urge trainees to eventually develop and use. As practicing clinicians, it is the approach we have personally and professionally developed and find most realistic, efficient, and effective. We have labeled it the "pragmatic therapeutic position."

We stress that this pragmatic therapeutic position is not what is commonly referred to as an eclectic approach, in which "one draws on several approaches when it 'feels right' " (Ivey & Simek-Downing, 1980, p. 7). Our pragmatic therapeutic position may draw upon several approaches; however, it is a systematic, reasoned program of counseling and psychotherapy grounded in primarily one major therapeutic position.

Brammer and Shostrom (1982) suggest that in one sense all therapeutic approaches are eclectic, and to a certain extent this is true. Many counselors and psychotherapists like to consider themselves eclectic (Garfield & Kurtz, 1974, 1977). They appear confused, however, about what eclecticism means (Swan, 1979; Thorne, 1973) and its therapeutic value. For example, although Corey (1982) recommends eclecticism as a framework for the professional education of beginning counselors, he notes the danger in this potentially undisciplined and unsystematic approach: it can be an excuse for either failing to develop a sound rationale for treatment or for systematically adhering to certain concepts, thus letting the practitioner pick and choose fragments from the various approaches that merely support personal biases and preconceived ideas.

Gathering baseline data

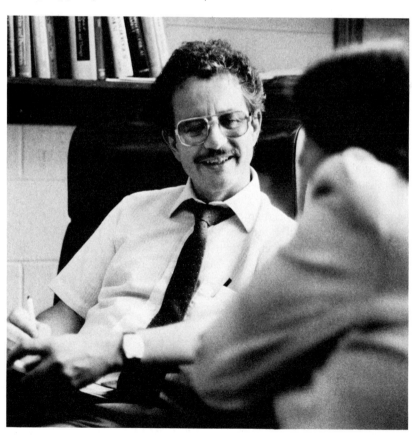

Shertzer and Stone (1974) formally define eclecticism as "the belief that a single orientation is limiting and that procedures, techniques, and concepts from many sources should be utilized to best serve the needs of the person seeking help" (p. 189). Our pragmatic therapeutic position accepts Shertzer and Stone's definition but adds a critical dimension; it thus has more structure than what might commonly be considered an eclectic orientation.

A truly effective therapeutic position must be more than a random borrowing of ideas from here and there. The effective therapist must have a conceptual framework (Dimond, Havens, & Jones, 1978) that enables him or her to *systematically apply* relevant concepts from other theories and then *integrate* them into a pragmatic therapeutic position. This position involves a practical set of procedures, yes, but guided by a basic theory. Unfortunately, many professionals who advocate eclecticism decline to theorize altogether, claiming that it is unwise to adhere too closely with a set of concepts or tested principles, or simply that specific theories are not useful.

Theory is necessary for effective therapeutic practice (unless the therapist and client are unusually lucky). Theory enables the practitioner to systematically study the therapeutic experience; it encourages clear, organized thinking, and helps the therapist predict, evaluate, and improve results (Brammer & Shostrom, 1982). A basic theory to operate from helps therapists understand clients' behaviors, how to change them for the better, and how changes are effected. "Without a theoretical orientation . . . action is vulnerable to over-simplified and glib imitativeness—even mimicry—and the use of gimmick" (Polster & Polster, 1973, p. 3). Thus, we strongly emphasize the importance of a basic theory in therapeutic practice, but pragmatic theory.

Earlier we discussed how we believe prospective counselors and psychotherapists should be trained. First, he or she should select and study thoroughly one basic theoretical approach that is backed by research and literature. Only after gaining a firm grounding in that approach should he or she systematically synthesize concepts from other relevant theoretical approaches. This developmental training process should give the practitioner both the external and internal elements of an effective pragmatic therapeutic position.

First, we ask that you explore the major therapeutic approaches in Part Two. Choose *one* that you find most compatible with your own personal theory of counseling. Work to understand in depth that approach in both theory and practice. Only then should you integrate other theoretical concepts. We'll now preview the means to implement this systematic synthesis and thus fully function from a pragmatic therapeutic position.

THE THERAPEUTIC PROCESS FROM A PRAGMATIC PERSPECTIVE

We have discussed how major approaches to counseling and psychotherapy can be classified by how much they emphasize specific domains of human functioning: feelings (affectively-oriented), actions (behaviorally-oriented), or thoughts (cognitively-oriented). Our ongoing review of the professional literature as well as our clinical training and experiences support this tripart classification.

Many conceptual schema propose the affective-behavioral-cognitive trichotomy as the most effective means of understanding clients' concerns and charting treatment directions. Similarly, Hutchens (1979, 1982) divides the major counseling theories into those that stress *feeling, acting,* and *thinking.* Likewise, L'Abate (1981), using different terms but a similar trichotomy, classified major psychotherapy theorists by their emphasis on *emotionality, activity,* or *rationality.* Selecting therapeutic strategies based on this type of classification system appears to maximize the probability of therapeutic success (Ward, 1983).

The therapeutic process proceeding according to a pragmatic therapeutic position has two major steps. The first is assessment, goal setting, and intervention according to the dominant therapeutic position a therapist has chosen and studied, be it affective, behavioral, or cognitive. Therapy focuses on one aspect of the client. Focusing on only one sphere of the client's functioning may not always be enough, however, or at least not the most efficient approach. For example, while affective and behavioral change *may* occur through cognitive change, a singular focus on thoughts may not bring about change in all three domains. Working with all three areas of the client makes successful, comprehensive therapy more likely.

Assessment, goal setting and *direct* intervention addressing the remaining two domains is the second step in a pragmatic therapeutic position. Cormier and Cormier (1979) report growing evidence that therapists use a variety of strategies in actual practice. Ellis (1982) supports this view in suggesting that the whole field of counseling and psychotherapy is becoming more comprehensive; however, it is "perhaps less overtly admitted by many practitioners of other leading schools" (p. 7). Krumboltz (1980) predicts that counseling will have a better "integration of thinking, feeling, and acting" (p. 466). It is this integration, or systematic synthesis, that is the essence of a pragmatic therapeutic position. This synthesis, though, is founded in an initial single therapeutic position. Figure 1-2 illustrates how assessment, goal setting, and intervention proceed according to a pragmatic theoretical position.

According to Figure 1-2, the affectively-oriented therapist's foremost focus is on assessing and changing how a client feels. The therapist then considers the client's behavioral and cognitive functioning in the

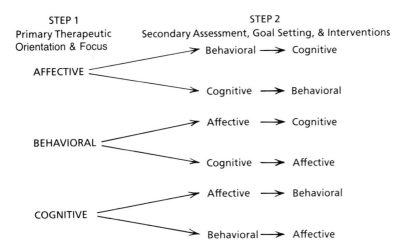

STEP 1
Primary Therapeutic
Orientation & Focus

STEP 2
Secondary Assessment, Goal Setting, & Interventions

FIGURE 1-2
The three pragmatic therapeutic positions

AFFECTIVE
→ Behavioral → Cognitive
→ Cognitive → Behavioral

BEHAVIORAL
→ Affective → Cognitive
→ Cognitive → Affective

COGNITIVE
→ Affective → Behavioral
→ Behavioral → Affective

order and degree determined by the therapist's assessment of the client's functioning and level of distress. Therapies based on the other two focuses follow a similar course.

In this manner, the therapist reaps the benefits of using one established approach to counseling and psychotherapy, yet by directly addressing the remaining two domains, overcomes the limitations of a singular focus.

These short cases illustrate a pragmatic therapeutic position. The cases follow the outline in Figure 1-2.

CASES

Affective/Behavioral-Cognitive

A woman with terminal cancer has only a few months to live. The therapist focuses on her *feelings* of loss and grief and tries to help her understand and express them so she can gain a greater acceptance of her impending death. To help the client overcome her depression, the therapist helps her plan out and then participate in satisfying *activities* to enhance her remaining days. The therapist and client also explore the *thoughts* she has about her situation ("It's not fair."). They then work to restructure the client's thinking ("Things are not always fair." "Some things can't be changed and to constantly ruminate over their unfairness only makes me miserable.")

Affective/Cognitive-Behavioral

A young man has confused feelings about his relationship with his fiancé. By attending to the client's *feelings,* the therapist conveys an empathic understanding of his concerns. By creating a climate of unconditional acceptance wherein no judgment is placed on how he feels, the therapist helps the client feel more like he wants to feel.

Therapy then shifts to exploring the client's *thoughts* about his relationship with his fiancé and the unrealistic expectations he has for it ("We must never disagree."). In addition, the therapist teaches the client more assertive *behaviors* to replace his normally dissatisfying passive responses to prevent disagreement at all costs.

Behavioral/Affective-Cognitive

A newly-divorced woman is very disturbed about being single again and making new friends with singles' interests. The therapist works with her to learn to *act* more outgoing and strike up conversations so she can meet people who have similar interests. The therapist also helps the client face her

feelings about new associations and work through her present emotional blocks. The client is then helped to *think* more positively about herself and her new life. This program encourages her to take risks and experiment with ways of being happy as a single person.

Behavioral/Cognitive-Affective

A middle-aged man has been very lethargic, approaching each new day dire and downcast. The therapist first helps the client develop a realistic program adding new and interesting *activities* to his daily routine. The emphasis then shifts to the client's *thoughts* about his life. Goals are set and therapeutic interventions undertaken to help him gain a

more positive perspective; objectively, he does have a number of potentially exciting things which he can enjoy if he chooses to. Finally, the client's *feelings* are addressed, although only to confirm the client's happier, more optimistic feelings stemming from other changes in his behaviors and thoughts.

Cognitive/Affective-Behavioral

A teenage boy is severely overweight and tells the therapist he snacks compulsively. The therapist helps the boy focus on *thoughts* such as "I must eat . . . ," "I must not be deprived . . . ," questioning their value. Simultaneously, the boy is taught to substitute more functional beliefs for them ("I can eat if I want to, but I'll pay the price," "I don't *have to* eat whenever I want to.").

The youth is then urged to explore his *feelings* about himself and how he would like to feel about himself. The therapist tries to help him accept his present state (alleviating his guilt and anxiety) but also induce a desire to change. Finally, the boy is taught to change his eating *behaviors* (balanced and regular meals with no snacking).

Cognitive/Behavioral-Affective

A young woman is mildly depressed because of a crisis in her life. She has a highly negative and self-defeating attitude towards herself, her present circumstances, and her future. She thinks "I'm no good," "Things are lousy in my life," "The future will be just as bad." The therapist helps the client change this self-defeating thinking by establishing a systematic program to counter it with more realistic and positive thinking.

The therapist then encourages the client to *behave* in ways that will disprove her negative thoughts. She is given tasks to accomplish in which her success will constantly contrast with her negative evaluations of herself and her life. Finally, the therapist and a medical doctor decide to moderate the client's *feelings* by having her take a mild tranquilizer to reduce her depression.

COUNSELING VERSUS PSYCHOTHERAPY

Counseling and psychotherapy are used equivalently throughout this book. Many professionals agree that no distinction exists between them and use the terms interchangeably, while others have sought to differentiate the two. Hansen, Stevic, and Warner (1982), reflecting much of current thinking in the latter view, describe counseling and psychotherapy as existing along a continuum.

> Let us concede that counseling and psychotherapy indeed exist along a continuum. Although they are at opposite ends of the continuum, they are related ways of helping people in need . . . the difference, then, is that counseling works toward helping people to understand and develop their personality in relation to specific role problems; psychotherapy aims at reorganization of

the personality through interaction with a therapist . . .
counseling does not attempt to restructure personality, but to
develop what already exists. (pp. 12, 13, 14)

Belkin (1980) states that counseling and psychotherapy differ only
in *degree* and *emphasis.* When the two are distinguished, this position
appears to be the most substantiated. (Aubrey, 1967; Bordin, 1968;
Brammer & Shostrom, 1982; George & Cristiani, 1981). Both Aubrey
(1967) and Bordin (1968), for example, distinguish counseling from psychotherapy by the degree of the client's disturbance: in counseling, clients
are "adequately functioning individuals" and in psychotherapy they are
"neurotic and pathological."

While this distinction is popular, it describes more what *should be*
rather than what *is* (Belkin, 1980). In practice, most cases are simply not
so clearly defined—neither in clients' personalities and problems nor in
actual treatment. Exactly where counseling ends and psychotherapy begins, if the two are viewed on a continuum, is not clear. The vagueness
becomes apparent when one considers the theoretical understanding and
skills that potential counselors and psychotherapists must acquire.

For initial training especially, trying to differentiate between counseling and psychotherapy in any way creates an unnecessary and false
dichotomy. Patterson (1973) addressed this point succinctly.

There seems to be agreement that both counseling and
psychotherapy are processes involving a special kind of
relationship between a person who asks for help with a
psychological problem (the client or the patient) and a person
who is trained to provide that help (the counselor or the
therapist). The nature of the relationship is essentially the same, if
not identical, in both counseling and psychotherapy. The process
that occurs also does not seem to differ from one to the other.
Nor do there seem to be any distinct techniques or group of
techniques that separate counseling and psychotherapy.
(pp. xii-xiii)

We call our therapeutic position pragmatic. We agree with Kirman
(1977) who makes the point that if a client has a problem, and seeks
help, it makes no practical difference whether practitioners call what they
are doing counseling or psychotherapy as long as they are properly trained
and certified.

When we perceive the helping process from the point of view of
the counselee, the differentiation between counseling and
psychotherapy becomes meaningless. We take from each helping
relationship what it has to offer though we may have hoped for

more. We give each helping relationship what we are able
regardless of the definition of role. (p. 22)

Throughout this book the terms counseling and psychotherapy will
be used synonymously, as will counselor, therapist, and the like.

The primary goal of any therapeutic endeavor is to help the client. Positive
change is most likely if the therapist operates from a well-conceived
framework. We have identified two elements of an effective therapeutic
position. The *external* element is a sound theoretical base emanating from
one of the major counseling approaches. The *internal* element, comprising
the therapist's personal values and experiences, coincides with the therapeutic position he or she develops.

    Descriptively, human functioning falls into three domains: the affec-
tive, behavioral, and cognitive. Likewise, the major approaches to counseling and psychotherapy are classified in a trichotomy as affectively-,
behaviorally-, or cognitively-oriented in terms of their *primary* focus for
assessment, goal setting, and intervention.

    We advocate two positions for counselors in training to sequentially
take: (1) choose and develop an expertise in one basic therapeutic position which has been documented and tested, and then (2) assume a
pragmatic therapeutic position, a systematic synthesis of therapeutic concepts emanating from one's basic position and incorporating others that
can directly address all three domains of a client's functioning. Developmental attainment of both these positions accrues the benefits of using
one established approach while overcoming any potential limitations imposed by a single focus.

    Part Two begins this developmental process by examining the
major affective, behavioral, and cognitive approaches to counseling and
psychotherapy.

SUMMARY

SUGGESTED READINGS

This chapter has addressed the importance of establishing a therapeutic
base from which to direct professional helping efforts. Others have offered different frameworks that complement, as well as contrast with,
our pragmatic therapeutic position. The following recommended resources are a sampling.

Brammer, L. M., & Shostrom, E. L. (1982). *Therapeutic psychology:
Fundamentals of counseling and psychotherapy* (4th ed.). Englewood
Cliffs, NJ: Prentice-Hall. The authors provide a fine review of the major
theories and therapeutic processes, synthesizing them within their own
conceptualization of how clients are best helped.

Garfield, S. L. (1980). *Psychotherapy: An eclectic approach.* New York: Wiley. This book describes specific client and therapist variables the author asserts are associated with successful therapeutic practice. Included is a fine summary of research in psychotherapy and discussion about evaluating the effectiveness of therapy.

Ivey, A. E., & Simek-Downing, L. (1980). *Counseling and psychotherapy: Skills, theories and practice.* Englewood Cliffs, NJ: Prentice-Hall. Ivey and Simek-Downing describe steps with which the practitioner can develop a general theory of counseling and psychotherapy. The authors seek to answer the question, "which theory for which individual under what conditions?"

Palmer, J. O. (1980). *A primer of eclectic psychotherapy.* Monterey, CA: Brooks/Cole. The author attempts to present a coherent eclectic approach to the process of counseling and psychotherapy, along with special applications to consider for working with adults, children, families, groups, and involuntary clients.

Patterson, C. H. (1980). *Theories of counseling and psychotherapy* (3rd ed.). New York: Harper & Row. This book offers an advanced treatment of the various approaches to counseling and psychotherapy. Particularly relevant is an excellent chapter on the convergences and divergences among the major theoretical orientations.

Part Two

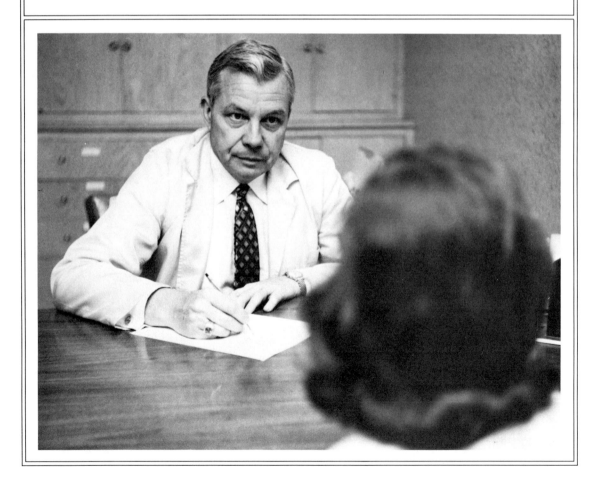

Theories of Counseling and Psychotherapy

This Part presents major theoretical approaches to counseling and psychotherapy that are most commonly used today. Note that no discussion of psychoanalytic theory is included. Historically, psychoanalysis has played an important part in the field of counseling and psychotherapy as a theory of personality. An understanding of Freud's basic ideas is helpful in fully comprehending the human condition. However, as a currently popular approach to counseling and psychotherapy, its use is waning compared with the orientations offered here. Our presentation of theoretical perspectives is thus selective. We have based it on an in-depth review of the professional literature, as well as questioning discussions with colleagues about their predominant approaches to working with clients.

In chapter 2, we investigate the affectively-oriented approaches to counseling and psychotherapy of existential therapy, person-centered therapy, and Gestalt therapy. Chapter 3 explores the predominant behaviorally-oriented approaches. Reality therapy also is presented in the behavioral camp. Chapter 4 reviews three representative cognitively-oriented approaches: rational-emotive therapy, cognitive therapy, and transactional analysis. Chapter 5 compares and contrasts the therapies presented in chapters 2, 3, and 4, and illustrates with a case how therapy with a client would vary depending on the approach used. The case illustration also provides further explanation and a clinical example of our pragmatic therapeutic approach.

We stress an important caveat: no theory is synonymous with particular *techniques*. More often than not, a therapist uses a wide range of different techniques depending on the client and what is happening during a particular session. Using a particular theoretical perspective in counseling and psychotherapy means applying its *principles* in practice.

In this section we ask that you focus on *theory*, on principles that help you better understand clients, identify what constitutes healthy human functioning, and conceptualize how a client can be helped through therapy. Techniques for implementing theoretical principles are presented in Part III.

It is our conviction that the view of human nature you possess from your already internalized personal philosophy of helping will determine the major external approach to counseling and psychotherapy you will ultimately choose and develop. This view of human nature forms the foundation for your interactions with clients. Along with a therapist's perceptions of therapeutic goals and the therapeutic process, it forms the theoretical basis for helping clients. We will analyze each of the theories in this section by considering three primary questions:

1.   How is human nature viewed?
2.   What are the goals of therapy?
3.   How is the therapeutic process ideally experienced?

2

Affectively-Oriented Approaches

Clients typically seek therapy because they "feel bad": they are anxious, depressed, demoralized, uptight, uncertain, strange, dissatisfied, confused. . . . What happens in therapy after the client describes these unpleasant emotions is in a large part a function of the therapist's conceptualization of emotion, which is, in turn, a function of his therapeutic orientation. This is significant for the client, since the way in which the therapist understands statements about feelings will dictate the particular subset of the client's past and present activities that will be considered relevant to assessment and to subsequent intervention.

(Woolfolk, 1976, p. 48)

The most distinguishing characteristic of affectively-oriented approaches to counseling and psychotherapy is their emphasis on underlying attitudes that govern all of a therapist's interactions with a client. Therapy focuses not on strategies or procedures but rather on the therapist creating a person-to-person climate with the client. Therapy is a special relationship in which the therapist seeks to know the client. *Knowing* the client as a person is more important than *knowing about* the client. The therapist seeks to change his or her external, objective perspective to an internal, subjective, and personal experience of the client (Boy & Pine, 1982; Kemp, 1971; Leaman, 1973; Rogers, 1975). Therapy is thus a human experience characterized by a human understanding of human existence (Patterson, 1969).

This humanity is the essence of affectively-oriented approaches. For this reason, they are often correctly described as falling within the humanistic psychology tradition. Shaffer (1978) identified five central themes of humanistic psychology.

1. The starting point for psychology in general is conscious experience. Humanistic psychology in particular emphasizes subjective reality, or the uniqueness of each person's experience.
2. The here and now—the immediate experience of the present moment—is stressed along with the wholeness and integrity of human behavior.
3. Humans are limited by both biological and environmental factors, yet, within the framework of these limitations, human freedom is always possible.
4. Human functioning cannot be reduced to drives, need satisfactions, or unconscious determinants.
5. People can never be defined as a product or as an entity; humans are continuously defining themselves.

Affectively-oriented approaches have deep roots in philosophy. This basis is epitomized by existential therapy, the first topic of this chapter. Existential ideas have been especially influential in developing other affectively-oriented approaches, notably person-centered therapy and Gestalt therapy. A discussion of these latter two will follow.

Existential therapy evolved from existentialism's view of the human condition and experience. Its primary focus is on feelings, the affective domain. The terminology of existentialism's major concepts illustrates this clearly: awareness, freedom, responsibility, meaning, alienation, being, aloneness, authenticity. Existentialism's roots can be traced to the 19th-century Danish philosopher Kierkegaard, but its development and popularization in the 20th century can be credited to Sarte (1946, 1956), Camus (1942, 1958), Heidegger (1962) and others. May (1958, 1961, 1969) was particularly influential in advancing existential thought among counselors and psychotherapists in the United States.

Existentialism as a movement evolved as a reaction against the steady encroachment of technology in which existential thinkers saw humans fast becoming like the machines they operate. They saw individuals as losing both their claim on human freedom and their ability for self-transcendence. Existential thinkers, each in his or her own way, sought to help humans in their search for meaning. The goal of existential therapy is to help clients learn who they are, who they desire to be, and what has true meaning for them. This awareness increases individuals' potential for making choices; that is, they become more aware of their freedom and their ability to take responsibility for the direction of their lives.

EXISTENTIAL THERAPY: A PHILOSOPHY OF WHAT IT MEANS TO BE HUMAN

The Human Condition

Existence, from the root *ex-sistere,* literally means "to emerge, to stand out." It is the existentialist's primary concern to describe humans as emerging and becoming in their entirety. There is general agreement that existentialism is the study of humankind's *being-in-the-world.* This fundamental concept posits that humans are in and act on the world while it simultaneously acts upon them. Any attempt to separate oneself from the world causes alienation and creates a false and arbitrary distinction. Consider the following:

> Two significant perspectives on any human situation are the subjective and the objective. They may or may not agree in the implications they suggest. No rule is adequate to decide between them. Only a living person ought to do that. The person who must make such decisions will be troubled, and ought to be troubled. That is why he is there. A rule and a machine applying it would not be troubled. It is important to the preservation of important human values that someone be troubled this way. I hope to reduce a secondary distress by the reassurance that such a person need not be troubled about being troubled. The uniquely human function is to be *concerned.* That concern is one of the most important human conditions. (Bugental, 1969, p. 53)

The objective view of the human situation has persons as objects; as things done to, the recipients of an action. The subjective view, by contrast, perceives persons as the subject of their own life; doers, those acting upon objects. Existentialists posit neither view alone as sufficient to clarify the existence of the individual nor the reality of his or her existence. Both the person and the experience must be studied. Bugental (1969), quoted previously, further stressed in this regard:

> To my way of thinking, the situation is clearly one for which we may borrow a concept from the physicists, the concept of complementarity. . . . So with the subjective and the objective perspectives of man: Each is important and helps us to understand more about ourselves and others than would either by itself. (p. 291)

Rollo May

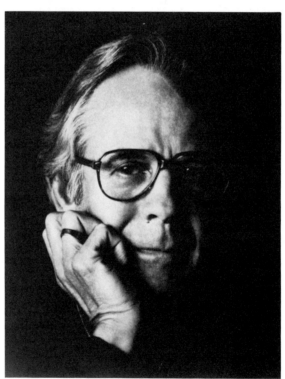

Existential philosophers look at the meaning of life and individuals' place in the world. They seek answers to questions of meaning: "What does that mean?" "Why did that happen?" "What really is?"

Rollo May (1953) was instrumental in taking many existential philosophical concepts and applying them to psychotherapy. He asserted that all individuals have an inborn urge to become a person; that is, they possess an innate tendency to develop their singularity, discover personal identity, and fully actualize their potential. To the extent that they fulfill these potentials, individuals experience the deepest joy that is possible in human experience, for nature has intended them to do so.

Becoming a person is not an automatic process, yet all humans have the desire to realize this potential. The process, however, is not always easy. It takes courage to become, and whether one wants to or not is a matter of choice and commitment. Humans experience a constant struggle within themselves. Although they want to grow toward maturity, independence, and actualization, they realize that growth is often a painful process. Hence, a struggle exists between the security of dependence and the delights and pains of growth (Corey, 1982).

Existential therapy is therefore concerned with human existence and the infinite possibilities of life. The often-used existential phrase "existence precedes essence" simply means that what clients do with their lives—the way they live—will determine what and who they are. Clients "become" through their actions and commitments to those actions. Choices are made between alternatives by exercising one's inherent free will and judgment. With this freedom to choose and act, however, comes responsibility. Clients themselves are responsible for their existence and their destiny.

Clients are also capable of self-awareness, that unique and distinctively human feature that allows them to think and decide. Awareness of the freedom and responsibility they possess can cause individuals to experience *existential anxiety.* Understanding that one *must* choose despite uncertain outcomes, causes this anxiety. Existential anxiety also arises from the awareness that one is mortal and will someday die. Awareness of eventual death, however, gives life significance because it becomes apparent that a person has only a limited time to actualize one's human potential. Existential guilt, then, results from failing to become what one is fully able to become.

Frankl (1959) proposed that the primary force in life is an individual's search for meaning and that each person must develop a purpose in life and create values that give life substance. This significance is discovered only through relationships with others. To analyze these relationships, the existentialist therapist looks at the *eigenwelt* (the individual and his or her body), the *midwelt* (other persons in the world), and the *umwelt* (the biological and physical world). Clients have problems when they are unable to create meaningful relationships. Specifically, a person may become separated or alienated from one's self and body, from others, or from the world. The central task of counseling and psychotherapy is to enable the alienated person to better understand himself or herself and what the world and relationships to that world are like. With greater understanding of the eigenwelt, the midwelt, and the umwelt, a person is able to freely act, rather than only be passively acted upon.

Authenticity as the Therapeutic Goal

Bugental (1965) proposed authenticity to be a "primary existential value" and a "central concern of psychotherapy." Three characteristics of authenticity are: (1) being fully aware of the present moment, (2) choosing how to live in that moment, and (3) taking responsibility for the choice.

Individuals experiencing problems have lost their sense of being, of who they are. The aim of therapy is to help them discover or rediscover their own being. If therapy is to be successful, clients must experience their existence as real and become fully aware of that existence so they can see options and potentials and can therefore change. The following excerpt is from a letter written by a client of an existential therapist. It vividly illustrates her attempts to discover who she is and then lead her life in a more authentic manner.

> Often now I find myself struggling deep within me with who I really am as a person and how I really feel. Emotions don't come easily to me even now. Feelings of love and hate are new to me, and often very scary. Many times I find it hard to reconcile myself to the fact that sometimes I can miss someone I care about one moment and then wish that they would go away the next. This inconsistency in myself, this dependency-independency struggle, is confusing to me at times. Sometimes I think that I would have been better off if I had remained as emotionally dead as I once was. At least then I didn't hurt so much. But I also know that I wasn't fully alive then either. (Corey, 1982, p. 64)

Existential therapists view persons in need of therapeutic help as individuals living restricted existences. Clients are seen as having limited awareness of themselves and are often vague about the nature of their distress. They may perceive few if any available options for confronting various life situations and frequently feel trapped or helpless. The central task of the therapist is confronting clients with their restricted existences and helping them become aware of their own part in creating these circumstances. The therapist might be seen as holding up a mirror to the client, or creating a climate in which the client can confront himself or herself. Clients come to see how they got the way they are and their potential to better their existence. In becoming aware of how they stifle their present existence, they can begin to accept responsibility for changing the future.

In writing about the therapeutic process, Jourard (1971) posited the importance of authenticity as a therapeutic goal for both therapist and client. Therapists, by being authentic and honestly open about themselves, invite clients to respond in a similarly authentic manner. "Manipulation begets counter-manipulation. Self-disclosure begets self-disclosure"

(p. 142). A therapist's modeling of authentic being will create a climate that fosters authenticity and growth in the client.

Jourard (1971) in his book *The Transparent Self* discussed his own growth in learning to be genuinely open within the therapeutic process:

> I wondered why I was so tense and exhausted. It soon became clear that my exhaustion came from withholding myself from my patient, from my own resistances to authentic being . . . With this realization, many recollections came rushing to me of patients who had begged me to tell them what I thought, only to be met by my cool, faultless reflection or interpretation of their question or else by a downright lie, e.g., "Yes, I like you," when in fact I found them boring or unlikable. Also, there came to me recollections of instances where I had violated what I thought were technical rules, for example, holding a weeping patient's hand or bursting out laughing at something the patient had said and of patients later telling me that when I had done these things, I somehow became human, a person, and that these were significant moments for the patients in the course of therapy. (pp. 145–46)

Attitude as Part of the Therapeutic Process

Specific procedures in the literal sense are not apparent in an existential therapist's practice. It is rather the therapist's *attitude* that enables clients to accomplish their goals. Dryfus (1971) stated this most explicitly:

> Existential counseling . . . is not a system of techniques but an underlying attitude toward counseling. . . . The method employed by the existentially-oriented counselor is . . . concerned with the immediate, existing world of the client at the moment. He is concerned with the raw data offered by the client. (p. 416)

This is not to say that attitude is the only "procedure" an existential therapist uses. Rather, the approach to procedures is focused by existential theory. Kemp (1971) pointed out in this regard that "technique follows understanding . . . the existential counselor's primary goal is to understand the counselee as a person, a being, and as a being-in-the-world. This does not mean that he has a low respect for technique, but rather the technique takes a legitimate place in a new perspective" (p. 18).

Apart from the predominant importance placed on attitude, existential questioning is usually central in helping clients attain therapeutic goals: To what degree am I aware of who I am? What am I becoming? Am I living life, or am I merely content to exist? To what extent am I accepting the freedom to choose my own way? How can I choose to re-create my present identity? How do I cope with the anxiety that comes from being aware of the choices I make?

How does one know if he or she possesses the appropriate attitude to function as an existential therapist? The following characteristics have been proposed by Kemp (1976) as indicating a minimal readiness:

1. The recognition that no person can be completely understood by the use of a rational thought and its products.
2. An awareness that information about John, however well-organized and sophisticated, does not assist us in understanding the essence of John.
3. The recognition and growing acceptance that there is a kind of truth unique to the person who expresses it. Although counselees' criteria and referents may seem objectively false, they are considered true if they follow logically from the counselees' perceptions of the matter.
4. An inquiring attitude regarding the significance of productive imagination and the function of symbols.
5. The ability to accept ambiguity. "Instead of accepting change as an academic concept, he must be willing and able to recognize and work with change in its serious dimensions and bewildering unpredictability." (pp. 139–40)

In reference to the excerpt from the client's letter cited previously, Corey (1982) had the following reactions as an existential therapist working with this woman:

1. React honestly to what the client is saying.
2. Share relevant, appropriate personal experiences similar to those of the client.
3. Ask the client to express her anguish over the necessity to choose in an uncertain world.
4. Challenge her to look at all the ways she avoids making decisions and to judge this avoidance.
5. Encourage her to examine her life since she began therapy by asking, "If you could magically go back to the way you remember yourself *before* therapy, would you?"
6. Tell her that she is learning that her experience is precisely the unique quality of being human: that she is ultimately alone, that she must decide for herself, that she will be anxious about being unsure of her decisions, and that she will have to struggle to define her life's meaning in a world that often appears meaningless.

A Case of Existential Therapy

The existential approach adds a focus and depth especially relevant to today's constantly changing society and its inherent "future shock" (Toffler, 1970, 1980). Existential therapy, unlike some other therapeutic approaches, does not view anxiety as dangerous or neurotic. Rather, anxiety is seen as a fundamental condition of existence. A function of therapy is to help clients accept anxiety as a part of their fundamental being. The value of this perspective is exemplified in a case offered by Bugental (1969).

The older woman smiled understandingly but with a trace of sadness at the girl as she said, "I certainly understand now why you did as you did, but you see I really have no choice in the matter. If I made an exception for you now, then I'd have to make an exception for everyone else who had good reasons for breaking the rules. Pretty soon the rules would be meaningless, wouldn't they? So, although I really am sorry about it, the situation is clear, and it calls for you to be restricted to campus for the next month."

The student looked appreciatively at the dean through her tears. "It helps to know that you understand, but somehow it just doesn't seem fair under the circumstances. This will mean I'll lose my job, and I don't know whether Dad will be able to keep me in school or not."

The dean was sympathetic but made it evident that she had no choice. She did promise to try to help the student find another job. The student left with confused feelings of gratitude and resentment. She was guilty for the resentment and told herself that she was unfair and probably selfish to feel it since the dean had been so understanding.

When the student was gone, Dean Stoddart sat back in her chair for a minute, herself swept by contradictory feelings. On the one hand, she felt a certain satisfaction that she had finally trained her feelings and her judgment to the point at which she could stand firm when the regulations required it. For so many years she had found herself carried away by her sympathies so that she almost never was able to combine understanding with constant application of the rules. She was always getting into hot water in those days, forever accused of being inconsistent or even of being undemocratic in having as many ways of administering the rules as there were people who came into her office.

Ruefully, Margaret Stoddart reflected that it had been a real struggle to be able to handle a situation as she had just handled this one. Yet, and here the irony came in, somehow she wasn't content. Somehow, she felt vaguely uneasy even as she reassured herself that she had done the job well. Later in the day, on the couch in my office, she found herself ruminating: "I don't know what it is that keeps bothering me about that interview. The student has probably forgotten it by now, but I feel restless whenever I think about it. And I keep thinking about it. It's like there's something I've overlooked, but I just can't think what it might be. . . .

Margaret Stoddart has completed her therapy with me, but her problem is still with her. Therapy did not solve it. It is the problem of being human. What therapy did do was very important, though. It helped Margaret confront her problem more directly. It did this in several ways. One of the very important ways was to help her recognize that it was appropriate for her to be troubled when she found herself in conflict between the rules on the one hand and the individual on the other.

The point of this is that Margaret had felt that it was an evidence that something was wrong with her to feel this conflict. She had had the image that if only she were as she should be, she wouldn't feel distress when she insisted that the rules must apply to an offending student, or she wouldn't feel misgivings when she decided to set the rules aside in another instance. She really believed that there was a right way to handle every case and that, if she were only the person she should be, she would know that right way. What therapy helped Margaret to recognize was that she would never get to such a point; indeed, that she should be suspicious if she ever found she was not concerned about her decisions. One of the most important things Margaret brought to her work was the very fact of her concern, her human feelings.

With the misgivings about those feelings reduced, Margaret could do a better job of being concerned about the issue that was valid: How much could she respect the individual while yet protecting the group? In this she asserted her own subjecthood while yet fostering others in doing likewise. (pp. 41, 42, 52, 53)

THE PERSON-CENTERED THERAPY OF PERSONAL POWER

Person-centered therapy, developed primarily by Carl Rogers, is closely related to the existential perspective, sharing many of its basic assumptions about humankind. While the roots of existentialism lie deep in philosophy, Rogers and his person-centered therapy have been most influential in implementing a point of view and making it relevant to many aspects of human life.

Rogers's early interests were in individual counseling and psychotherapy. He developed a systematic theory of personality and applied it to counseling individuals, calling it *client-centered therapy* (Rogers, 1951). During the 1950s Rogers and his associates conducted extensive research to test how valid the underlying hypotheses of client-centered therapy are in both the process and outcomes of counseling and psychotherapy. On the basis of this research, his theories were further refined (Rogers, 1961).

Client-centered ideas have spread to a variety of fields far from their point of origin. They have been applied to education (Rogers, 1969); personal growth in a group (Rogers, 1970); families and couples (Rogers, 1972); administration, minority, interracial and intercultural groups; and international relations (Rogers, 1977). Because of its ever-widening scope of influence, especially in the politics of power—how persons obtain, possess, share, or surrender *power* and *control* over others and themselves—Rogers has retitled his approach as it pertains to the therapeutic relationship the *person-centered* approach. He describes how this evolution occurred:

> This new construct has had a powerful influence on me. It has caused me to take a fresh look at my professional life work. I've had a role in initiating the person-centered approach. This view developed first in counseling and psychotherapy, where it was known as client-centered, meaning a person seeking help was not treated as a dependent patient but as a responsible client. Extended to education, it was called student-centered teaching. As it has moved into a wide variety of fields far from its point of origin . . . it seems best to adopt as broad a term as possible: person-centered. (Rogers, 1977, p. 5)

Rogers has not presented his person-centered approach as fixed and complete. He has never been content with the status quo and has constantly sought to reshape and refine his ideas as new information becomes available.

An Inherent Acceptance of Human Potential

When Rogers first began developing his approach, a common belief was that human beings were by nature irrational, unsocialized, and destructive to themselves and others. Rogers rejected this negativistic view, instead promoting an abiding faith in people's ability to develop in a positive and constructive manner if given an environment of respect and trust.

One of the clearest, most direct statements of the person-centered perspective was offered by Rogers (1957) in response to writers who had addressed his "view of man":

> My views of man's most basic characteristics . . . include certain observations as to what man is not, as well as some description of who he is.
>
> I do *not* discover man to be well-characterized in his basic nature by such terms as fundamentally hostile, antisocial, destructive, evil.
>
> I do *not* discover man to be in his basic nature completely without a nature, a *tabula rasa* on which anything may be written, nor malleable putty which can be shaped into any form.
>
> I do *not* discover man to be an essentially imperfect being, sadly warped and corrupted by society.

> In my experience I have discovered man to have characteristics which seem inherent in his species, and the terms which have at different times seemed to me descriptive of these characteristics are such terms as positive, forward-moving, constructive, realistic, trustworthy. (p. 199)

It is not difficult to see the attraction of this positive view of humanity. For persons accustomed to thinking of themselves in negative terms, the idea that they could take charge of their lives, make decisions, and act upon the world was a happy realization.

Accompanying this positive view of humans' potential is an equally important emphasis on persons' interactions with their environment. The environment according to Rogers is not an objective reality, perceived in the same way by everyone, but rather a subjective, personal reality, unique to each individual. Rogers (1959) asserted that "man lives essentially in his own personal and subjective world, and even his most objective functioning, in science, mathematics, and the like, is the result of subjective purpose and subjective choice" (p. 191). "Every individual exists in a continually changing world of experience of which he is the center" (Rogers, 1951, p. 483).

An individual's sense of self emerges from interactions with the environment. Rogers (1951) defined the self as "an organized, fluid but consistent conceptual pattern of perceptions of characteristics and relationships of the 'I' or 'me,' together with values attached to these concepts . . . which emerge as a result of evaluational interactions with others" (p. 498). How individuals adapt to life is always related to their self-concepts. Life situations are always: (a) assimilated into one's self-structure, (b) ignored because they are inconsistent with the sense of self, or (c) perceived distortedly because they are not harmonious with self-perceptions (Belkin, 1980).

Psychological maladjustment comes from denying or distorting life situations; significant experiences consequently are not accurately organized into the self-structure, creating an incongruence between self and experience. Psychological adjustment exists when experiences are accurately assimilated on a symbolic level into one's self-structure. Optimal adjustment is synonymous with complete congruence of self and experience or complete openness to experience. Improvement in psychological adjustment progresses toward this end (Meador & Rogers, 1979).

The Self-Actualizing Individual

The therapeutic goal of person-centered therapy is to help clients become fully functioning persons, not merely assist them with solving problems.

Before clients can begin working toward this end, they must unmask their true selves and experience elements of their personalities that have been hidden. Only then can individuals become themselves, no longer content to automatically conform to others expectations and deny honest feeling.

> Below the level of the problem situation about which the individual is complaining—behind the trouble with studies, or wife, or employer, or with his own uncontrollable or bizarre behavior, or with his frightening feelings, lies one central search. It seems to me that at bottom each person is asking, "Who am I, *really*? How can I get in touch with this real self, underlying all my surface behavior? How can I become myself?" (Rogers, 1961, p. 108)

A person emerges by becoming increasingly more self-actualized. Rogers (1961) described the self-actualizing person as exemplifying four characteristics: (1) openness to experience, (2) trust in one's organism, (3) possession of an internal locus of evaluation, and (4) willingness to become a process.

Openness to experience means perceiving reality without distorting it to conform to a preconceived picture of self. The opposite of rigidity and defensiveness, openness to experience implies a greater awareness of reality as it exists outside oneself. All trees are not green, not all men are stern fathers, not all women are supportive mothers, many "either–or" situations contain varying shades of gray. A person who is open to experience can respond to a new situation *as it is* rather than distorting it to match a preconceived pattern.

A second characteristic of a person in the process of becoming self-actualized is an increased sense of self-confidence. With openness to experience comes a greater access to available information about a situation. With more immediate awareness of both satisfying and unsatisfying consequences, a person can more quickly correct mistaken choices. Individuals' sense of trust and self-governance thus emerges.

Related to self-trust, an internal locus of evaluation entails looking to oneself when making choices, decisions, or evaluative judgments. Approval or standards by which to guide one's life are sought less from others. The individual recognizes that "I am the one who chooses" and "I am the one who determines the value of an experience for me."

The final characteristic of the person in the process of becoming self-actualized is a grasp of the distinction between process and product. Most individuals who enter therapy want to achieve some fixed state (product) in which the presented problem is solved and one's life situation is more satisfying. Clients soon come to realize that growth is a continuing process.

The following excerpt from one client at the end of counseling provides a rather personal description of what it means to become more of a person:

> I've tried out many new behaviors and I find myself having become more sensitive and feeling. I realize that I haven't yet finished the job of fully understanding and reorienting myself, but that's only confusing, not discouraging, now that I realize that growth is a continuing process. I still get angry and upset sometimes, but I find myself feeling a deep sense of encouragement when I'm able to take positive action, where in the past I had sat idly by.

The development of person-centered therapy represents a personal demonstration by Rogers of the process of becoming self-actualized. The approach has been constantly changing and growing; always a process, never a product. It has three main phases.

Phase I: *Nondirective.* In this phase the therapist accepts and trusts the client in a permissive and nonintervening climate. The therapist's main technique is helping the client clarify personal experience in order to gain insight into oneself and one's life.

Phase II: *Reflective.* This phase centers on reflecting the client's feelings and avoiding personally threatening situations with the client in the therapeutic relationship. The Reflection technique enables the client to match up his or her ideal self-concept with the real self-concept.

Phase III: *Increased Personal Involvement.* Although consistent with all past work, this phase is characterized by increased personal involvement of the therapist. To emphasize the present, the therapist takes on a more active, expressive role. There is even more emphasis on attitude as opposed to skills. The therapeutic thrust is now on experiencing oneself as a person. Therapy focuses on the client's experiencing and the expression of the therapist's experiencing. The client grows by learning to use the experience of the present moment.

Early formulations of the person-centered approach stipulated that therapists were to refrain from introducing their own values and biases into the counseling relationship. They were to forgo commonly used procedures such as setting goals, giving advice, interpretation, and the like. More recently, these prohibitions have been lifted and therapists are encouraged to participate actively in the therapeutic process. Focus has shifted from techniques to the therapist's attitudes about the counseling relationship. The aim is to create a climate in which clients feel fully accepted. The therapeutic relationship then is the critical variable, not what the therapist chooses to say or do.

The Therapeutic Process: Necessary and Sufficient Conditions

Given that individuals have an innate capacity to change their maladjustments to psychological health, to become more self-actualized, the responsibility for developing personal potential is the clients'. The person-centered therapist facilitates a therapeutic climate in which the client, who knows himself or herself best, can assume personal responsibility for his or her being. Power and control are placed clearly in the hands of the client:

> The politics of the client-centered approach is a conscious renunciation and avoidance by the therapist of all control over, or decision-making for, the client. It is the facilitation of self-ownership by the client and the strategies by which this can be achieved; the . . . locus of decision-making and the responsibility for the effects of these decisions . . . is politically centered in the client. (Rogers, 1977, p. 14)

Rogers (1961) summarized the essence of the person-centered approach in one sentence: "If I can provide a certain type of relationship, the other person will discover within himself the capacity to use that relationship for growth and change, and personal development will occur" (p. 33). What are the qualities and characteristics of this relationship? It is not an intellectual relationship; the therapist does not help the client by sharing knowledge. Explaining the client's thoughts and behaviors and prescribing actions that should be taken are of little lasting value. The relationship that helps the client to discover his or her capacity to use that relationship for change and growth has six necessary and sufficient conditions (Rogers, 1967):

1. Two persons are in psychological contact.
2. The first, whom we shall term the client, is in a state of incongruence, being vulnerable or anxious.
3. The second person, whom we shall term the therapist, is congruent, or integrated in the relationship.
4. The therapist experiences unconditional positive regard for the client.

5. The therapist experiences an empathic understanding of the client's internal frame of reference and endeavors to communicate this experience to the client.

6. The communication to the client of the therapist's empathic understanding and unconditional positive regard is to a minimal degree achieved. (p. 73)

Rogers has stated that no other conditions are necessary for constructive personality change to occur. If these conditions are present to any degree, then a relationship develops that the client feels is safe, secure, and supporting (though not necessarily supportive), and the therapist is perceived as dependable and trustworthy. This is the type of relationship that fosters change and growth. Through such a therapeutic relationship the therapist often grows as much as the client. The relationship that Rogers calls for affects all partners in it.

The person-centered therapist thus seeks to convey certain attitudes or qualities to clients. Three primary attitudes that come directly from the six aforementioned conditions are congruence, empathic understanding, and unconditional positive regard.

Of the three, congruence is the most critical, according to Roger's most recent writings. Congruence is communicated by a counselor who is genuine and real in the therapeutic relationship. There are no contradictions between what the therapist says and what he or she does. Negative as well as positive feelings are openly expressed. This open expression, and acceptance, of feelings facilitates honest communication with the client.

Conveying congruence may entail the therapist expressing a wide range of feelings: anger, happiness, boredom, frustration and more. This communication is not an indiscriminate self-sharing, but rather an appropriate self-disclosure. Therapists must be responsible for their own feelings and be aware of feelings that distance them from their clients.

The second attitude to be conveyed by the therapist is that he or she accurately understands the client's private world and can formulate some of its significant fragments. The therapist strives to sense the client's inner world of private personal meanings as if they were his or her own, but only vicariously. This empathic understanding enables the client to explore his or her feelings freely and deeply, thus comprehend himself or herself more completely. The therapist often goes beyond recognizing obvious feelings to help clients sense vaguely experienced affects.

Empathic understanding is not evaluative, nor is it simply communicating objective knowledge. Instead, it is a deep and subjective understanding of the client with the client; a sense of personal identification. The therapist shares in the client's subjective world, yet maintains a distinct identity. Rogers (1975) reaffirmed the critical importance of empathic understanding in stating, "Research evidence keeps piling up, and it points strongly to the conclusion that a high degree of empathy in a relationship is possibly the *most* potent and certainly one of the most potent factors in bringing about change and learning" (p. 3).

The third attitude that therapists need to communicate to clients is sincere, unconditional caring for them as persons. Therapists seek to value and accept their clients with no stipulations. Their attitude is "I accept you as you are," not "I'll accept you when." Clients' past behaviors don't matter; they are viewed as persons with potentials. Excerpts from a letter to Rogers (1976) vividly contrasts unconditional positive regard with conditional regard:

> I am beginning to feel that the key to the human being is the attitudes with which the parents have regarded him. If the child was lucky enough to have parents who have felt proud of him, wanted him, wanted him just as he was, exactly as he was, this child grows into adulthood with self-confidence, self-esteem; he goes forth in life feeling sure of himself, strong, able to lick what confronts him. . . . But the parents who like their children—if. They would like them if they were changed, altered, different; if they were smarter or if they were better, or if, if, if. The offspring of these parents have trouble because they never had the feeling of acceptance. These parents don't really like these children; they would like them if they were like someone else. . . . I am coming to believe that children brought up by parents who would like them "if" are never quite right. They grow up assuming that their parents are right and that they are wrong; that somehow or other they are at fault; and even worse, very frequently they feel they are stupid, inadequate, inferior. (p. 101)

Rogers's adherence to the critical importance of the therapist attitudes of congruence, empathic understanding, and unconditional positive regard is not absolute. Rogers stressed that these attitudes exist on a continuum, and only the fully actualized therapist can communicate them to clients. Because therapists are human, they cannot be fully congruent, empathic, or accepting. The person-centered approach posits that the *more* the therapist is able to communicate these three attitudes, the *more* likely it is that successful therapeutic outcomes will occur.

Applying the Person-Centered Approach

We have already stated that the relationship between counselor and client is the critical change component in person-centered therapy. In this framework, therapeutic procedures consist of the therapist communicating the attitudes of acceptance, understanding, and respect to the client. Procedures or techniques *per se* are gimmicks that depersonalize the relationship. Whatever the therapist expresses must be honest. If procedures are applied consciously, then the therapist lacks congruence and is not acting genuinely.

Certain elements of therapy, however, are emphasized within this approach. One element is the immediacy, the "here and now" of the client's existence. The client's feelings in the present moment provide the primary focus in therapy. A second, related element is the emotional aspect of the therapeutic relationship. Intellectually, clients may know what their real situation is, but because they respond emotionally, this knowledge does not help to change behavior. Emphasis on these elements and the necessary and sufficient conditions described earlier constitute the core of the counselor's reponsibility in the following transcript, originally presented in *Client-Centered Counseling: A Renewal* (Boy & Pine, 1982).

In it, the counselor essentially responds to the client by reflecting her perceptions of his experience. Her reflections are in the form of statements that the client might make to himself. Through such reflections, a therapeutic climate is established in which the client feels he is accepted and understood, and that the counselor perceives him and his feelings from *his* internal frame of reference.

The client is a 58-year-old man in a cardiac rehabilitation program. He suffered a major coronary two years ago. In the beginning, the client, although talkative, was depressed and unaware of many of his feelings about his heart attack. This transcript is from his sixth session with the counselor.

Co: Hi, Edward, how are things?

Cl: O.K.

Co: You know that Wednesday you and I won't meet because we are going to have our first group counseling session [with other heart patients].

Cl: Yes

Co: I'm really counting on you to help carry the ball because I know you are really interested. For a lot of new group members this will be a strange experience.

Cl: I hope they can open up. I hope there will be a good outcome from the sharing in the group—maybe relaxation physically and mentally. If you talk about it, it's not so bad as if you hold it inside.

Co: You feel better now talking about your feelings.

Cl: Yes—really. Sometimes I feel uncomfortable talking to people about my heart attack because it seems like I'm crying on their shoulders. I don't know whether they feel that way.

Co: But that's how it makes *me* feel.

Cl: Maybe it's my imagination but it seems after I tell someone about my heart attack they seem to protect me more—they take over.

Co: They feel sorry for me and I don't want pity.

Cl: Right! I guess that's it. I don't like to tell people because I don't want pity—yeah. I lowered myself when I got my heart attack.

Co: I'm not clear on what you mean, Edward.

Cl: I mean I blamed myself for my heart attack. I think I still do. I didn't know enough about heart attacks and what to look for.

Co: Maybe if I knew more about heart attacks I could have prevented mine. This makes me feel regretful and upset.

Cl: Yeah. I had the feeling I overworked myself when it was not necessary.

Co: Maybe if I hadn't been a slave to my work I wouldn't have abused my body so much.

Cl: Yes, like when I was on a job with a jackhammer, breaking concrete, and I found myself out of breath and tight in the chest. Now if I had been more educated I'd have known these were symptoms. But no.

Co: I wish I could have done something to prevent it.

Cl: Yes, but since I've been talking to you I've gained an awful lot. Even *with* my heart attack I didn't lose anything—in fact, I believe I've gained. Now I'm looking at what is here today. I realize I can really help people.

Co: So you really feel now—

Cl: Instead of helping with plumbing I'm helping *people* now. This is the switch I've made because I'm leading church groups now. Maybe I kind of knew it in the past—but I never put it into practice before!

Co: I have a chance now to work and share with people. I have a new way of living and I really love it.

Cl: Yes. Now I go and meet people. I used to feel odd because there were a lot of words I don't pronounce right, but now I can say, "Hey, I'm me, I don't pronounce this word right—so what!"

Co: So what! I'm me!

Cl: So, I've overcome this.

Co: I've developed a lot of self-confidence.

Cl: Very much so. And I want to share the beauty I'm getting now. I can't keep it to myself.

Co: The meaning I'm getting out of life . . . what I hear you saying is you're so full of love for people you really want to share it.

Cl: Yes. I have to go on their home ground though. I see so much beauty in life and people overlook it.

Co: And I want them to appreciate life as I do now. I want to help.

Cl: Before, I didn't have time to appreciate what's around.

Co: Life was going so fast because I kept so busy.

Cl: Yes, I was so busy I couldn't keep up and my body couldn't take it. Now there is so much beauty and I want to share it. So many people reject the beauty around them.

Co: Uh, huh.

Cl: I'm living now in a different world. I have a different approach to everything.

Co: This is what you want to share.

Cl: Yes, I'm enjoying myself. I'm enjoying life.

Co: And I'm so grateful I've had this second chance. I'd have missed so much.

Cl: Yes, when you asked me once, "How do you feel about dying?" Well, I'm just starting to live.

Co: I know that. I can feel that in you.

Cl: I'm starting to appreciate life. I want to give a lot. I don't have any money to give—but I've got much more important things to give.

Co: You do have a wealth to give.

Cl: Because if I see someone who needs help—

Co: Edward, did you just hear what I said to you?

Cl: Yes. You said I've got wealth.

Co: Do you believe that?

Cl: Yes, there are a lot of things I can share with others.

Co: I think you have a whole treasure box of things you can give.

Cl: Yes, and I'm not going to die until I can give those things in my treasure box away and someone can multiply them. In this way, I'm not ready to die. This is when I get scared to die. I don't want to run out of time. I think the future looks brighter, the family is much closer. They don't nag me as much to be careful.

Co: Uh, huh.

Cl: I feel pretty lucky.

Co: Things at home are better. I'm not being treated like a sick person . . . the way that they used to treat me.

Cl: Right. It was so aggravating and it used to depress me. I resented it and I'd want to fight it like we've talked about.

Co: But now that I've talked about my feelings with my family, instead of holding them inside, things really do seem to be much better and we are all happier together.

Cl: Amen to that!

Co: I'm happy you are feeling good about the changes that are going on inside of you, Edward. It's really exciting for me to be experiencing your growth.

Cl: O.K., Elaine—I look forward to seeing you next week. (pp. 155–57)

No other approach to counseling and psychotherapy has become more popular in less time than Gestalt therapy in the 1960s and early 1970s. Dynamic, dramatic, intensive, and absorbing, Gestalt therapy as advanced by Frederick (Fritz) Perls uses a set of experiential procedures that rapidly move clients to a deeper understanding of themselves and their concerns.

GESTALT THERAPY: REINSTATING GROWTH THROUGH GREATER AWARENESS

Human Nature

The Gestalt view of human nature is influenced heavily by existential philosophy. Passons (1975) identifies eight assumptions forming the framework for Gestalt therapy that clearly point out its existential underpinnings:

1. Individuals are composite wholes made up of interrelated parts. None of these parts—body, emotions, thoughts, sensations, or perceptions—can be understood outside the context of the whole person.
2. Individuals are also part of their own environment and cannot be understood apart from it.
3. Individuals choose how they respond to external and internal stimuli. They are actors, not reactors.
4. Individuals have the potential to be fully aware of all their sensations, thoughts, emotions, and perceptions.
5. Individuals are capable of making choices because of this awareness.
6. Individuals have the capacity to govern their own lives effectively.
7. Individuals cannot experience the past and the future, they can only experience themselves in the present.
8. Individuals are neither basically good nor bad.

In many ways, these eight assumptions are so clearly existential that it would be difficult to distinguish them as having a Gestalt therapy focus were they not identified as such. The Gestalt view of human nature, like existentialism, considers individuals to be continuously interacting with others and with the world, striving for authentic encounters, becoming more aware and actualized as life is lived meaningfully in a manner that fulfills one's potential. This may sound similar to the person-centered therapeutic viewpoint as well; however, there is one striking difference. Rogers describes the process of self-actualization as striving to become all that one is capable of becoming. The process is future-oriented. The Gestalt position is fully present-oriented. As the Gestalt therapist Kempler (1973) states, "Becoming is the process of being what one is and not a process of striving to become" (p. 262).

The primary importance of the present is likely the most significant concept in Gestalt therapy. Because the past is gone and the future has not yet arrived, only the present has significance. Perls (1969) described anxiety as "the gap between the now and the later." To Perls, individuals who stray from the present and become preoccupied with the future will experience anxiety. In putting themselves in the future, persons often experience "stage fright;" they become filled with "catastrophic expectations of bad things that will happen" (p. 30). Others contemplate the wonderful things that the future may bring, but do nothing in the present to make these things possible. Rather than living in the present, they try to fill the gap between the now and the later with resolutions, plans, and visions (Corey, 1982).

Similarly, "unfinished business" from one's past can interfere with effective living in the present. Unexpressed feelings such as guilt, grief, resentment, anger, alienation and the like are associated with distinct memories of specific events. Because they have never been fully experienced consciously and resolved, they linger in the background and are carried into the present in ways that interfere with effective living. Unfinished business persists until an individual faces and deals with the unexpressed feelings (Corey, 1977).

Enhancing Awareness of the Present Moment

Perls (1969) proposed the primary goal of therapy was "to make the patient *not* depend upon others, to make the patient discover from the very first moment that he can do many things, *much* more than he thinks he can do" (p. 29). Instead of relying on themselves and their own capacity for self-regulation, individuals get caught in trying to maintain an externally imposed self-image. Rather than using their energy to interact with and assimilate their environment, they direct their energy toward playing roles. As these roles demand more and more energy, individuals have less energy to devote to fulfilling the needs of self. Because these needs never go away, these persons are continually anxious, which in turn leads to inappropriate and unsatisfying behaviors (Hansen, Stevic, & Warner, 1982).

Perls contended that the average person uses only a fraction of his or her potential. Finding out how one prevents oneself from realizing that potential provides the means of making life richer. Awareness, by and of itself, is seen as curative (Corey, 1977). With awareness, clients learn to face and accept denied parts of their being and become aware of subjective experience and reality. They become unified and whole and true to themselves. The need to play roles dictated by an externally imposed self-image disappears.

Most persons are able to stay in the present for only a short while. Perls found that his clients were inclined to find ways to interrupt their flow in the present. Instead of experiencing their feelings in the "now," they would often talk about them as if they were someone else's. Perls sought to help these individuals fully experience the present with vividness and immediacy rather than merely talk about it. He would encourage the client by asking "what" and "how," but not "why" questions. Questions such as "What is happening now?" "How are you feeling now?" "What are you experiencing as you relate this incident to me?" facilitate dialogue about the present. "Why" questions, by contrast, lead only to rationalizations and self-deceptions and away from the immediacy of the present moment.

It is important to understand that Gestalt therapy does not ignore the past or the future but considers them important only as they relate to significant aspects in the client's present functioning. Should a past event, for example, seem to have a significant bearing on present attitudes or behavior, it is brought into the present through direct experiencing in the here-and-now. Rosen (1972) cited an excellent example of this process:

> As an example of direct experiencing, not talking about problems, a patient who says that he has trouble expressing his hostility may be asked to say something hostile to each member in the group, or to the therapist in an individual session. He and the therapist, and others, if present, can directly experience his difficulty in doing this, and can also experiment with appropriate focusing on the patient's voice, posture, response of others, etc. what are the factors involved in this difficulty. Finally, he may be urged to try again using his newly gained awareness. He may observe, when asked "What are your hands saying when they clasp one another?" that they are holding one another for reassurance. When asked to say what he feels when he holds them apart he may experience his fear more intensely. He may be directed to try saying to someone "I'm afraid and also furious at you for. . . ." If timing is good and he feels safe he may then have a different experience in expressing his anger, perhaps more clearly and forcefully than ever before in his life. (p. 96)

A Set of Powerful Therapeutic Procedures

Ivey and Simek-Downing (1980) exemplify the process of Gestalt therapy as a "set of powerful techniques for enhancing awareness of interpersonal experiencing" (p. 278). They maintain that Gestalt therapy's major contribution is methodological rather than theoretical. Gestalt therapeutic procedures are a means of bringing existential experience alive. This methodological focus is a clear, concise way of conceptualizing the clinical practice of Gestalt therapy. A sample of these very potent therapeutic procedures (some of which are more characteristic of group encounters) as described by Levitsky and Perls (1970) are outlined below.

Levitsky and Perls describe the "rules" and "games" of Gestalt therapy. These rules include the *principle of the now* (using the present tense), the *I and thou* (addressing someone directly rather than talking about him or her to the therapist), *using "I" language* (substituting "I" for "it" when talking about the body and its actions), *the use of an awareness continuum* (concentrating on the "how" and "what" of experience rather than on the "why"), and *asking clients to convert questions into statements*.

The games include:

1.   The Game of Dialogue. The Gestalt therapist pays close attention to splits in personality function. One main division is between the "top dog" and the "underdog." The top dog represents righteousness, demands, authoritarianism, and bossiness. The top dog seeks control with "shoulds" and "oughts" and manipulates with threats of catastrophe. The underdog manipulates by playing the passive victim; defensive, apologetic, and powerless. This passive side avoids assuming responsibility and constantly seeks excuses. The therapist has the client play both roles by carrying out an oral dialogue between the two parts. This dialogue brings the conflict into the open so that the client can become aware of these antagonistic roles. Corey (1977) cited some common conflicts that can be illuminated with the dialogue procedure: parent versus child, responsible versus impulsive, puritanical versus sexy, aggressive versus passive. The *empty chair* technique is often used to carry out the dialogue game. An example of the Gestalt approach later in this chapter illustrates this procedure.

2.   Making the Rounds. In this procedure the therapist requests a person in a group to say something or do something to everyone else in the group. For example, an individual who expresses a desire to be more open with others would be asked by the therapist to share something personal with each person present. In doing so, the individual is forced to take the risks and confront the fears inherent in self-disclosure. By experimenting with a new behavior, openness with others, the individual can learn and grow.

3.   "I Take Responsibility." In this procedure, clients are asked to follow each statement about themselves with ". . . and I take responsibility for it." The experience helps clients become more personally aware of and accountable for their feelings, rather than projecting their feelings onto others. For example, a client might say "I'm angry at what you did . . . and I take responsibility for my anger."

4. I Have a Secret. The client is asked to think of a personal secret that causes him or her shame or guilt and, without sharing it, imagine how others might react to it. This procedure is an excellent means of dealing with irrational fears in particular because it illumines reasons for not revealing certain secrets.

5. Playing the Projection. Clients who express a perception that is a projection are asked to play the role of the person involved in the projection in order to discover their conflicts in this area. In playing the "projection game," the therapist asks the client who is saying "I hate you" to play the role of the hated person in order to determine whether the hate comes from an inner conflict of the client.

6. Reversal. As in playing the projection, a client plays a role in the reversal technique. The client acts out a behavior that is the opposite of what he or she would normally do. Reversal gives clients an opportunity to experience the very things that they feel fearful and anxious about, thus becoming aware of parts of themselves that have been denied or submerged. With awareness comes greater acceptance of certain personal attributes that have been denied.

7. Rehearsal. Like reversal, rehearsal involves playing a new role. Perls believed that many clients experience stage fright and anxiety because they fear they will not play their social roles well. Rehearsal provides an opportunity to rehearse a new role in therapy that a client would like to try outside of therapy. The rehearsal strengthens the client's belief that the new behavior can be carried out in the "real world."

8. Exaggeration. This procedure focuses on developing greater awareness of subtle signals and cues individuals send through body language. Movements, postures, and gestures often communicate significant meanings, yet may be incomplete. The client is requested to exaggerate a movement or gesture repeatedly, which usually intensifies the feeling attached to the behavior and makes its inner meaning clearer. Likewise, should the client make an important statement in a casual way, indicating that he or she doesn't recognize its importance, the client is asked to repeat it again and again with increasing loudness and emphasis.

9. May I Feed You a Sentence. In listening to or observing a client, the therapist may conclude that a particular attitude or message is being implied. The therapist then says "May I feed you a sentence? Say it and try it on for size. Say it to several people here." The therapist then proposes the sentence and the client tests out his or her reaction to it. Typically, a Gestalt therapist does not simply interpret for, or to, the client.

Although there is an interpretive element in "May I Feed You a Sentence," the client must still make the experience personal through active participation. If the sentence "fed" is truly key, the client will spontaneously develop the idea.

Fritz Perls

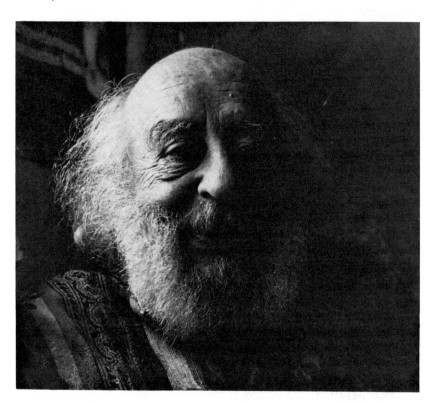

Perls himself made a major impact on counseling and psychotherapy through his exciting and very active therapeutic style. Gestalt writers (Kempler, 1973; Latner, 1973; Polster & Polster, 1973) and Perls (1969) all emphasized the therapist's personality as the vital ingredient in therapy. Perls (1969) referred to the use of techniques and set procedures as "phoney therapy" if therapists' personal qualities as an instrument in therapy are ignored. Thus, the counselor–client relationship must be fully developed before introducing rules and games as outlined above. Further, the more clients are prepared for these therapeutic procedures, the more likely they are to gain increased self-awareness and progress. Passons' (1975) general guidelines in this regard are valuable considerations:

1. Clients will get more from Gestalt exercises if they are oriented and prepared for them.

2. To derive maximum benefit from Gestalt approaches, the therapist must introduce certain techniques at the right time and in the appropriate sequence.

3. Therapists should learn which experiments are best practiced in the session itself and which can be best carried out outside the session.

4. The therapist should not suggest techniques or procedures that are too advanced for a client.

To Passons' points we add that the best way to learn about Gestalt procedures is to experience them yourself. Personal experimentation and learning will help ensure that you will employ these procedures with respect, care, understanding and expertise.

Experiencing the Present: A Case

Much of Perls's major therapeutic activity was conducted in workshops. These workshops were not therapy groups; rather, participants volunteered to work with Perls individually. The group did not interact except that when a volunteer came to a therapeutic realization, he or she was sometimes asked to express it to those present. The following excerpts are from Perls's encounter with Carol, a workshop participant. The use of the empty chair and game of dialogue procedures are prominent throughout as Carol's therapy.

CAROL: I'm trying to decide whether to divorce my husband or not, and have been for ten years.

FRITZ: It's a real impasse, yah! a real unfinished situation. And this is typical of the impasse. We try *everything* to keep the status quo, rather than to get through the impasse. We keep on with our self-torture games, with our bad marriages, with our therapy where we improve, improve, improve, and nothing changes, but our inner conflict is always the same, we maintain the status quo. So talk to your husband. Put him there.

CAROL: Well, I feel like I've been—I've found out some things, Andy, and I found out who you—are to me, and I love you in some ways. You know, I didn't love you when I married you, but I do love you now, in some ways, but—I feel like I'm not gonna be able to grow up if I stay with you, and I don't want to be a freak.

FRITZ: Change seats.

CAROL: That's not fair, Carol, because I love you so much, and we've been together for so long . . . and I want to take care of you . . . I just want you to love me, and—

FRITZ: I don't understand. First, he says he loves you, and now you say he wants—he needs love.

CAROL: Yes. I—I really need—I guess I do need love.

FRITZ: Is it a trade? A trade agreement—love versus love?

CAROL: I need you.

FRITZ: Ah! What do you need Carol for?

CAROL: Because you're exciting . . . I feel dead without you . . . You're a *drag*, Andy. I can't *feel* for *both* of us . . . I'm scared of leaving, too, but—we're just scared. We both need love. I don't think I can give it to you.

FRITZ: Can we start with resentments. Tell him what you resent about him.

CAROL: Ohh, I resent your being such a burden on my back. I resent—every time I leave the house, I have to feel guilty about it. I feel guilty for—

FRITZ: Now that's the lie. When you feel guilty, you actually feel resentful. Scratch out the word guilty, and use the word *resentful* instead, each time.

CAROL: I resent not being able to feel free. I want to move. I want—I resent . . . I resent your nagging at me . . .

FRITZ: Now tell him what you appreciate in him.

CAROL: All right. I really appreciate—your taking care of me, and your loving me, 'cause I'm—I know nobody else could really love me like you do. I resent your—

FRITZ: Now let's scratch out the word "love," and put in the real words instead.

[The encounter continues on another but related path and later returns to the question of the marriage.]

FRITZ: Now tell this—talk like this to Carol, "Carol, shit or get off the pot."

CAROL: I've been telling her.

FRITZ: Let's have it again.

CAROL: Ohhhhh. (laughs) Oh, Carol, when are you gonna make up your *mind*? What are you gonna do? Do *something,* for Christ's sake. You're just a dull, monotonous rattle—on and on with your goddamn fantasy world. Prince *Charming*. You're not getting so pretty any more. You never were. Take you away, shit. Nobody's gonna come and take you away. Get up and go, if you're gonna go.

FRITZ: Change seats.

CAROL: Yeah, but at least I know what I've got here. It's not so bad really, you know, if I just look at things. Stop being so dramatic about it, it's really not bad at all. I'm very lucky. Eugghhlhch! (laughter)

FRITZ: Say this again.

CAROL: Eugghhch! / Fritz: Again. /
       Eyahhgh! / Fritz: Again. /
       Eyagghh! So reasonable. Oy, vey! You've been so *reasonable*. Well you sure did a *boner*.

FRITZ: Change seats again.

[Again the encounter continues, until finally Carol asks Perls for help in understanding, if not deciding for her. His summary reply to her ends the encounter.]

FRITZ: This would be telling. I can tell you only this much: It is possible to get through the impasse. If I would say how, I would be "helpful," and it would be of no avail. She has to discover it, all on her own. If she really gets clear, "I'm stuck," she might be willing to do something about it. She is pretty close to realizing, at least that she is stuck in the marriage. She doesn't realize yet that she is stuck with her self-torture, in her game. "You should/you should not; you should/you should not; yes/but; but in case this happens/then; why doesn't Prince Charming come/but Prince Charming doesn't exist." All this verbiage, what I call the merry-go-round of the being stuck whirl, the real whirl. I think you got a good example. The only solution is to find a magician with his magic wand. And this doesn't exist. All right. (Perls, 1969, pp. 167–172)

Affective approaches put the person into primary focus. The human capacity for self-consciousness, choice, and decision-making have a central place in the therapeutic process. Individuals are viewed as possessing the potential for awareness and freedom to shape their own lives. These approaches all seek to highlight the joys of living, the moment-to-moment excitement of existence, and the beatitude of simply "being" (Belkin, 1980).

AFFECTIVE APPROACHES: THEORETICAL ANALYSES

Therapy evolves through an encounter between the counselor and client and the subsequent relationship that develops. As subjective aspects of experience, all events, whether external or internal, are judged from the perceptual frame of reference of the observer—the client. It is the client who constructs what is real for him or her at a given moment. Therapy is geared toward helping clients reclaim their responsibility for choosing the quality of their lives. Insight and awareness are sought through direct experience. Priority is placed however, on feelings, on affective awareness over intellectual understanding. Gestalt therapy particularly emphasizes this, viewing talking about feelings as means to avoid experiencing them.

Affectively-oriented therapists place secondary emphasis on therapeutic practices and procedures. The therapists' basic attitudes and personal characteristics are the critical components in helping clients. One's philosophy and ability to relate to clients are what really count. It is through the realness of the therapeutic relationship that clients come to realize the power within themselves to change the direction of their lives. Corey's (1977) commentary stresses the predominent strengths of an affective therapeutic orientation:

> In my judgment, one of the major contributions . . . is its emphasis
> on the human-to-human quality of the therapeutic relationship.
> This aspect of the approach lessens the chances of dehumanizing

psychotherapy by making it a mechanical process. Also, I find the philosophy . . . very exciting. I particularly like the emphasis on freedom and responsibility and the person's capacity to redesign his or her life by choosing with awareness. From my viewpoint, this model provides a sound philosophical base on which to build a personal and unique style of the practice of therapy because it addresses itself to the core struggles of the contemporary person. (p. 51)

Of the affectively-oriented approaches considered in this chapter, existential therapy has been the most criticized, primarily for its seeming lack of pragmatic purpose. Patterson (1973) particularly questions the therapeutic practices of the existential therapist:

One must still ask how the existential therapist operates, how he interacts with clients, how he participates in the therapeutic relationship. . . . If the therapeutic relationship is defined as an encounter, what does this mean? What does it mean to say that the therapist is authentic? If he is concerned with the mode of being-in-the-world of the client, how does he gain access to this world? And when he understands the client's mode of being-in-the-world, what does he do with this understanding? (p. 423)

Patterson's querying comments point out the lack of a systematic statement of existential therapy's principles and procedures for conducting psychotherapy. Others have also accused existential therapy of lacking rigor in methodology. Those who prefer an approach based on research contend that its concepts are not empirically sound, its definitions not operational, its hypotheses not testable, and its practice not proven by research on both process and outcome.

While many of the underlying concepts of existential therapy are for some abstract and difficult to apply in practice, it must be remembered that existential theorists were philosophers, not psychotherapists (Corey, 1982). Beginning existential therapists should be philosophically-oriented and able to translate philosophy into practice through their own personality and innovative practice; they must be willing to understand clients first and find relevant techniques that follow.

While it may not be possible to present a strict set of existentialist practices that applies to counseling and psychotherapy, the more easily understood person-centered and Gestalt therapies have their roots in existential philosophy. The person-centered approach especially has incorporated the essential components of existential thought (Patterson, 1973; Shertzer & Stone, 1974). Similarly, Gestalt therapy is placed by a number of writers within the existential tradition (Belkin, 1980; Ivey & Simek-Downing, 1980; Morse & Watson, 1977). Although person-centered and

Gestalt therapies maintain a philosophical consistency, their therapeutic methodology differs drastically.

Person-centered therapy developed out of Rogers's work over the past four decades. Evolving through experience, the approach has undergone many changes since its inception. Rogers has willingly offered his therapeutic concepts as testable hypotheses and submitted them to research. Even Rogers's critics have given him credit for his support of research and his openness to changing his theories when research suggested change was called for.

Present-day person-centered therapy is the dominant approach of most entry-level training programs in counseling and psychotherapy. It offers the beginning therapist a "safe" model of therapy from which to practice. Person-centered therapists typically reflect content and feelings, clarify messages, help clients begin to use their own resources, and help them find their own solutions. Direct influencing is not an expected part of the approach. The potentially harmful effects of more forcefully facilitating immediate and radical change thus cannot come into play. For the beginning practitioner, a person-centered orientation offers more realistic assurance that clients will not be psychologically harmed through mistakes or inexperience of the therapist. (Corey, 1977)

The beginning therapist must be cautioned, however, that person-centered therapy is much more than merely mirroring back to a client what he or she has just said (an unfortunately common misperception). The approach is based on a set of attitudes that the counselor brings into the counseling relationship. Genuineness, positive regard, and empathic understanding are the components of therapeutic success according to Rogers, not specific therapeutic techniques. Therapist authenticity is so vital to the success of the approach that whoever practices it must feel comfortable with its existential underpinnings and truly incorporate them into himself or herself. Otherwise, that counselor is not practicing person-centered therapy.

The major limitation of the person-centered approach lies in what it omits, rather than what it advocates. Corey (1982) explains:

> I see the model as an excellent place to begin a counseling relationship, for unless trust is established and attitudes of respect, care, acceptance, and warmth are communicated, most counseling interventions will fail. But it is not a good place to remain as the counseling process develops. Although I see the core conditions that Rogers describes as being necessary for client change to occur, I also see the need for the knowledge and skills of counselors to be applied in a more directive manner than is called for in the person-centered model. (p. 94)

Despite such potential limitations, it is clear that the person-centered approach will be used by many prospective counselors. The optimistic attitude of its underlying philosophy and its simplicity have a broad appeal. Rogers's application of the approach to education, business, industry, and international relations as well as from counseling and psychotherapy clearly attests to this.

Gestalt therapy is the most provocative of the affectively-oriented approaches, with its powerful procedures and excitingly active style. The lively manner with which past, current, and future concerns are all brought to life in the present at a therapy session is particularly promising. Clients are helped to actually experience their feelings rather than simply talk about them. The result is heightened awareness that can enable a client to assume more personal responsibility for his or her life. Gestalt therapy refuses to accept helplessness as an excuse for not changing. The confidence clients gain from facing the confrontations in Gestalt therapy can create a pervasive optimism that spreads into all aspects of their lives.

It is easy to become swept up in the excitement of Gestalt therapy. But holding to a Gestalt perspective, it is important to also consider the polarities of the approach. There are limitations. Patterson (1973) addresses one limitation:

> **What is the source of the success of Gestalt therapy? The prior question, of course, is, is it effective? Other than Perls' statement of his personal skill, there is no explicit claim for the effectiveness of the method. And Perls' skill was never evaluated by research. (p. 375)**

Shepard (1970) cautions against assuming that Gestalt therapy is any type of "instant cure" on the basis of the dramatically quick results observed in the brief demonstrations for which Perls is famous. Real progress may require a great deal of time, including advances and retreats. The flashes of insight and good feeling following a brief workshop encounter often fade, leaving no permanent change or improvement if not followed by more therapy. Corey (1977) expressed concern about clients accepting an "I do my thing, and you do your thing" lifestyle. Gestalt therapy (at least as described by Perls) does stress responsibility for oneself but also denies responsibility to others. Corey saw this as a dangerous position to maintain, since, realistically, clients' behavior does effect the feelings of others and clients are thus partially responsible for others.

Finally, the most often expressed limitation of Gestalt therapy lies within its practitioners. There is a real danger that a therapist will view the total approach as merely a set of procedures and not consider its existential foundation, the critical importance of the personality of the practitioner of the procedures. The therapist who hides behind Gestalt "rules and games" cannot model authentic behaviors. As Jourard (1971) noted, "Manipulation begets counter-manipulation" (p. 142).

Ivey and Simek-Downing (1980) conducted a skills analysis, comparing the work of Rogers and Perls as representative of their respective therapeutic practices. Rogers's primary skills were in attending and listening, whereas Perls tried to actively influence clients with directives, confrontive feedback, and interpretations. Rogers heavily emphasized conveying empathy, warmth, and positive regard. In contrast, Perls was seen as remote from clients; his respect for them became evident only when they became truly themselves. Both therapists tried to have genuine encounters with their clients, although Rogers tended to wait patiently for the relationship to develop and Perls preferred to make things happen. Perls was most concerned that clients develop their own meanings and find their own directions in life. He never hesitated, however, to offer an opinion, interpretation, or directive to clients proposing what they should do within the therapeutic encounter. Ivey and Simek-Downing in their analysis made special note that Perls's directives almost always centered on telling clients what to do *in the session*; outside the therapy session, his directive was to "do your own thing").

We will examine these skills differences in more depth in Part III. Affective approaches' concepts may seem abstract and difficult to completely comprehend at first. More exposure and time create a more concrete picture. We encourage you to further explore these approaches through the following suggested readings.

SUGGESTED READINGS

Existential Therapy

Buber, M. (1970). *I and thou*. New York: Scribner's. Buber offers an existential exploration of the nature of the human condition in poetic terms.

Frankl, V. (1959). *Man's search for meaning*. New York: Washington Square Press. Frankl posits the importance of a search for personal meaning as the primary human motivator. His basic theme is expressed in his statement, "He who has a why for living can bear almost any how."

Jourard, S. (1971). *The transparent self*. (rev. ed.). New York: Van Nostrand Reinhold. Perhaps more than anyone, Jourard has expounded on the value of openness as opposed to concealment of persons' real selves. In this book, he shares his views on a wide variety of topics ranging from marriage, love, the need for privacy, education, psychotherapy, and more.

Sarte, J. (1946). *No exit*. New York: Knopf. Existentialism is often perceived as too complex because of its wide and varied vocabulary. Sarte presents a description of the existential problems of three persons in this moving play. The analogies to us all are readily realizable.

Shaffer, J. (1978). *Humanistic psychology.* Englewood Cliffs, NJ: Prentice-Hall. An excellent introduction to existential concepts as they apply to education, psychology, psychotherapy, and personal growth.

Person-Centered Therapy

Boy, A. V., & Pine, G. J. (1982) *Client-centered counseling: A renewal.* Boston: Allyn and Bacon. The authors offer a renewed and revitalized look at client-centered therapy. The necessity as well as effectiveness of a personal approach in enhancing self-concept is emphasized.

Rogers, C. (1951). *Client-centered therapy.* Boston: Houghton Mifflin. Rogers' early work on the implications and theory of client-centered therapy.

Rogers, C. (1961). *On becoming a person.* Boston: Houghton Mifflin. This is probably Rogers's best known work. It is a compilation of Rogers's ideas on education, therapy, communication, family life, and more.

Rogers, C. (1970). *Carl Rogers on encounter groups.* New York: Harper & Row. A short, easy-reading book that provides an excellent introduction to encounter groups. It considers not only the process and outcomes of such groups, but also expounds upon how change occurs from a personally experienced viewpoint.

Rogers, C. (1977). *Carl Rogers on personal power: Inner strength and its revolutionary impact.* New York: Delacorte. Rogers emphasizes the implications of centering power with the person in this particularly pointed volume.

Gestalt Therapy

Fagan, J., & Shepard, L. (Eds.) (1970). *Gestalt therapy now.* Palo Alto, CA: Science and Behavior Books. Original articles on the theory, techniques, and applications of Gestalt therapy contributed by Perls and others make this "must" reading.

Latner, J. (1973). *The gestalt therapy book.* New York: Julian Press. The author examines the role and function of the therapist in employing a Gestalt therapy framework in clinical practice.

Passons, W. (1975) *Gestalt approaches in counseling.* New York: Holt, Rinehart and Winston. Passons offers many clear and concise examples of applications of Gestalt procedures. The book provides a particularly fine treatment of the importance of preparing clients to experience Gestalt procedures.

Perls, F. (1969). *Gestalt therapy verbatim.* Moab, Utah: Real People Press. Gestalt therapy is explained by Perls himself using transcripts of his work with clients. His commentary and theoretical points clearly posit the power of this approach in advancing positive client change.

Perls, F. (1969). *In and out of the garbage pail.* Moab, Utah: Real People Press. In a playful and poetic manner, Perls reflects on his life and on the origins and continuing development of Gestalt therapy.

3

Behaviorally-Oriented Approaches

Insight is not action. Understanding the underlying causes of individual problems does not necessarily change one's everyday life.

(Ivey & Simek-Downing, 1980, p. 217)

Whereas affective approaches to counseling and psycho-therapy focus primarily on how clients *feel* and how they can become more aware of feelings, particularly about themselves, behaviorally-oriented approaches focus on an observable ability to *act*. Understanding feelings is not enough for clients to change their lives.

This chapter addresses two behaviorally-oriented approaches: behavior therapy and reality therapy. After introducing relevant behavior therapy principles on human nature and therapeutic goals, we will discuss three of its major aspects: classical conditioning, operant conditioning, and observational learning. We will then address behaviorally-oriented reality therapy, which has a more philosophical basis, yet still emphasizes action as opposed to thinking or feeling. Both approaches offer unique ideas and applications to the behaviorally-oriented practitioner.

BEHAVIOR THERAPY

The descriptor behavior therapy has been used to label many specific practices and procedures that use learning theory principles to constructively change human behavior (Rimm & Masters, 1979). Because behavior therapy embraces diverse practices and procedures, Kazdin (1978) contends that there is often disagreement on its assumptions and features. He lists five characteristics that unify the heterogenous approaches in behavior therapy:

1. The present influences behavior, as opposed to historical determinants.
2. Observation of overt behavior change is the main criterion by which treatment should be evaluated.
3. Treatment goals are concrete and objective in order to make replication of treatment possible.
4. Basic research is a source of hypotheses about treatment and specific therapy techniques.
5. Target problems in therapy are specifically defined, so that treatment and measurement are possible.

Behavior therapy has been distinguished from other psychotherapeutic approaches by its reliance on the scientific method (Thoresen & Coates, 1980). The concepts and methods used by behavior therapists are stated explicitly, tested empirically, and revised continually. Assessment and treatment are interrelated for they occur simultaneously. A sound research base is critical in effective treatment. Behavior therapy has expanded dramatically in the past few decades as a result of its scientifically demonstrated effectiveness in helping individuals deal with a wide range of problems.

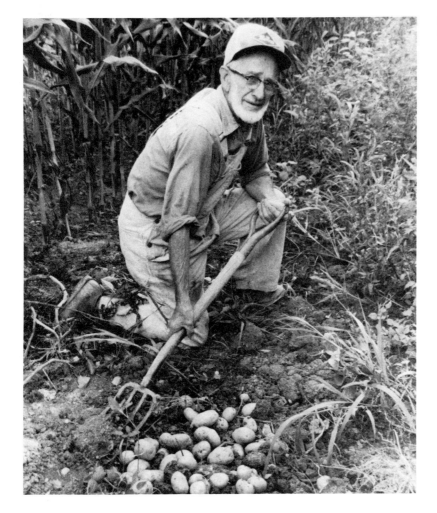

People are a product of their experience

Human Nature

Behavior therapists consider the human personality as developing from consistent patterns of action (Chambless & Goldstein, 1979). Individuals are neither inherently self-actualizing nor self-denigrating: They have equal potential for proceeding in either direction in their lives. Persons become what and who they are through the skills they have learned or not learned.

Behavior therapists see individuals as a product of their experience. Hosford (1969) posited that human beings begin life like a Lockean *tabula rasa* on which nothing has been written or stamped. Individuals react to stimuli they encounter in their environment. Heredity and interaction with environment produce behavior. Personality is formed from positive and negative habitual patterns of learned behavior. Maladaptive behaviors do not differ from adaptive behaviors in the way they are acquired. Behavior is maladaptive or adaptive only because persons label it as such (Shertzer & Stone, 1974).

Clients facing problems in their lives either lack skills or are applying learned skills inappropriately. Thus, behavior therapy involves learning, and its goals and process are intimately linked with learning theory.

Therapeutic Goals

Specific and objectively stated learning objectives constitute the essential therapeutic goals of behavior therapy.

> If counseling can be said to have a single goal, it is to help each individual take charge of his or her own life. In order to assume control of one's own life one needs two major types of skill: the ability to make decisions wisely and skills for altering one's own behavior to produce desirable consequences. . . . A counselor's job then becomes one of arranging appropriate learning experiences so that people develop these skills. (Krumboltz & Thoresen, 1976, pp. 4–5)

Behavior therapists view establishing therapeutic goals and evaluating goal attainment as highly structured endeavors. Because clients generally enter therapy as a result of some acute stress, treatment that does not offer immediate help is viewed as potentially permitting the problem to worsen, to the client's detriment. The essential structure of therapy is formed by agreed-upon goals for change. Bandura (1977) identifies goals as behavioral standards against which individuals assess the consequences of their own actions. Kazdin (1975) asserts that any statement of therapeutic goals requires an answer to the question, "What behavior is to be changed in the stimulus conditions specified?" (p. 66). Building upon the thrust of both these writers, Stuart (1980) proposes that the goals of therapy consist of:

1. Specification of some target behaviors.
2. Specification of the conditions under which these behaviors are to be emitted.

3. Specification of some measure of personal and/or social change that is expected to result from the emission of the target behaviors under the specified conditions. (p. 144)

Goals thus comprise what is to be done, under what conditions, with what results.

A critical component in goal setting in behavior therapy is the precision with which therapeutic goals must be established. As Haley (1977) declared, "Problems, whether one calls them symptoms or complaints, should be something one can count, observe, measure, or in some way know one is influencing" (pp. 40–41). Goals must be refined to the point that they are clear, concrete, understood, and agreed upon by both the therapist and client as specific behaviors to be increased or decreased in frequency and/or duration. Assessment begins with a baseline measure of clients' original behavioral repertoire and is used throughout therapy to determine the degree to which therapeutic goals are being progressively attained.

Our discussion of the therapeutic process in behavior therapy considers three major learning paradigms: classical conditioning, operant conditioning, and observational learning. Representative intervention strategies with case excerpts accompany each paradigm to illustrate its application to clinical practice. In each presentation, you should note how specifically therapeutic goals are established, monitored, and evaluated throughout the process.

BEHAVIORAL CONNECTIONS: CLASSICAL CONDITIONING

Behavior therapists most often use the terms *stimulus* and *response* when speaking about human learning. The classical conditioning perspective states that a client's response to any given stimulus can usually be predicted, depending on how that stimulus and response were connected in previous experiences.

Classical conditioning involves connecting or pairing an unconditioned stimulus (US) with a conditioned stimulus (CS). The presence of a US automatically evokes an unconditioned response (UR). If the US is paired with a CS with sufficient intensity and/or over a long enough period of time, then that CS will come to elicit a conditioned response (CR) that is the same as the UR. For example, suppose the taste of milk makes you ill. In and of itself, there seems to be no reason for this to occur. Perhaps, however, as a child, you became nauseous (UR) after sipping some sour milk (US). The normally neutral stimulus of milk (CS) was paired with sour milk (US) and thus came to be connected with the noxious response of nausea (UR and then CR). While the glass of milk you have in your hand now is not sour, the connection learned as a child and maintained as an adult is between milk and nausea. Thus, milk has been conditioned to elicit a "natural" immediate response of nausea. One proven and very popular intervention strategy derived from classical conditioning is systematic desensitization.

Learning a specific skill can be a goal of behavior therapy

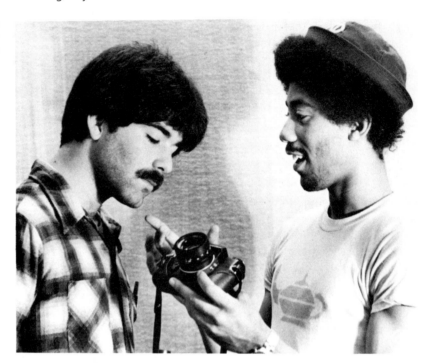

Disconnecting and Reconnecting: Systematic Desensitization

Systematic desensitization is a behavioral intervention procedure developed by Wolpe (1958) that was originally used to eliminate or reduce maladaptive emotional responses such as fear or anxiety. Operating from a classical conditioning perspective, Wolpe proposed that people become fearful and anxious in particular situations because they have associated fear with these situations in the past. For instance, a person might have experienced anxiety from an actual life-threatening encounter, such as witnessing at close range a bank robbery. As a result of this pairing, the individual later connects these frightening feelings with banks and trys to avoid them.

Wolpe (1958) used the term *reciprocal inhibition* to describe the form of classical conditioning that underlies systematic desensitization. In reciprocal inhibition, a relaxing response is paired with an anxiety-producing stimulus so that a new bond develops between the two, with the anxiety-provoking stimulus no longer eliciting an anxiety response. Bugg (1972) explains this learning principle:

> The essential principle of reciprocal inhibition is that an organism cannot make two contradictory responses at the same time. Behavior therapy assumes that anxiety responses are learned behaviors and may be extinguished by reconditioning. If a response that is contradictory to anxiety results in a more pleasant state or more productive behavior for the subject, the new response to anxiety-evoking stimuli will gradually replace the anxiety response. (p. 823)

According to Wolpe, fear and anxiety responses reflect excessive sympathetic nervous system activity, which readies the body for emergencies. He suggested that anxiety can be eliminated or inhibited by having a client imagine or engage in activities causing parasympathetic nervous system activity (returning the body to a normal, stable state), such as relaxation or assertion, while imagining the feared situation or approximations of that situation. The procedure is termed systematic because of the step-by-step manner in which a client is desensitized to the feared stimulus. Wolpe suggests that it is inappropriate to initially pit the inhibiting response such as relaxation directly against the image of the anxiety-producing event. If this was prematurely attempted, anxiety would be too great and relaxation would not occur. Instead, the therapist and client together develop a hierarchy of events, with the anxiety-inducing event at the top and a situation or event related but remote from the anxiety-inducing event at the bottom. The hierarchy is gradually climbed so that the client is exposed to closer and closer approximations of the feared event while relaxing. If done properly, the client can eventually imagine the feared event without anxiety. After this therapy, the client is able to encounter the actual feared situation with little or no anxiety.

Research findings (Rosen, 1976) show the value of presenting clients with a "therapeutic rationale" for desensitization. Rimm and Masters (1979) propose that while it helps to tell clients *that* systematic desensitization is effective, it is more beneficial for therapists to explain *why.* They suggest the following explanation:

> At the beginning of treatment, we are going to get you really relaxed. Then you are going to imagine scenes related to your fear, starting with ones that are only a little frightening, and working your way up. Because I will be introducing the scenes in a *graduated way,* and because you will be relaxed when you imagine them, before long you are going to be able to imagine situations related to [phobic object], and actually feel

comfortable at the same time. And if you can *imagine* [phobic object] and still feel calm, they when you come across an actual [phobic object] out there in the real world, you will find you are not afraid anymore. It is really helpful if people understand why desensitization works, so do you have any questions about the logic or rationale of what we are going to be doing? (p. 46)

Progressive Relaxation

Jacobson (1938) is credited with initially developing the progressive relaxation procedure. A client can usually learn the rudiments of progressive relaxation in a 30-minute session, but careful training and planning are necessary if relaxation is to be induced upon command. Wolpe and Lazarus (1966) suggest six sessions, with 20 minutes devoted to relaxation training, plus the client spending two 15-minute periods each day practicing independently.

The first step in progressive relaxation training is asking the client to get as comfortable as possible. An easy, casual manner combined with a sense of assured confidence from the therapist will greatly help the client begin to relax. The next step is asking the client to close his or her eyes and take a few deep breaths, exhaling slowly each time.

Then tell the client in a soft, soothing voice, "We are going to do something that you should find enjoyable. We need to go at a pace you find comfortable, so if we're going too fast or too slow, please let me know and we'll adjust the pace accordingly. Usually I'll be aware of how you are doing as I can observe your responses and will time what I'm doing to where you are. First, would you make a fist with your right hand and hold it tight—good—tighter—1, 2, 3, 4, 5. Now, let go and relax. Notice the difference between the relaxation and the tension. Feel the comfort as you let your hand open and relax."

Very often, naive clients, when asked to tense one body part such as a fist, proceed to tense other parts of the body automatically. For example, while making a fist, the client might be observed gritting the teeth, tensing the neck muscles, or squinting. This tension interferes with relaxation induction. Therefore, if the client tenses multiple body parts, point this out, and ask the client to consciously try to tense *only* the specified area.

Normally, the client then repeats the tension–relaxation cycle with each body part, twice. The goal is to make the client acutely aware of the difference between tensed and relaxed states. Each time, the therapist asks the client to: (a) tense the body part, (b) hold the tension for a 5-second count, (c) let the tension go and relax, and (d) concentrate on the difference between tension and relaxation. A suggested order to continue with relaxation induction of body parts after the right fist would be:

left fist

right arm

left arm

chest

back

shoulders

neck

face

midsection

thighs

calves

feet

After completing the last tension–relaxation cycle, the client can then be taught "cue-controlled relaxation" (Russell & Sipich, 1973), following instructions such as, "Now you are going to try to become even more relaxed. Notice your breathing. [pause] Each time you begin to exhale or let out a breath, say the word 'relax' (or 'calm' or 'peace') to yourself so that the word will become a cue for deep, deep relaxation."

The therapist can initially prompt by saying "relax" just as the client exhales. The therapist repeats this cue two or three times and then turns control over to the client with, "Now say 'relax' to yourself, just as you start to exhale." This skill is then practiced for 2 to 3 minutes.

The relaxation procedure is now complete. In the first two or three sessions, the client should be guided through the entire procedure, including cue-controlled relaxation. In later sessions, it usually suffices to have the client practice an abbreviated version, involving three to five body parts especially susceptible to tension, followed by a few minutes of cue-controlled relaxation. This training does not require more than 8 to 10 minutes and has been found to be adequate and effective (Rimm & Masters, 1979).

Constructing the Hierarchy

The hierarchy is a graded series of situations or scenes that the client is asked to imagine while relaxed. The scenes should depict realistic, concrete situations relevant to a specific fear that the client has experienced or anticipates. It is usually helpful to develop an imaginary anxiety scale. Wolpe and Lazarus (1966) suggest: "Think of the worst anxiety you have ever experienced or can imagine experiencing, and assign to this the number 100. Now think of the state of being absolutely calm, and call this 0. Now you have a scale. On this scale how do you rate yourself at this moment?" (p. 73). This type of scale accomplishes two things: The counselor and client both understand how anxious the client is at any time in the past or present, and the beginning and end points of an anxiety hierarchy are established. Through questioning and further analysis, the situations relevant to the client's fear or anxiety can be included.

Stedman (1976) describes hierarchy construction with his use of systematic desensitization to assist a school phobic 9-year-old:

> I began desensitization designed to counteract Alice's specific anxieties experienced in the school situation. Deep muscle relaxation proved successful. Establishment of a hierarchy at first took the form of items involving reading, but it was soon noted that Alice became anxious when called upon to perform any unfamiliar, complex academic task in front of the teacher and the class. Also, because of her absence from school, she had missed a number of music lessons and now suffered acute anticipatory anxiety with regard to performing on the recorder in music class. Thus, a later hierarchy, focusing on music but designed also to counteract anxiety over performance of unfamiliar school work, was established. . . .

Excerpts from Music Class and Academic Hierarchy

1. I am at home at night thinking about sitting in music class watching the others play their recorders. . . .

5. I am in music class with the teacher by herself. I am playing an easy familiar tune on my recorder, and the teacher looks pleased. . . .

9. I am in music class with the teacher by herself. I am playing a hard tune on which I make many mistakes, and the teacher looks slightly displeased. . . .

14. I am in music class with the teacher and all the students. I am playing an easy tune in front of the class, with the teacher watching me. . . .

18. I am in front of the music class, playing a fairly hard tune on which I make many mistakes, and several students smile and laugh. . . .

22. I have played poorly in front of the music class, and the teacher corrects me after class for a poor performance. . . .

26. I am in reading class, and the teacher calls on me to stand up and read. I stumble over words, while several students laugh at me and the teacher looks impatient. . . .

29. I am in reading class, and the teacher calls on me to stand up and read. I stumble over words, and the teacher asks me to sit down and comments that I should know the work. The whole class laughs. (pp. 284–285)

The Desensitization Procedure

Once a relaxation response has been learned and the hierarchy developed, the client and therapist are ready to begin the actual desensitization procedure. The client is asked to sit with eyes closed and to relax as much as possible using cue-controlled relaxation. When relaxed, the client is asked to visualize as clearly as possible the hierarchy scene the therapist describes and to put himself or herself in it. The client is asked to raise a finger when the scene is clearly visualized and to signal again if anxiety is experienced while visualizing the scene. If no anxiety is signaled after 10 seconds, the client is instructed to stop imagining the scene. The client's level of anxiety is assessed, even in the absence of a signal. Some clients habitually fail to report small increments of anxiety, and over several hierarchy scenes these increments could swell to levels that would interfere with treatment. This assessment is accomplished by simply asking the client where he or she "is" on a 10-point anxiety scale (Rimm & Masters, 1979). If no anxiety is signaled, no increase in rated anxiety is reported, and no signs of anxiety are apparent after an interval of 30 to 40 seconds, the same scene is given to the client again. The client then proceeds on to the next scene in the hierarchy if no anxiety is experienced.

Cormier and Cormier (1979) present a dialogue between a client and counselor in the scene presentation of a systematic desensitization procedure. The dialogue illustrates the counselor's responses to both a non–anxiety-provoking scene and a scene that elicits client anxiety:

COUNSELOR: Joan, after our relaxation session today, we're going to start working with your hierarchy. I'd like to explain how this goes. After you've relaxed, I'll ask you to imagine the first item on the low end of your hierarchy. That is, the more pleasant one. It will help you relax even more. Then I'll describe the next item. I will show you a way to let me know if you feel any anxiety while you're imagining it. If you do, I'll ask you to stop or erase the image and to relax. You'll have some time to relax before I give you an item again. Does this seem clear?

CLIENT: I believe so.

COUNSELOR: One more thing. If at any point during the time you're imagining a scene you feel nervous or anxious about, just raise your finger. This will signal that to me. OK?

CLIENT: OK.

COUNSELOR: Just to make sure we're both on the same track, could you tell me what you believe will go on during this part of desensitization?

CLIENT: Well, after relaxation you'll ask me to imagine an item at the bottom of the hierarchy. If I feel any anxiety, I'll raise my finger and you'll ask me to erase the scene and relax.

COUNSELOR: Good. And even if you don't signal anxiety after a little time of imagining an item, I'll tell you to stop and relax. this gives you a sort of breather. Ready to begin?

CLIENT: Yep.

COUNSELOR: OK, first we'll begin with some relaxation. Just get in a comfortable position and close your eyes and relax. . . . Let the tension drain out of your body. . . . Now, to the word *relax,* just let your arms go limp. . . . Now relax your face. . . . Loosen up your face and neck muscles. . . . As I name each muscle group, just use the word *relax* as the signal to let go of all the tension. . . . Now, Joan, you'll feel even more relaxed by thinking about a pleasant situation. . . . Just imagine you're sitting around a campfire on a cool winter night. . . . You're with some good friends, singing songs and roasting marshmallows. . . . Now I'd like you to imagine you're sitting in English class. It's about 10 minutes before the bell. Your mind drifts to math class. You wonder if anything will happen like getting called on [presentation of item 3 in hierarchy]. . . . (Joan's finger goes up). . . . OK, Joan, just erase that image from your mind. . . . Now relax. Let relaxation flood your body. . . . Think again about being in front of a campfire. (Pauses for about 40 seconds for relaxation.) Now I'd like you to again imagine you're sitting in English class. It's almost time for the bell. You think about math class and wonder if you'll be called on [second presentation of item 3 in the hierarchy]. . . . (At 30 seconds, Joan has not signaled.). . . . OK, Joan, now just erase that image and concentrate on relaxing. (Pauses about 40 seconds.) OK, again imagine yourself sitting in English class. It's just a few minutes before the bell. You think about math class and wonder if you'll be called on [third presentation of item 3]. (At 30 seconds, no signal. . . . Since the last two presentations of this item did not evoke anxiety, the counselor can move on to item 4 or can terminate this scene-presentation session on this successfully completed item if Joan is restless.) (pp. 455–456)

BEHAVIORAL CONTINGENCIES: OPERANT CONDITIONING

Operant conditioning, in its various forms, is probably the single most popular behavioral learning paradigm (Belkin, 1980). In classical conditioning, the pairing or connecting of stimuli determines a client's actions; in operant conditioning, the reinforcement that *follows* an action determines whether that action will be repeated. Thus, learning through operant conditioning is the opposite of learning through classical conditioning. Operant learning occurs because of what happens after a particular action; classical learning occurs in response to a stimulus in the environment. In operant conditioning an individual must first act in a certain manner. The probability that the action will be repeated or not repeated is contingent upon whether the action is reinforced, punished, or ignored.

There are four basic contingencies possible in the operant learning paradigm: reward, escape, punishment, and omission (Rachlin, 1970). A reward, or positive reinforcement, tends to *increase* the probability that the action it follows will recur because the reward is pleasurable. Escape or negative reinforcement also *increases* the probability that an action will recur because the action is followed by the removal of, or escape from, an aversive consequence. Punishment *decreases* the probability that an action will recur because the action is followed by painful or aversive consequences. Omission or extinction also *decreases* the probability that an action will recur because there is no reinforcement after the action.

Contingency management is the name given to the use of operant conditioning principles as a behavioral intervention strategy with clients. Rimm and Masters (1979) defined contingency management as "the contingent presentation and withdrawal of rewards and punishments" (p. 155). The ultimate success of any contingency management program, however, is determined by the kind of contingencies used and how they are applied. We will now consider these valuable tools for effecting client change.

Positive Reinforcement

The terms reinforcement and reward are often used synonymously, and to a considerable extent they do overlap in meaning. A *positive* reinforcer is an event, behavior, privilege, or material object that will increase the probability of occurrence of any behavior upon which it is contingent (Premack, 1965; Skinner, 1953). A smile or a compliment from another person is an event that is likely to act as a reinforcer and increase the probability that an individual will in the future act in the same manner that elicited the smile or compliment. It is important to emphasize the "likely"—although a therapist can often anticipate what will act as a reinforcer for a particular client, he or she cannot be certain until it is observed that the contingent presentation of the speculated reinforcer does, indeed, affect the client's actions (Rimm & Masters, 1979).

Positive reinforcement is probably the most widely used and successful of operant principles. The therapist who wants to use positive reinforcement should consider these relevant questions: What behaviors should be reinforced? What type of reinforcer should be used, and how frequently? Should the positive reinforcer be combined with another technique, such as punishment or extinction?

Negative Reinforcement

Negative reinforcement also strengthens and increases the likelihood that an action will recur. Many persons incorrectly equate negative reinforcement and punishment because both involve aversive events. Negative reinforcement refers to an increase in the performance of an action when that action results in escaping from or avoiding an aversive event. Thus, adding a positive event or terminating a negative event both have the same effect on an individual's actions: they increase the frequency of the actions on whose occurrence they are contingent. For example, a teacher may yell at students to be quiet. If the students do in fact become quiet after the teacher yells at them, they have negatively reinforced the yelling, and the teacher will probably yell again in similar circumstances.

Negative reinforcement can be used effectively either alone or with other techniques for increasing adaptive behavior. Because negative reinforcement involves aversive events, it is best used only when positive alternatives alone are found ineffective, and should be used simultaneously with techniques that teach more appropriate actions.

Punishment

Punishment means presenting or withdrawing an event following an action to reduce the future performance of that action. Of all the behavioral learning principles, punishment has been the most publicized, which is unfortunate because it has given the public a one-sided view of behavior therapy. It is especially regrettable that many examples reported in the press are a product of persons lacking adequate training and use contingencies that would not be sanctioned by experienced behavior therapists (Groden & Cautela, 1981).

There are three basic forms of punishment: response cost, overcorrection, and time-out. Response cost refers to the contingent removal of a reinforcer after inappropriate behavior. Examples of response cost are plentiful in everyday life: library and traffic fines, pay deductions for lateness, and other penalties.

Overcorrection refers to two consequences in sequence following an undesired behavior (Foxx & Azrin, 1973). The first is restitution, in which an individual must correct the effects of the misbehavior; the second consists of extensive rehearsal of the correct behavior. Overcorrection has found its way into the judicial system in recent years. In nonviolent crimes, such as malicious destruction of community property by youth, the youth have been not only required to pay for the damage done but also to serve on work projects cleaning up the community.

Time-out, or, more appropriately, time-out from reinforcement, refers to removing all positive events for a specified time. To effect a time-out, an individual is isolated for a period in an area that contains no positive or potentially reinforcing elements. Sending a child to his or her room for misbehavior might be intended as a time-out, but if the room is full of toys and games, or a TV set, remaining there hardly constitutes a time-out from reinforcement. Time-outs are best accomplished by withdrawing major rewards such as social attention (for example, by ignoring), but as just noted, if alternative sources of reinforcement are available, the time-out is not effective.

Most behavior therapists use punishment as little as possible and only when nonpunishing procedures are apparently insufficient. A number of behavior therapists have sought to develop effective, nonaversive procedures for treating even the most problematic behavior problems and have made much headway (Repp & Deitz, 1974).

Extinction

All actions learned through operant conditioning must be reinforced at least occasionally if they are to recur. Behavior reduction resulting from the absence of reinforcement is known as extinction. Extinction is similar to time-out in that in both situations behavior is changed because of a lack of consistent reinforcement. They differ, however, in one basic way: "In extinction, reinforcement is withheld for a particular behavior, while in time-out the client is denied access to all sources of reinforcement through either transferring him or her to a nonreinforcing situation or removing the source of reinforcement from the present situation" (Benoit & Mayer, 1976, p. 208).

Benoit and Mayer (1974) point out critical questions counselors must consider before deciding whether extinction is appropriate: Are the reinforcers of the behavior to be extinguished known? Can these reinforcers be withheld? Have alternative behaviors been identified? Can the subject tolerate an increase in the negative behavior? Benoit and Mayer also note the importance of distinguishing between simply ignoring an action and extinguishing it. Extinction requires that the reinforcement for a particular action be withheld. It may well be, as they suggest, that the reinforcement for a specific action is not always apparent. For instance, an individual may be getting pleasure out of some fantasy associated with an action rather than any observable overt response.

Answering the kinds of questions Benoit and Mayer ask will help a therapist decide if extinction can be used or whether an alternative is necessary. It is especially important to note that in employing extinction, negative behaviors are likely to intensify before they decrease in frequency. Consider, for example, a parent trying to reduce a child's tantrums. Extinction is used to remove reinforcement, in this case the parent's responding with attention to the child's tantrum. At first, the child's rate and intensity of tantrums will increase because the behavior has provided reinforcement in the past and the child likely knows from experience that it is just a matter of time until the parent can stand no more! The parent must be able to withstand the pressure if extinction is to be successful.

Extinction is always more effective when combined with other techniques that stimulate and simultaneously reinforce alternative appropriate actions. Unless the client can identify a new means of deriving reinforcement, he or she is more likely to continue old ways, no matter how maladaptive or unreinforcing.

Contingency Contracting: An Operant Intervention

Of all the interventions in behavior therapy, the use of operant conditioning principles in a contingency management program is certainly backed by the most empirical research. Contingency management in which the contingencies are clearly formalized in advance between counselor and client is called *contingency contracting*. This intervention strategy has been used effectively with a wide range of problem behaviors. In and of itself, contingency contracting implies little more than clearly identifying specific behaviors and their contingent consequences.

In a contingency contract the desired, or target, behavior and the contingencies for achieving it or not achieving it are specified. The positive contingencies can be called *rewards;* the negative, *sanctions* (Stuart, 1971). For example, a contingency contract for a smoker might include:

TARGET BEHAVIOR: To reduce cigarette smoking from 60 cigarettes a day to 40 cigarettes a day for the next week.

REWARD: If less than 40 cigarettes have been smoked that whole day, $5.00 will be contributed to buying new clothes on the weekend.

SANCTION: If more than 40 cigarettes have been smoked that day, $5.00 will be contributed to the American Cancer Society.

Some behavior therapists have requested clients to deposit a valuable possession or money with the therapist (Boudin, 1972; Mann, 1972). If the client achieves the target behavior, some or all of the money or the possession are returned. If the contract terms are not met, the therapist turns over the possession or the money to someone else—often a group disliked by the client, such as a liberal having to contribute to a staunch conservative group. Mahoney and Thoresen (1974) caution, however, that clients may be reluctant to agree to contingency contracting involving deposits of money or possessions because of the very real risk of loss.

Cormier and Cormier (1979) describe six features of an effective contingency contract:

1. The contract terms should be clear to all involved parties. The target behavior to be achieved should be realistic and clearly specified. For example, a contract designed to increase contacts with new persons should specify something like "Initiate a conversation to last at least 3 minutes with 2 new persons each day" rather than "meet more people." Weathers and Lieberman (1975) noted that "novices in contracting are inclined toward writing vague, general terms using the ambiguity to ease the negotiation. . . . [The result is that] each party can interpret a vague statement in ways agreeable to himself. This serves only to postpone the conflict" (p. 209).

2. The contract should include a balance of rewards and sanctions appropriate to the desired target behavior. The client always should be rewarded for sufficiently achieving the contracted target behavior. Some sanctions may be necessary to maintain the potency of a contract (Mann, 1972), although occasionally an effective contract may include only rewards (Vance, 1976). Whether or not sanctions are included is best determined on an individual basis, since individual clients will respond differently to the use of a sanction as a motivational device.

3. The contract should emphasize the positive. A bonus clause often provides an additional inducement to attain the target behavior.

4. The contract should involve another person, who has a positive rather than a negative role, to help administer rewards for desired behaviors and ignore undesired behaviors. Generally, it is not a good practice to have persons other than the therapist punish the client for failing to comply with the contract terms. Clients have been found to respond negatively, not positively, to aversive environmental pressure (Hackett, Horan, Stone, Linberg, Nicholas, & Lukaski, 1976).

5. The contract should be in writing and signed by involved parties. A written contract minimizes ambiguity and increases the chance of the client achieving the target behavior.

6. The contract should include a recording system (a progress log) that specifies the behavior to be observed, the amount (frequency or duration) of the behavior, and the rewards and sanctions to be administered. If possible, the recording system should be verified by at least one other person. Kanfer (1975) notes that a recording system provides a means of keeping clients informed of their progress while carrying out the contractual agreement. A progress log is one example.

Figures 3–1 and 3–2 respectively illustrate a contingency contract and a progress log. The contract and log include the six features of an effective contract, with each characteristic noted in the righthand column of Figure 3–1. The progress log is used to keep track of the desired behavior and its duration. A third person assists with the contract by verifying the progress log. This surveillance by another person has been shown to influence the results of contingency contracting (Jones, Nelson, & Kazdin, 1977).

A major part of the success in contingency contracting depends on how the contract is negotiated and then implemented. Initially, it is critical that all of the contract terms are negotiated by all parties involved—client, therapist, verifier, and any other significant individuals. The central feature of a contract is that *all* concerned parties specify the terms (Cormier &

FIGURE 3–1
Contingency Contract.
From *Interviewing Strategies for Helpers: A Guide to Assessment, Treatment, and Evaluation,* by W. H. Cormier and L. S. Cormier. Copyright © 1979 by Wadsworth, Inc. Reprinted by permission of the publisher, Brooks/Cole Publishing Company, Monterey, California.

	Name of person making contract____ *Sara* _____	
	Name of other persons____ *Jane (Roommate)* _____	
	Date____ *June 10, 1977* _____	
Goal to contract:	*To increase my daily exercise at home from zero to 10 minutes daily.*	(Target behavior) (Criterion level)
Action steps carried out by me:	*I agree to do 10 minutes of exercises each day in the morning after getting out of bed and to keep track of the amount of daily exercise on my log sheet.*	(Terms of contract)
Action steps carried out by others:	*Jane will do exercises with me and will verify my log sheet.*	(Participation clause for other persons)
Rewards carried out by me:	*For each day that I do 10 minutes exercise I will either watch 30 extra minutes of TV or read in my favorite book 30 extra minutes.*	(Positive consequences-self-administered)
Carried out by others:	*Jane will give positive feedback after 10 minutes of exercise and will see that I have 30 minutes quiet time to read or watch TV at night.*	(Positive consequences administered by others)
Bonus:	*If at the end of one week I have done 10 minutes of exercise each day, I will spend $5.00 any way I want to.*	(Additional positive consequences for nearly flawless completion of contract)
Sanctions (optional) carried out by me:	*For each day that I do not do 10 minutes exercise I will not watch TV or read my favorite book that day.*	(Sanctions—self-administered)
Carried out by others:	*For each day I do not do 10 minutes exercise, Jane will ignore this and say nothing.*	(Sanctions—other administered)
Date contract will be reviewed:	*July 10, 1977* Signed **Sara M.**	(Client signature)
	Jane P.	(Other person's signature)

Cormier, 1975). A contract differs from a rule or proclamation, in which only one person defines the terms. Contract negotiation implies that the terms are specified without the threat of explicit or subtle coercion (Weathers & Lieberman, 1975). The advantage of the contract is that the terms are more likely to be acceptable to everyone who will implement them (Williams, Long, & Yoakley, 1972).

Before the contract takes effect, the therapist should make sure the client is specifically committed to the *actions,* not the promises in the contract (Kanfer & Karoly, 1972). Both oral and written commitment (a signature on the contract) are valuable (Cormier & Cormier, 1979). Requesting that the client rehearse the contracted-to behaviors in a coun-

Name			Sara		

Behavior being observed_____ *Daily physical exercises*

Verification source_____ *Jane*

Week	Date	Amount/ Frequency of Behavior	Reward Used (or) Sanction Used	Verified By
1	June 11	10 min.	30 min. TV	J.P.
1	June 12	10 min.	30 min. reading	J.P.
1	June 13	10 min.	30 min. reading	J.P.
1	June 14	15 min.	30 min. reading	J.P.
1	June 15	10 min.	30 min. reading	J.P.
1	June 16	10 min.	30 min. TV	J.P.
1	June 17	15 min.	30 min. TV plus $5.00 for a record (bonus)	J.P.
2	June 18	10 min.	30 min. TV	J.P.
2	June 19	10 min.	30 min. TV	J.P.
2	June 20	5 min.	no TV	J.P.
2	June 21	10 min.	30 min. reading	J.P.
2	June 22	10 min.	30 min. reading	J.P.
2	June 23	5 min.	no reading	J.P.
2	June 24	10 min.	30 min. reading but no bonus	J.P.

FIGURE 3-2

Progress Log. From *Interviewing Strategies for Helpers: A Guide to Assessment, Treatment, and Evaluation,* by W. H. Cormier and L. S. Cormier. Copyright © 1979 by Wadsworth, Inc. Reprinted by permission of the publisher, Brooks/Cole Publishing Company, Monterey, California.

seling session before trying them "in the real world" can help the client carry out the actions more easily. Rehearsing in a therapy session also motivates the client to implement the contract regularly and systematically (Cormier & Cormier, 1979). Further, as Kanfer (1975) observed, the effectiveness of a contract often depends on the degree that the contract is used for "everyday conduct."

There are several ways to encourage clients to adhere to the terms of a contingency contract. First, clients are more likely to carry out the agreement if rewards are maximized and costs are minimized (Weathers & Liberman, 1975). As these writers assert, the contract must do more than simply meet the "status quo"; advantages that exceed the status quo must be available to the client. Second, contract terms will be implemented with greater consistency if they are reasonable and do not require too much of the client's time, effort, or achievement. If the contract asks too much or fails to reward the client for small steps of progress, the client is likely to become discouraged and abandon the effort (Cormier & Cormier, 1979). The therapist should help a client develop a contract that uses abilities the client already has and provides reinforcement for gradual levels of improvement (Weathers & Lieberman, 1975). Third, the contract should be reviewed periodically to determine whether it is being carried out or if revisions in it are necessary. Finally, the therapist should encourage and reinforce the client as the contract is being used. Support and regular review by the therapist will increase the probability that clients will initiate and maintain contract terms (Cantrell, Cantrell, Huddleston, & Wooldridge, 1969).

SEEING IS BELIEVING: OBSERVATIONAL LEARNING

Classical and operant conditioning are the more traditional principles of learning theory. The use of observational learning in behavior therapy is a relatively recent development (Bandura, 1969; 1971). Classical and operant conditioning require an overt, observable response by a client for learning to occur. By contrast, observational learning or *modeling* principles propose that persons learn not only by actually doing but also by watching the behavior of models, either in the real world or through various media. Completely new and novel behaviors can be learned simply by observation. For example, it is easier and more efficient to teach a beginner the forehand stroke in tennis by showing a film of a skilled tennis player than by rewarding each discrete portion of the stroke that is actually performed.

In its simplest form, modeling is learning by example. If the example is positive, then positive behavior will be the likely outcome; if, on the other hand, the example is negative, then undesirable behavior will result (Belkin, 1980). The child who models his or her parents' cooperative behaviors is likely to cooperate with others. It is a well-documented fact that children of abusive parents, for example, are likely to be abusive toward their own children (Kempe & Helfer, 1980).

There are a number of basic functions that modeling serves (Rimm & Masters, 1979). By observing a model, a client can learn new, more appropriate behavior patterns, and modeling may serve an *acquisition* function. This observational learning effect refers to integrating new patterns of behavior based on watching a model demonstrate the behavior. Even more likely, observing a model's behavior in various situations provides social *facilitation* of appropriate behaviors. The client is induced to perform learned behaviors that he or she has not been applying or has been applying inappropriately. Clients often misunderstand how to use correctly many previously learned behaviors. Modeling may lead to the *disinhibition* of behaviors that the client has avoided because of fear or anxiety. And, through disinhibiting behaviors, modeling may promote the *direct extinction* of the fear associated with the person, situation, or object toward which the avoidance behavior had been directed.

Bandura (1969, 1977) delineated four component processes involved in observational learning: attention, retention, motor reproduction, and motivation. *Attention* is the activity of the observer in focusing on what is modeled. For example, it might be very difficult for a client to attend to a model when feeling very anxious. In such cases, the therapist may have to introduce relaxation procedures before modeling can be used

(Cormier & Cormier, 1979). One way to help a client attend is to point out or cue the client about what to look for before the model is presented.

Retention is how the client is able to organize and code what has been modeled or demonstrated. The ability of individuals to describe behavior in words often enhances retention significantly (Rimm & Masters, 1979). For instance, while a client is watching a model display appropriate social skills, the therapist might urge the client to orally describe specifically what is occurring: "She is leaning forward when she is talking, clearly listening with interest, periodically making direct eye contact with him, and showing an obvious enjoyment in the conversation by smiling and nodding her head."

The third component of the modeling process is *motor reproduction,* which refers to the ability of the client to reproduce, rehearse, or physically practice the modeled behavior. Rehearsing what has been observed is often best and most easily accomplished by having the client play the model's role in a counseling session. The client can practice the model's actions while the therapist adopts a complementary role.

The final component of the observational learning process is *motivation.* A therapist can motivate by giving the client a reason for using a modeled behavior. For example, the therapist can explain how the demonstrated behavior will benefit the client. Motivation can also be enhanced if a client successfully performs the modeled behavior, which is best accomplished by repeated practice of small, successive steps (Cormier & Cormier, 1979).

The four components of the observational learning process—attention, retention, motor reproduction, and motivation—are developmental. Attention is requisite to retention. Likewise, retention is needed before motor reproduction can occur, and so on. Thus, all phases of the process are vital to actual learning. The process can be enhanced further, however, by the characteristics of the model and by how the modeling procedure is presented.

Models: An Inexhaustible Supply

Although models are virtually limitless in their availability, several general categories of models are generally used in therapeutic situations. The most common type is the *live model.* The therapist is the most accessible model for most clients. Through actual behavior during sessions, a therapist can teach self-disclosure, risk taking, openness, honesty, compassion, respect, self-acceptance, tolerance and courage. In addition to modeling desirable behaviors, therapists can also adversely influence clients' actions by modeling lack of regard and respect for self or others, fear, rudeness, and rigidity. Therapists can be models for their clients for better or worse (Corey, 1982).

Models can also be *symbolic.* The use of films, videotapes, and other representational devices can be vehicles for modeling specific behaviors. In reviewing the research on the use of symbolic modeling, Bandura (1969) reported that symbolic modeling was successful in a variety of applications. One such application used filmed models who were able to encounter certain frightening circumstances without suffering negative consequences. Such symbolic modeling enabled clients to decrease or eliminate certain fears.

Multiple models can give the observer a great number of alternative ways to act, for they display a variety of appropriate and successful styles of behaving. Multiple models may give more cues to a client and have a greater impact that a single model because the client can draw from the strengths exhibited by each model.

Modeling

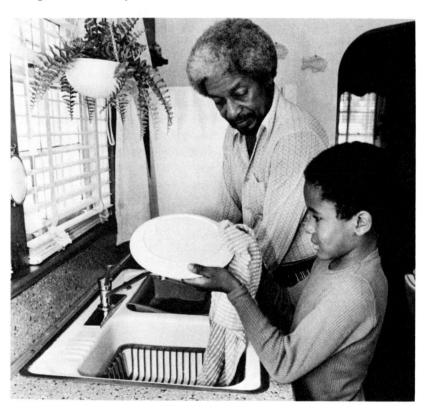

The "Ideal" Model?

The characteristics of a model will directly effect the success of observational learning efforts. The "ideal" model may not be the one most persons would consider ideal, however. Research indicates that modeling is more effective when the model and the client are quite similar (Bandura, 1971). A model who is similar to the client in age, sex, race, and attitudes is more likely to be imitated than a model who is unlike the client. Models at a moderate level of prestige and status are more likely to be imitated than those at a lower level. However, the status level of the model should not be so high that the client views the model's actions as unrealistic for herself or himself to emulate.

Kazdin (1973; 1974) proposes that a coping model is very often better than a mastery model. That is, a model who shows some fear or anxiety, makes errors in performance, and shows some degree of struggle or coping while performing an activity will be less threatening and more realistic than a model who performs flawlessly. Clients have been found to identify more readily with a coping model, or what Marlett and Perry (1975) refer to as a "slider" model, who displays gradual improvement during a complex series of modeled behaviors. For example, anxious clients may model new behaviors more quickly if they observe timid models gradually attain calmness rather than perform fearlessly at once. Modeled behaviors should be attuned to the perspective of the client and not be beyond their immediate reach (Cormier & Cormier, 1979). Models who share, yet overcome, similar handicaps are therapeutically beneficial when viewed by clients as having mutual concerns and like histories (Rosenthal, 1976).

Developing Decision-Making: A Session with Stan

In a sense, modeling is the most simple and obvious method to teach clients more adaptive ways of acting. Seeing and hearing directly, especially with the therapist acting as the model, can bring home the message much more effectively than through other forms of learning. The following case illustrates this.

Stan is a 35-year-old school teacher experiencing difficulties in many aspects of his life because he cannot effectively evaluate situations and then make appropriate decisions that are in his best interests. His impulsive actions or avoidance of acting at all have resulted in a rather confused and unsatisfactory lifestyle, especially socially.

Cormier and Cormier (1979) suggested therapists implementing modeling as an intervention strategy keep the following guidelines in mind:

1. Tell the client what to look for before the modeled demonstration.
2. Select a model who is similar to the client and who can demonstrate the goal behaviors in a coping manner.
3. Present the modeled demonstration in a sequence of scenarios that minimize stress for the client.

4. Ask the client to summarize what he or she saw after the demonstration.

Typically, after watching the desired behaviors modeled, the client practices the behaviors. Modeling is a prerequisite for rehearsal when the behaviors are not in the client's present skills repertoire. For Stan, the goal of this session is behavior acquisition. The therapeutic rationale is simple: Stan wants to make more satisfying decisions, but doesn't know how. Without a modeled demonstration, Stan would have difficulty practicing something virtually unknown to him. The therapist, through modeling, gives Stan some new skills he can use during rehearsals of the desired decision-making behavior and then later outside the session.

[To begin, the therapist provides a therapeutic rationale for Stan to help him understand why they will be using this intervention strategy.]

THERAPIST: We had agreed that today we would begin working on developing more effective decision-making skills. The procedures we will employ I have used with other clients who have found them to be most beneficial and I think you will also. We will talk about the various components of effective decision-making and then practice the necessary skills in some role-play experiences here in our session. It will give you a chance to practice making decisions without having to worry about the actual consequences. As you acquire more decision-making skills in this way, it will be easier for you to implement them on your own. How does this all sound to you?

STAN: It sounds OK. I like the idea of having an opportunity to practice here.

[The therapist then offers an overview of how they will proceed and instructs Stan as to what to look for before the modeled demonstration (the *attention* component of the modeling process). Notice as well that the therapist asks Stan to select someone from his everyday environment to serve as the model. Stan is urged to select someone he regularly interacts with, the assumption being that he will choose someone in similar circumstances and with common interests. He does.]

THERAPIST: Great. What we'll do is go over one part of the decision-making process at a time. We'll work on each until you feel confident with the skills involved in it and then move on to the next component.

STAN: Fine.

THERAPIST: Let's start with how you might first determine what alternatives are available to you when faced with a decision. What is something that you were faced with recently?

STAN: Well, I was at home the other evening alone and just sat there sort of frozen unable to decide what to do.

THERAPIST: OK. Is there someone who you are friendly with that you might have been able to call and discuss what you might have done? Someone who you have some common interests with?

STAN: Yeah. My friend Chuck.

THERAPIST: Great. Let's role play you and Chuck having a conversation about what you might do on Saturday evening. You play the role of Chuck and I'll be you. In observing me play you, try to identify how many different alternatives I come up with and the skills I employ to arrive at the conclusions I do (Again, the *attention* component). I'll start. (as Stan) Hi, Chuck. What are you planning to do this Saturday evening?

STAN (as Chuck): I haven't really given it a lot of thought. Maybe go to the Yankees game. They're home against Boston. Would you like to come?

THERAPIST (as Stan): Thanks. That's a possibility. Actually, I was trying to think of all the different alternatives available before deciding what specifically I'm going to do. Got any other ideas?

STAN (as Chuck): Well, there's a party at Mary's house for the office crowd. Jim Jacobs is transferring to another office.

THERAPIST (as Stan): That's another alternative that might be fun. Anything else you can think of?

STAN (as Chuck): There's always the Mandarin Cafe. It's a fairly good place to meet other singles.

THERAPIST: Another good idea. I guess some of the things I've been thinking of were the Dog Track, going into the city, or asking a few people over for dinner.

STAN (as Chuck): Well, which is it going to be? What about a decision?

THERAPIST (as Stan): Right now, all I'm trying to do is think of all the possible alternatives.

STAN (as Chuck): Well, why not the Yankees-Boston game. It's sure to be your best choice. The other things you could likely do almost any time.

THERAPIST (as Stan): That's probably true, but right now I'm not concerned about whether which alternative is the best or worst. I'm just trying to think of all the possible choices that are open to me.

[The therapist then stops modeling decision-making skills via the role-play and emphasizes again to Stan what to look for, providing further instruction on this first phase of a decision-making process.]

THERAPIST: Let's stop for a moment. What I was trying to do was to attempt to come up with every way I could to spend Saturday evening, if I were you. The skill of generating potential alternatives is called brainstorming—the more choices the better. And at this point of the decision-making process, I was only trying to generate alternatives, not evaluate them.

[The therapist then asks Stan to review what he saw during the modeled demonstration (the *retention* component of the modeling process).]

THERAPIST: What did you notice about what I did during our role-play?

STAN: Well, I noticed that you tried to get me as Chuck to suggest as many ideas as I could before you offered any. That seemed to work well as far as generating more alternatives. Also you weren't looking to go along with the alternative that appeared most attractive at first glance, but rather wanted to come up with as many as possible before evaluating any of the potential choices. Coming up with all the possibilities we did made me realize how little thought I give to brainstorming.

[The therapist now asks Stan to review what he will attempt to do to reproduce and rehearse the skills that were just modeled for him (the *motor reproduction* component of the modeling process).]

THERAPIST: Very observant on your part, Stan. Let's switch roles now. This time we'll give you an opportunity to rehearse what you just learned for yourself. You be yourself and I'll be Chuck. Would you briefly review what skills you're going to try to employ during the next role-play?

STAN: First, I'm not going to make a snap decision. I'm going to try to be patient and come up with as many alternatives as possible. Further, I won't worry about whether an alternative is so great or just mediocre. Quantity, not quality, is my present concern.

THERAPIST: A great way to put it.

[The process is repeated again, this time with Stan playing himself. Stan's ability to successfully perform the modeled behavior just demonstrated to him will have a direct effect on his motivation to continue (*motivation*, the fourth component of the modeling process). Also note that the therapist is proceeding through the decision-making process by modeling one step of that process. Successful reproduction of the skills in that step will be accomplished prior to continuing to the next step and new skills. Thus, Stan's motivation will be further enhanced.]

REALITY THERAPY Behavior therapy in its strictest sense proposes that human beings are neither self-actualizing, nor self-denigrating. As human beings, they simply have equal potential for proceeding in either direction; their learning experiences and the skills they do or do not acquire determine who and what they become. Many practitioners find they desire a more directional philosophy of human nature, yet firmly believe in the major behavioral principles and practices; especially that *action* is the primary medium for facilitating successful treatment.

For the therapist desiring such a compromise, reality therapy, like behavior therapy, is a basically active, directive, didactic, and concrete approach that uses a contract. The therapist's main task is to encourage clients to face reality and judge their present behavior. Action is the primary focus, not attitudes, insight, the past, or unconscious motivation (Corey, 1982). Reality therapy, however, unlike behavior therapy, includes what might be considered a basic existential assumption, that a "growth force" impels human beings to strive for a "success identity."

The Importance of Identity

Glasser and Zunin (1979) posit the reality therapy perspective on human nature in stating:

> We believe each individual has a health or growth force. Basically people want to be content and enjoy a success identity, to show responsible behavior and to have meaningful interpersonal relationships. (p. 315)

Reality therapy, like the person-centered approach in chapter 2, is largely the product of a single person, Dr. William Glasser. He believed people are mainly motivated by trying to fulfill one basic need: the need for *identity*. According to reality therapy, it is most useful to consider identity in terms of a "success identity" versus a "failure identity." Other persons are significant in forming identity. Having love and acceptance is directly related to a success identity; lacking love and acceptance is related to a failure identity. According to Glasser (1965), the basis of reality therapy is to help clients fulfill the basic psychological needs, which include "the need to love and to be loved and the need to feel that we are worthwhile to ourselves and to others" (p. 10). In doing so, individuals are able to develop a success identity.

Glasser (1965) has stated that all clients who enter therapy have been unsuccessful in meeting their needs, and in trying to do so they often select ineffective behaviors that virtually assure failure. In this regard, he asserted:

> In their unsuccessful effort to fulfill their needs, no matter what behavior they choose, all patients have a common characteristic: *they all deny the reality of the world about them.* Some break the law, denying the rules of society; some claim their neighbors are plotting against them, denying the improbability of such behavior. Some are afraid of crowded places, close quarters, airplanes, or elevators, yet they freely admit the irrationality of their fears. Millions drink to blot out the inadequacy they feel but that need not exist if they could learn to be different; and far too many people choose suicide rather than face the reality that they could learn to solve their problems by responsible behavior. Whether it is a partial denial or the total blotting out of all reality of the chronic back-ward patient in the state hospital, the denial of some or all of reality is common to all patients. (p. 6)

The key to individuals fulfilling their psychological needs and thus developing success identities is *responsible behavior;* behavior that leads to the satisfaction of personal needs without depriving others of the ability to fulfill their needs (Glasser, 1965). Responsible behavior results in the formation of a success identity; irresponsible behavior results in the formation of a failure identity.

Asserting Responsible Action

The basic therapeutic goal of reality therapy is to help clients develop and maintain a success identity through responsible action. As Glasser and Zunin (1979) state:

> Identity change follows change in behavior. To a great extent, we are what we do, and if we want to change what we are, we must begin by changing what we do and undertake new ways of behaving. (p. 315)

Clients, as they develop a personal sense of responsibility, become increasingly more able to alter their behaviors, to arrive ultimately at more acceptable and satisfying standards that, in turn, enable them to gratify their needs. Glasser (1965) states:

> *To be worthwhile we must maintain a satisfactory standard of behavior.* To do so we must learn to correct ourselves when we do wrong and to credit ourselves when we do right. If we do not evaluate our own behavior, or, having evaluated it, if we do not act to improve our conduct where it is below our standards, we will not fulfill our need to be worthwhile and we will suffer. (p. 12)

Reality therapy attaches values to clients' behaviors, assessing success or failure against these values. Responsibility is the foundation: a value in itself against which other values are assessed. Responsible behavior is the therapeutic "yardstick":

> Reality therapy differs from conventional therapy in that it labels behavior as either responsible or irresponsible (not the person as mentally ill) . . . Responsibility is considered the basic concept of reality therapy and is defined as the ability to meet one's needs without depriving others of the ability to meet theirs. Realistic behavior presumably occurs when an individual considers and compares the immediate and remote consequences of his actions. (Rachin, 1974, p. 46)

Reality therapy has been described as a "common-sense approach to counseling" (Ivey & Simek-Downing, 1980). It advocates finding out what clients want and need and examining their present assets and failures, and also considers environmental factors that must be addressed if needs are to be satisfied. People live in a *real* world; they must face that world, accepting its limitations as well as its positive offerings, and learn to live adaptively with both.

A Process of Teaching and Learning Responsible Behavior

Glasser (1965) contended that teaching (and clients learning) responsibility is the core of reality therapy. Reality therapists teach clients better ways to fulfill their needs by exploring their understanding of reality and then showing them how to act responsibly within the context of that reality. In order to effectively teach clients, Glasser (1965) asserts that the therapist must first become involved with the client, for "unless the requisite involvement exists between the necessarily responsible therapist and the irresponsible patient, there can be no therapy" (p. 25).

Glasser (1965) focuses on the therapist's role in becoming involved with clients in stating:

> One way to attempt an understanding of how involvement occurs is to describe the qualities necessary to be a therapist. The more a person has these qualities, the better he is able to use the principles of reality therapy to develop proper involvement.
>
> The therapist must be a very responsible person—tough, interested, human, sensitive. He must be able to fulfill his own needs and must be willing to discuss some of his own struggles so that the patient can see that acting responsibly is possible though sometimes difficult. . . . The therapist must always be strong, never expedient. He must withstand the patient's requests for sympathy, for an excess of sedatives, for justification of his actions no matter how the patient pleads or threatens. Never condoning an irresponsible action on the patient's part, he must be willing to watch the patient suffer, if that helps him toward responsibility. . . . Finally, the therapist must be able to become emotionally involved with each patient. To some extent he must be affected by the patient and his problems and even suffer with him. (pp. 26–28)

After becoming involved with a client, the reality therapist points out to the client the unrealistic aspects of her or his irresponsible behavior. The therapist does not make direct value judgments and decisions for the client, but rather tries to help them realistically appraise their own behavior. Questions such as "What are you doing—and does this behavior get you what you desire?" are asked. If a client chooses to argue that her or his concept of reality, one that is maintaining a failure identity, is correct, Glasser (1965) suggested, "We must be willing to discuss his opinions, but we must not fail to emphasize that our main interest is his behavior rather than his attitude" (p. 34).

Glasser summarizes the therapeutic process of reality therapy, stating:

Developing a therapeutic involvement may take anywhere from one interview to several months, depending upon the skill of the therapist, his control over the patient, and the resistence of the patient. Once it occurs, the therapist begins to insist that the patient face the reality of his behavior. He is no longer allowed to evade recognizing what he is doing or his responsibility for it. When the therapist takes this step—and he should start as soon as involvement begins—the relationship deepens because now someone cares enough about the patient to make him face a truth that he has spent his life trying to avoid: *he is responsible for his behavior.* Now, continually confronted with reality by the therapist, he is not allowed to excuse or condone any of his behavior. No reason is acceptable to the therapist for any irresponsible behavior. He confronts the patient with his behavior and asks him to decide whether or not he is taking the responsible course. (p. 33)

One Client's Experience with Reality Therapy

Glasser and Zunin (1979) present the case of a 30-year-old woman complaining of difficulties in many areas of her life. We present excerpts from this case here to illustrate some of the basic concepts of reality therapy as a behaviorally-oriented approach.

During the initial visits the therapist concentrated on creating a meaningful therapeutic involvement. This was done in part by being personal, warm, friendly, and concerned about her difficult current life situation. Initial emphasis was placed on exploring this woman's strengths, potentials, and attributes. An exploration of her current life was made with particular attention to the activities she enjoyed. These were activities with her husband, family, friends, children, hobbies, and so forth. This discussion not only served to enhance the therapeutic involvement but also provided the woman with an enhanced self-esteem and an increased understanding of her strong qualities and reinforced the fact that she had something to offer herself and others at this point in life. It was important to the therapist that he not allow her to paint a picture of herself as only disorganized, lonely, desperate, and dissatisfied.

An intensive inquiry into her current activities in a detailed fashion was made during the initial phase of therapy. this included a detailed understanding of her interaction with her husband when they are together and their behavior toward each other, her interaction with her friends and her children, and her behavior regarding participation in organizations, religion, school and so forth.

As therapy progressed, she was assisted directly in understanding that there were many alternatives available to her and that these alternatives would be explored and discussed. Individuals in situations like this often, as a result of their inner conflicts, have an inability to see alternatives, thinking there is "really no choice." Her inner suffering certainly indicated serious inner conflict and certainly each side of the conflict was a result of many factors. Her suffering, the therapist surmised, would not disappear without a change in her behavior. She was assisted in understanding that her attitude, thinking, and personality would follow, and not precede, a change in behavior. She was assisted in understanding that, to a large extent, we are what we do and if we want to change what we are, we must begin by changing what we do and undertake new directions of behavior.

She was repeatedly confronted with her alternatives and guided toward assuming responsibility for decisions. At the same time, her ambitions were mobilized and she was assisted and directed in exploring her interests in a meaningful and constructive manner. . . . Discussion of feelings of hopelessness, depression, or loneliness were continually converted into questions regarding her behavioral activities, attitudes, and modes of interaction.

As therapy progressed, this woman was assisted in making specific value judgments about all aspects of her behavior. "Is what you are doing in this particular situation getting you what you want—if not let's talk about what you can do to change this situation to enable you to get what would be more satisfying to you." The making of plans to alter her specific behavior took a relatively long period and the therapist thought it was desirable to write out with the patient during the therapy sessions some of the plans, or have the patient write as they were talking. The woman was guided in making specific value judgments, which not only took into consideration her feelings, for example, about having an affair, but legal, sociological, moral, and humane issues as well. . . .

After the patient made value judgments about specific aspects of her behavior and was assisted in plan making . . . she was then faced with making a commitment to follow through with the plan . . . if the plan failed at any point, rather than exploring the reasons for failure, or the excuses for failure, the therapist in a nonjudgmental but a warm and caring way proceeded to make a new plan with the patient rather than focus on why the old plans failed. . . .

During the course of the therapy, the therapist repeatedly emphasized that he was interested in dealing with the present, particularly with her present attempts to succeed and to deal with her problems in a mature and effective manner. With this woman, it was necessary for the therapist to assure her that he would stay with her until the problems she came for were resolved. Any resort by the patient to "I can't" in discussing situations was appropriately converted to "you mean you won't or you don't want to—let's explore the pros and cons." Until this woman realized she was responsible for her own behavior and that she was not in an irreconcilable or irreversible situation, no therapeutic progress occurred. She finally realized and acknowledged that, in fact, she was responsible for her behavior. . . . Thus, the patient was assisted in understanding her capacity for more worthwhile behavior within her immediate surroundings. Her ultimate choice to change those surroundings and her decision to change her behavior and her subsequent maintenance of her decisions were the therapy. (pp. 334–337)

A Caveat: The Reality Therapist

Corey (1982) describes how many of Glasser's readers have developed a distorted notion that the reality therapist functions as a moralist. Glasser (1972) asserts that his principle of the critical importance of evaluating behavior had been frequently misunderstood. In clarifying his position, he disavowed the role of the reality therapist as a moralist:

Some people accept and others reject reality therapy because they misunderstand this principle. Both groups believe the reality therapist acts as a moralist, which he does not; he never tells anyone that what he is doing is wrong and that he must change. The therapist does not judge the behavior; he leads the patient to evaluate his own behavior through his involvement and by bringing the actual behavior out in the open. (p. 119)

BEHAVIORAL APPROACHES: THEORETICAL ANALYSES

Learning can be defined as changes in behavior that are not due to native response tendencies, maturation, or temporary states of the organism (i.e., fatigue or drugs) (Hilgard & Bower, 1966). Therapy is obviously concerned with behavior change and therefore involves learning and learning theory. Counseling and psychotherapy thus might be considered an application of principles of learning theory (Patterson, 1973).

While this reasoning may appear acceptable, the actual situation is not as simple as such logic might suggest. The affectively-oriented approaches in chapter 2, for example, have not developed from learning theory, nor do they use its principles. Although it would appear that any approach must be consistent with learning theory principles, most approaches do not systematically evaluate their processes or outcomes from this point of view (Patterson, 1973).

Corey (1982) described the initial reaction of many of his students to behavior therapy. Their responses mirror common misconceptions of counselors and psychotherapists in the present but especially of the past. He notes:

> I have found that students sometimes approach behavior therapy with a closed mind, thinking that it is associated with a strictly deterministic and scientific approach to human behavior. Some students make the mistake of perceiving the behavior therapist as a technician and researcher who treats people like laboratory animals. It is clear that, although contemporary behavior therapy rests on a scientific view of human behavior that calls for a structured and systematic approach to counseling and therapy, this does not mean that factors such as the importance of the therapeutic relationship or the potential of clients to choose their own way are diminished. (p. 163)

It is interesting to note that what has often been cited as the greatest fault of behavior therapy often proves to be its greatest advantage in the clinical setting, namely, its direct dealings with the symptom (Belkin, 1980). The vast majority of clients seek therapy because of specific *behaviors*. Rarely do individuals request immediate help to acquire greater insight or achieve self-actualization; they want to solve a specific, symptomatic problem. These problems are most readily related to how they act or fail to act. Thus, behavior therapy, with its primary emphasis on action and therefore the presenting symptom, provides a practical bonus to the therapist (Belkin, 1980).

With this focus on action, however, behavior therapy has been criticized for its lack of emphasis on the human qualities of the client. Some critics suggest that the behavioral perspective reduces the complexity of human life to simple equations that, although they may adequately explain an individual's overt actions, do not sufficiently account for motives of actions, accompanying feelings and emotions, and similarly less tangible factors. Sprinthall (1971), for example, argues that behavior therapy "virtually ignores developmental stages: stages of moral development, personal development, epistemological development—so much so that we may have inadvertently left the human being out of the process" (p. 66).

These criticisms have been called by behavior therapists unfair and unfounded biases. As Lazarus (1977) states:

> Behavior therapy and behavior modification have acquired a bad press. To receive funding, many hospitals and community agencies have had to drop the label *behavior* from their program proposals. In several quarters, the term *behavior modification* is

an adrenalin-raiser that evokes unfortunate stereotypes. One grows weary of explaining that behavior therapists do not deny consciousness, that they do not treat people like Pavlovian dogs, that they are not Machiavellian and coercive, that aversion therapy (except in the hands of a lunatic fringe) has always been a minor and relatively insignificant part of our armamentarium, and that we are not ignorant of the part played by mutual trust and other relationship factors among our treatment variables. (p. 553)

It is fully valid to state that behavior therapists do focus on specifics and employ a systematic approach to the counseling process. They perceive less value in the more global approaches to helping clients. While therapists of other orientations might assume that they understand what a client means in stating, "Life has no value for me," the behavior therapist seeks to help that client concretely define what she or he is attempting to communicate so that realistic therapeutic goals can be developed and worked toward. How can a goal of achieving "greater value in life" be attained? How can it's attainment be assessed? Behavior therapists work with their clients to set clear, concrete goals that can be readily recognized and evaluated. The behavior therapist might ask the client bemoaning a lack of value in life, "What *specific* aspects of your life do you find unsatisfactory? How do you see *these certain factors* causing you problems? What *specifically* would you have to see happening in your daily life to evaluate your circumstance more positively?"

This emphasis on the specific and systematic is likely the most valuable contribution of behavior therapy. Its theoretical principles and therapeutic procedures can be readily subjected to experimental verification. Thus, behavior therapy is continually evolving and improving. This criterion has been used to produce very desirable treatment results as well. Behavior therapy places a premium on careful assessment and validation of treatment outcomes. It is not enough for practitioners to merely make clinical "observations" that their interventions are promoting favorable client outcomes. Rather, they are challenged to demonstrate that what they are doing is working (Corey, 1982).

The behavior therapist's main task then is to work with clients to design therapeutic intervention programs through which specified target behaviors will be modified. This chapter has looked at the major theoretical principles and some accompanying therapeutic procedures of learning theory with which to accomplish this task. The basic concepts of classical conditioning, operant conditioning, and observational learning have been described and an intervention strategy emanating from each offered to amplify their practical therapeutic value. The behaviorally-oriented reality therapy is a compromise for individuals committed to an existential view of human nature but who need to first and foremost focus on specific and concrete *action.* Much more information and many more interventions are available and we encourage you to pursue them through the suggested readings at the end of this chapter.

SUGGESTED READINGS

Behavior Therapy

Adams, H. E., & Unikel, I. P. (Eds.). (1973). *Issues and trends in behavior therapy.* Springfield, IL: Thomas. This book offers not only clinical but also experiential and practical applications of behavior therapy concepts.

Alberti, R. E., & Emmons, M. L. (1978). *Your perfect right: A guide to assertive behavior.* San Luis Obispo, CA: Impact. The authors provide a brief and to-the-point explanation of the theory and guidelines for the practice of assertion training.

Bellack, A. S., & Hersen, M. (1977). *Behavior modification: An introductory textbook.* Baltimore: Williams & Wilkins. A fine introduction to topics such as social-skills training, self-management techniques, token economies, and more.

Gambrill, E. (1977). *Behavior modification: Handbook of assessment, intervention, and evaluation.* San Francisco: Jossey-Bass. Gambrill reviews behavioral research and therapy from an operant perspective.

Goldstein, M. R., & Davison, G. C. (1976). *Clinical behavior therapy.* New York: Holt, Rinehart and Winston. Insights into behavior therapy particularly as practiced within a clinical setting are expounded upon in this easy-reading volume.

Kanfer, F. H., & Goldstein, A. P. (1980). *Helping people change.* (2nd ed.). New York: Pergamon Press. A comprehensive account of contemporary behavior therapy. A superb resource for identifying specific techniques.

Krumboltz, J., & Thoresen, C. (Eds.). (1976). *Counseling methods.* New York: Holt, Rinehart and Winston. A case study book that covers a wide range of client issues. It offers a "cookbook" of behavior therapy procedures.

Skinner, B. F. (1953). *Science and human behavior.* New York: Macmillan. The primary spokesperson for operant conditioning provides an overview of his methods and how they might be applied to a wide array of situations ranging from individual change to changes in the larger society.

Skinner, B. F. (1971). *Beyond freedom and dignity.* New York: Bantam. Skinner presents his ideas about human nature from a behavioristic perspective. Behavioral technology in society, punishment and its alternatives, freedom, and values are among the issues addressed.

Williams, R., & Long, J. (1979). *Toward a self-managed life-style.* (2nd ed.). Boston: Houghton Mifflin. Behavioral procedures are all too often thought of as being applied to others. The authors illustrate applications of individual self-change strategies.

Reality Therapy

Bassin, A., Brater, T. E., & Rachlin, R. L. (Eds.). (1976). *The reality therapy reader.* New York: Harper & Row. A multitude of authors including Glasser consider the foundations of reality therapy. A broad range of applications are covered ranging from individual to marital to group therapy.

Glasser, W. (1961). *Mental health or mental illness.* New York: Harper & Row. Glasser's initial book describing in easy-to-understand language his views of how human beings function.

Glasser, W. (1965). *Reality therapy.* New York: Harper & Row. This book outlines the basic concepts of reality therapy and offers illustrations of the approach in actual practice.

Glasser, W. (1976). *Positive addiction.* New York: Harper & Row. This book examines Glasser's ideas on addiction, postulating that it can be powerfully positive and strengthening or negative and weakening.

Glasser, W. (1981). *Stations of the mind: New directions for reality therapy.* New York: Harper & Row. In this work, Glasser considers perspective as a critical theoretical clinical concept and applies it to reality therapy.

4

Cognitively-Oriented Approaches

Epictetus, the first century Stoic philosopher stated:
"Men are disturbed not by things, but by the views which
they take of them."

The central assumption of the cognitively-oriented approaches to counseling and psychotherapy is that "learned misconceptions (or faulty beliefs, or mistaken ideas) are the crucial factors which must be modified or eliminated before psychotherapy can be successful" (Raimy, 1975, p. 186).

Unlike affective and behavioral approaches, cognitive approaches posit that cognitions are the most important determinents of human emotions and behaviors. Simply stated, individuals feel and act on what they think. Specific events and/or other persons cannot make an individual feel or act in any way; the individual must initiate his or her own emotions and behaviors—cognitively. Therefore, external events can contribute to but do not directly cause emotional or behavioral reactions. Rather, it is individuals' internal events, their perceptions and evaluations of external events, that are direct and powerful sources of emotional and behavioral reactions (Walen, DiGiuseppe, & Wessler, 1980). Cognitive interventions focus on modifying feelings and actions by changing clients' patterns of thought.

What are commonly considered the major cognitively-oriented approaches to counseling and psychotherapy most popular today include cognitive therapy (Beck, 1976), cognitive behavior modification (Meichenbaum, 1977), rational-emotive therapy (Ellis, 1962; Ellis & Grieger, 1977), and rational-behavior therapy (Maultsby, 1975). Although it is incorrect to designate any individual as the founder of the cognitive therapy movement, Albert Ellis was a pioneer and has been one of its most prolific proponents. Ellis's rational-emotive therapy is the initial focus of this chapter. It is followed by a discussion of Beck's cognitive therapy, a more structured approach than Ellis's. Beck is a leading authority on depression and its analysis and treatment through cognitive therapy. Finally, we will consider an approach not always placed in the cognitive camp, but whose emphasis, though interactional, is clearly cognitive: transactional analysis.

RATIONAL-EMOTIVE THERAPY

Given that individuals feel and act on what they think, rational-emotive therapy (RET) posits that certain types of thoughts result in extreme emotional distress and problematic behaviors. Consequently, individuals must learn to analyze their thoughts to better cope with potentially distressing events. If extreme distress is a product of distorted thinking, then the best way to conquer problems is to change one's thinking. RET does not suggest such change will come easily, especially when a person is faced with

Albert Ellis

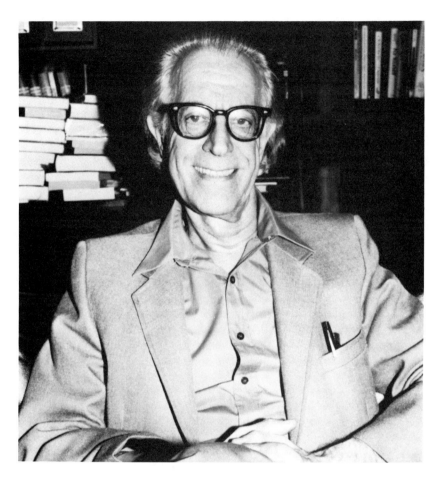

disappointing and frustrating life circumstances. Irrational beliefs are usually changed only by actively and persistently identifying, challenging, and revising one's thinking.

A Cognitive Conceptualization of Human Nature

Albert Ellis, founder of RET, described his approach's basic beliefs about human nature:

> It assumes, naturally, that virtually everything people do includes very important learning elements. We have a strong innate or biological tendency, for example, to walk on the ground rather than (as monkeys have) to swing from trees. But we still learn, by the helpful teachings of others *and* by our own self-practice, how to walk better, faster, straighter, or longer. We innately tend to

suckle at our mother's breasts and later to eat nonliquid kinds of food. But we also learn bigger and better breast-sucking; and we learn to eat a tremendous variety of foods that we rarely would imbibe during our first few years of life. So biological inheritance *and* self- and social-learning tendencies combine to make us human and to provide us with our main goals and satisfactions, such as our basic values of staying alive and of making ourselves happy or satisfied in many ways while remaining alive. Because of our innate and acquired tendencies, we largely (although not exclusively) control our destinies. And we do so by our basic values or beliefs—by the way that we interpret or look at the events that occur in our lives. (Ellis, 1977, p. 5)

The first and most basic principle of RET is that cognitions are the most important determinants of human emotion and behavior. The second major principle of RET is that dysfunctional emotional states and behavioral patterns result from dysfunctional thought processes. Some characteristics of dysfunctional thinking are: overgeneralization, oversimplification, exaggeration, faulty deductions, unproven assumptions, illogic, and absolutistic notions. The term used to describe these cognitive errors is "irrational beliefs" (Walen, et al., 1980). RET hypothesizes that certain specific types of irrational beliefs account for most human emotional disturbance and dysfunctional behaviors. In this regard, Ellis (1971) states:

> Practically all "emotional disturbance" stems from *demanding* or *whining* instead of from *wanting* or *desiring*. People who feel anxious, depressed, or hostile don't merely *wish* or *prefer* something, but also *command, dictate, insist* that they achieve this thing. Typically, . . . they *dictate* that life and the world be easy, enjoyable, and unfrustrating; and they *manufacture* overrebelliousness, self-pity, and inertia when conditions are difficult. (p. 168)

Thus, whenever individuals begin to feel and act extremely disturbed, the disturbance usually begins with a desire that gets blocked in some way. The wish itself is appropriate and harmless, but disturbance and dysfunction come about when the desire escalates into an absolute demand (e.g., "I must have my way!"). Such a demand can usually be recognized by cue words such as *must, have to, should, ought,* and *need.*

A second and similarly irrational belief relates to "awfulizing" or "devastation" cognitions, which exaggerate the negative consequences of a situation. Ellis (1971) proposes:

> Just about every time you feel disturbed or upset—instead of merely displeased, frustrated, or disappointed—you are stoutly

> convincing yourself that something is *awful,* rather than
> inconvenient or disadvantageous. . . . When you *awfulize* or
> *catastrophize* about reality, you are setting up an unverifiable,
> magical, unempirical hypothesis. (p. 168)

Therefore, when individuals experience extremely upsetting emotions, they are viewing bad circumstances as much more than just bad, rather, as "the end of the world" (e.g., "I can't go on living now that my spouse has left me."). These exaggerated devastation cognitions can be identified by individuals' use of such words as *horrible, terrible, awful,* and *unbearable.*

Finally, the third major irrational belief postulated by Ellis relates to individuals' evaluations of their self-worth. Ellis (1965) states:

> Perhaps the most common self-defeating belief of a highly
> disturbed patient is his conviction that he is a worthless,
> inadequate individual who essentially is undeserving of self-
> respect and happiness . . . particularly because they find it almost
> impossible to separate their selves from their performances and
> therefore insist that if their *deeds* stink *they* likewise must be
> highly odiferous. I maintain that no matter how inefficient their
> *products* are, they are still an ongoing *process,* and their process
> or being simply cannot be measured as can be its products. (p. 1)

Individuals are not their behavior. Ellis proposes that there is a great difference between being a "bad person" and *acting* badly. Thus, instead of a client saying "I am a bad parent," it is correct to say "I have been doing some bad parenting." The former is clearly an overgeneralization because it is virtually impossible to find anyone who commits *only* negative parenting acts. Human beings are far too intricate to be judged as a totality (Walen, et al., 1980).

The ABCs of RET

Ellis developed a simple schema to illustrate the role of cognitions in emotional and behavioral disturbance. He calls this schema the ABCs of RET. Ellis (1979) proposes the major goal of RET to be "minimizing the client's central self-defeating outlook and acquiring a more realistic, tolerant philosophy of life" (p. 205). Therefore, showing clients how they can change the beliefs that cause their disturbances and dysfunctions is the heart of RET. Clients' comprehension of the ABC framework helps them understand this process and goal.

In this framework, A stands for the *activating experience,* usually some obnoxious or unfortunate environmental disturbance. C stands for the emotional and behavioral *consequences;* those reactions that propel persons to seek counseling and psychotherapy. Most people tend to consider that A directly causes C; the circumstances one encounters causes certain feelings and actions. RET challenges this equation as naive and insensible to what people *think* about specific circumstances; their B, or belief system. Individuals' belief systems have two parts: rational and irrational. It is these latter irrational beliefs—demands, devastation, and self-hatred—that are the focus for the therapeutic process.

Clients, when they believe that A (the activating experience) is directly responsible for C (emotional and behavioral consequences), are either ignoring or more likely unaware of the presence and impact of their cognitions. In seeking therapy, these individuals are very likely experiencing quite debilitating and distressful consequences. The therapist's primary task is to teach them that their problems result not from A alone but from their misperceptions about A. While this basic objective may sound simple enough, it is often difficult for clients to grasp. Walen, DiGiuseppe, and Wessler (1980) explain this further:

> Our everyday language is filled with examples antagonistic to this concept. How often do we say or hear phrases such as "*He* made me so mad!" or "*It* has got me so upset!" More correctly, we could say, "*I* made me mad" and "*I* got me upset." How strange these sound to our ear! Yet the common ingredient in the corrected statements implies an important concept: that we are responsible for our emotions. Thus, emotions are not foisted upon us or injected magically into us, but result from something we actively do. Specifically, emotions result largely from what we tell ourselves. Clients come to therapy firmly believing that A causes C, and this belief is reinforced by virtually every important person with whom they come in contact. You, the therapist, will be teaching quite a revolutionary idea: that B causes C. (p. 14)

Expanding the ABCs

The ABC model of RET serves as a goal statement in helping to explain to clients the cognitive source of their emotional distress and maladaptive behavior. In expanding the model to ABCDE, clients learn how they can reduce distress and modify maladaptive behavior. D stands for *disputation*, the process through which clients learn to challenge and debate with themselves about their irrational thinking. Seeing and clarifying A, B, and C is an assessment procedure, important for both the therapist and the client. Until the therapist is able to pinpoint the connection between B and C, it cannot be conveyed to the client. Unless clients comprehend the connection, they will not understand the value or relevance of changing their beliefs. Changing beliefs is the essence of the therapeutic process and occurs at D, the disputation.

Walen, DiGiuseppe, and Wessler (1980) offer an outline (modified here) for disputing irrational beliefs once the A, B, and C have been identified:

1. Point out to clients that as long as they hold on to their irrational belief, they will experience distress. This step helps clients develop the motivation to change their beliefs.
2. Provide a rational belief and ask clients how they might feel and act if they held it. In this step, the therapist models a more helpful belief.
3. Once clients acknowledge that they would feel better and act more adaptively with this new belief, use this feedback to encourage them to give up their irrational belief.
4. Ask how valid the irrational belief is and how functional it is for clients to maintain it with questions such as "Where does it say that you *must* do . . .?" "How is it *the end of your world* if this occurs?" "How does your current belief help you feel or act better?"
5. Once clients admit that their irrational beliefs are not valid, are dysfunctional, and do not help them feel or act better, ask them to give up their irrational beliefs and make a commitment to maintain more rational beliefs.

After successfully disputing their false beliefs, then, at E, clients will experience a new emotional and behavioral *effect;* they will feel and act more adaptively based upon rational beliefs.

Case Illustration: The Active Directive Therapist

Most RET therapists take an active, directive approach to therapy. The therapist structures the sessions, the client provides content. Wessler and Wessler (1980) described the structure of typical RET session as encompassing certain tasks for both the client and the therapist. The therapist, however, must create a climate in which these tasks can be presented and processed. The primary tasks of the RET therapist posited by Wessler and Wessler (1980) follow.

1. Establish a relationship with the client, but don't spend a great deal of time developing a particular kind of relationship. Simply, strive to give the client confidence in therapy and to talk freely about himself or herself.
2. After an initial rapport is established, identify the problem. You can inaugurate this by asking, "What problem are you seeking help with?" or a similar question. Most clients define their difficulties in

terms of A or C of the ABC model, and the client must be helped to see and confirm the potential connection between A and C. (Probing for Bs comes later.)

3. The third task is goal setting. The ultimate goal of RET is changes in C—emotional and behavioral consequences. The client's response to the question, "How would you like to feel and act differently than you feel and act now?" can define therapeutic goals. Also try to obtain a commitment from the client to actively work to achieve the agreed-to goals.

4. Explain RET and the cognitive hypothesis of emotional and behavioral disturbance, showing the influence of irrational beliefs on C. A long theoretical discourse is not advocated; rather, give a brief orientation to the basic ABC model emphasizing the influence of irrational beliefs in particular.

5. Given the specific As and Cs presented by the client, work to uncover irrational beliefs. *Beliefs are defined as irrational only if they have dysfunctional consequences for the client, not because they contain certain cue words such as* must, awful, *and the like.* This point is important to remember because many beginning RET therapists often look at what the client is thinking only and not at the total ABC picture. Why change a belief if it creates no problems?

6. Dispute irrational beliefs and replace them with more rational beliefs by using the disputation procedure.

7. End the session with a homework assignment. RET is a cognitive-learning approach. A major tenet in RET, therefore, is that unless the client puts his or her rational beliefs into practice, the effects of therapy will have meaning, or last. Homework might be a reading, writing, listening, imagining, or an action assignment. Its goal is to strengthen the client's comprehension of the basic principles of RET and applying them to everyday life.

Not all these tasks are included in every session. As therapy progresses, rapport building and orientation are emphasized less, goals are achieved or altered, and new problems arise. Ultimately, the therapist's task is to help the client become his or her own therapist; able to identify, challenge, and change beliefs so that more satisfying consequences happen more often. The following excerpt from a therapy session illustrates how a therapist might determine a client's self-defeating irrational beliefs and use a disputation process to help the client to more satisfying emotional and behavioral effects.

The client is a young college student who feels that he is being bullied by his parents, especially his father. He's become extremely sensitive to his father's neurotic behavior toward him and makes himself so

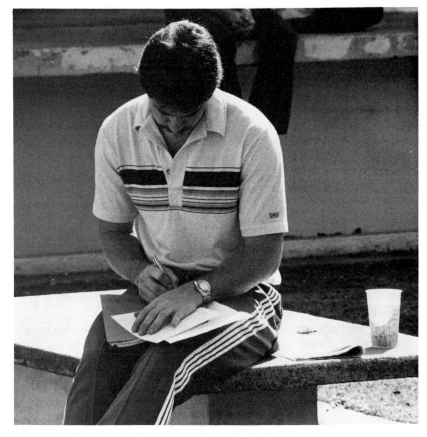

Writing can be homework in RET

angry that he hasn't been able to maintain his studies. The session is already underway and the preliminaries of rapport building, problem identification, and goal setting have earlier been discussed. The excerpt begins immediately after the client has been given a brief orientation to RET by the therapist.

THERAPIST: Let's do an ABC analysis of your situation with your father. A, your father says something critical to you, and C, you feel extremely angry. What might be some of the Bs you might be thinking to yourself?

CLIENT: When I get angry at him?

THERAPIST: Right. Look for any demands on him or the situation you might be making.

CLIENT: Well, I should not have to be in a situation where someone is being so critical of me for no good reason.

THERAPIST: That's a good thought to be in touch with. But is that an anger-provoking belief. It sounds more like a "poor-me" thought.

CLIENT: Maybe you're right.

THERAPIST: Poor-me beliefs make you sad, not angry.

CLIENT: Well, my father should be more positive.

THERAPIST: That sounds like it. Anger beliefs are usually demands directed outward, at someone or thing. It's "he must." He must not criticize me, he musn't say rotten things about me. Any others you can think of now?

CLIENT: (Relates a brief story of a recent incident)

THERAPIST: OK, stop there. What might be the irrational belief here, the demand in that instance?

CLIENT: Well, even though he and my mother are treating me that way—they *are* treating me that way. That's just the way it is and there's nothing I can do at the moment to change that.

THERAPIST: That might be a more rational belief and if you held that you'd likely not get angry. But for now, what is the irrational belief? Again, look for a demand statement you are thinking to yourself about their actions.

CLIENT: Well, that they should treat me fairly!

THERAPIST: Right. Your parents, and particularly your father should, ought to, must treat you fairly and squarely. This is where the anger is coming from. From the theory we know that irrational demands will result in anger. Your belief is that your father must treat you fairly. He must not neurotically and unjustly criticize you.

CLIENT: I also have a lot of demands for myself. I mustn't take this crap from him. I'm a fine son and have acted only in ways that he should be proud of me for. I really feel like just hauling off and socking him right in the jaw sometimes.

THERAPIST: Something similar to that might be good to think to yourself if you weren't in a rage, but were merely determined to try to change what could be changed. If you did those things assertively, you could do them more effectively and efficiently. But let's go back to where we were—we've got an A, a B, and a C.

CLIENT: OK.

THERAPIST: Earlier you set as your goal for therapy getting rid of the intense feelings of anger that you have towards your father. Now that we've identified your anger and the beliefs creating it, let's look at the D of our ABCDE framework: disputation. To dispute your irrational belief, those demands, you want to ask yourself two questions. First, how does it help you in any way to maintain those demands?

CLIENT: Well, obviously it doesn't. They only keep me angry and that anger I want to get rid of.

THERAPIST: Right. So they're very dysfunctional beliefs. They hurt, not help you. And they don't seem to have had any effect on your father's actions either, except maybe making him more critical. The second question you want to ask yourself is, "Where is the evidence that my father *must* act fairly toward me?"

CLIENT: Well, I think that he should. I think it would be stupid just to sit and happily take his crap.

THERAPIST: If you're asking, "Are you trying to get me to feel nothing or to just joyfully accept his abusive behavior," I'd say "Of course not, that's unreal." But as you just noted, getting so intensely angry is very dysfunctional for you. For that reason, I think it would be best to get rid of your rage and bring it down to where you can say, "I don't like this and I'm going to do what I can about it. I'm going to work my butt off to change this situation." What has your anger done for you so far? It's got you so unraveled that you are unable to concentrate on your studies.

CLIENT: You're right. I just couldn't get some of the really rotten things he's said to me off of my mind and my work in school has simply eroded as a result.

THERAPIST: OK. So let's go back to our disputation. Ask yourself, "Why must my father be nice to me?" Remember, not why would it be better if he was nice, but why *must* he absolutely and unequivocally be nice; the demand.

CLIENT: I don't know. At college, I see so many people living at home and doing well. They're running around with the family charge card and doing whatever they want to, and their parents fully support them both financially and psychologically.

THERAPIST: I completely agree that it would be a lot better if your parents and your father in particular were less critical and more supportive toward you. But why *must* he be that way? Is there a law that all fathers must support their children at all times?

CLIENT: Why *must* he be supportive? (pause) I think he should, that's why!

THERAPIST: Again, not why it would be better, but why does he *have to* be?

CLIENT: Just because I want him to. (laughs)

[The therapist forces the client to try to come up with the answers himself rather than answering for him.]

THERAPIST: That's right. "He has to do everything I want." Where's that going to get you? Where has that gotten you in the past?

CLIENT: Hmmm.

THERAPIST: I agree with you completely that it would be great if your father fully supported you. It would make for a much more pleasant home life for you. Your life would even be better if your parents waited on you hand and foot and provided for every desire you expressed. We could prove that. We could do an experiment and prove the reasons why it would be better if your father was more supportive. But the question is "Why *must* he be supportive?"

[The therapist never disputes the desirability of the client's claim that it would be more advantageous to have what he wants (a very rational belief) *merely the demand*.]

CLIENT: OK, so he doesn't have to.

THERAPIST: You say that sounding somewhat half-hearted.

CLIENT: Well, it does help me to think that it's not really my fault that he acts the way he does. And the idea that he doesn't *have to* be supportive and fair is true. I mean it would definitely make life sweeter if he was, but for sure my demanding that he be doesn't make him so.

THERAPIST: Beautiful! And if that's the B, the belief you hold about your father's criticism of you, will you be so enraged all the time? How will you feel at C, the consequences?

CLIENT: Well, I wouldn't be happy, but I don't feel as mad right now as I have. In fact, I really see him more clearly for what he is, a neurotic who's acting neurotically.

THERAPIST: Sounds like the disputation we just did helped you to arrive at a more rational belief about the activating experience and now you have a more functional and satisfying E, or effect. You are not as angry and find yourself more in control of how you feel and act. So that you can continue to maintain what we did in the session and enhance your efforts here, I'm going to give you a book to read before we get together again next week; *Overcoming Frustration and Anger* by Paul Hauck. Reading it will reinforce what we did in the session today.

CLIENT: OK. You know, I really do feel better. I mean just by changing what I was thinking from "He must be less critical!" to "That's unfortunately just him and the way he is."

THERAPIST: Great! Proof of the value of the ABCDE process for you.

BECK'S COGNITIVE THERAPY

Beck's cognitive therapy conceives of human nature and approaches therapy similar to RET. Beck developed his approach independently of Ellis, although the influence of RET is apparent in many of his writings (Rimm & Masters, 1979). Both cognitive therapy and RET conceptualize human behavior and emotion as an ABC paradigm. Both stress the role of faulty or irrational thinking in causing negative emotions. And both stress the here and now (including homework) and relatively short-term therapy.

Differences between cognitive therapy and RET lie more in emphasis than basic assumptions. Cognitive therapy is more diagnostically oriented and explicitly relates particular patterns of thought to specific categories of psychopathology, most notably depression. Beck is recognized as a leading authority on depressive disorders; however, his analysis of the cognitive content of various disorders such as a common phobia like the fear of flying (Beck, 1976) reflects the specificity of his approach. This specificity is also seen in his analysis of the thought patterns associated with different emotional states, including anxiety, sadness, anger, and euphoria.

The therapeutic process advocated by cognitive therapy is somewhat more structured than RET. Cognitive therapy does not view ideas as rational or irrational, but rather refers to the term *"rule."* Beliefs or rules are a problem only when they are *too* absolute, *too* broad, *too* extreme, or *too* arbitrary. Individuals' basic rules give rise to unhealthy thoughts or beliefs about themselves or possible visual images, which are called *automatic* thoughts, because of the habitual way they are acted upon. Much of therapy via Beck's approach involves helping clients ferret out their automatic thinking and, ultimately, their personally-held basic rules, and then test these rules both logically and empirically.

Cognitive therapy is best illustrated by how it deals with depression. Behaviorally and affectively, depression is manifested by a variety of symptoms such as crying, continual sadness, suicidal threats, and loss of appetite. Cognitive therapy sees these symptoms as a direct result of certain cognitions of the depressed person.

The Cognitive Triad: Human Nature and Depression

The central tenet of the cognitive therapy view of depression is that idiosyncratic, distorted conceptions of depressed persons are central to developing and maintaining their depressive symptoms. Particularly important are the thoughts associated with the "cognitive triad" (Beck, 1967). This cognitive triad consists of three major themes of depressed individuals: (1) a negative view of the self, (2) a negative view of the world, and (3) a negative view of the future (Beck & Shaw, 1977). Beck (1963, 1964) analyzed verbatim recorded interview material of depressed and nondepressed persons in psychotherapy. The reports of the depressed clients consistently indicated they saw themselves as "losers." Depressed clients' reports also indicated specific idiosyncratic negative *content* not present in the reports of nondepressed clients. This content formed the basis for Beck's cognitive triad:

A negative view of self. Depressed individuals show a marked tendency to view themselves as deficient, inadequate, or unworthy, and to attribute their unpleasant experiences to a physical, mental, or moral defect in themselves. Furthermore, they regard themselves as undesirable and worthless because of their presumed defect and tend to reject themselves (and to believe others will reject them) because of it.

A negative view of the world. Depressed persons' interactions with their environment are interpreted as representing defeat, deprivation, or disparagement. They view the world as making exorbitant demands on them and presenting obstacles which interfere with the achievement of their life goals.

A negative view of the future. The future, for depressed individuals, is seen from a negative perspective and revolves around a series of negative expectations. Depressed persons anticipate that their current problems and experiences will continue indefinitely and that they will increasingly burden significant others in their lives.

Beck (1963, 1964) further noted the *way* that depressed persons interpret their life. Depressed clients tend to distort their experiences: they misinterpret specific irrelevant events as personal failure, deprivation, or rejection; they tend to greatly exaggerate or overgeneralize any event that reflects negatively on themselves; they also tend to persevere in making indiscriminate, negative predictions of the future. Depressed clients' cognitions reflected a *systematic bias* against themselves. Because of this overemphasis on negative data, to the relevant exclusion of positive data, the label "cognitive distortion" came to be most appropriate when describing the thinking of depressed persons (Beck & Shaw, 1977).

Burns (1980) identifies and describes ten cognitive distortions that form the basis for most all depression. These are defined in Figure 4–1.

FIGURE 4–1

Definitions of Cognitive Distortions. From FEELING GOOD: The New Mood Therapy by David D. Burns, M.D. Copyright © 1980 by David D. Burns, M.D. By permission of William Morrow & Company.

1. ALL-OR-NOTHING THINKING: You see things in black-and-white categories. If your performance falls short of perfect, you see yourself as a total failure.

2. OVERGENERALIZATION: You see a single negative event as a never-ending pattern of defeat.

3. MENTAL FILTER: You pick out a single negative detail and dwell on it exclusively so that your vision of all reality becomes darkened, like the drop of ink that discolors the entire beaker of water.

4. DISQUALIFYING THE POSITIVE: You reject positive experiences by insisting they "don't count" for some reason or other. In this way you can maintain a negative belief that is contradicted by your everyday experiences.

5. JUMPING TO CONCLUSIONS: You make a negative interpretation even though there are no definite facts that convincingly support your conclusion.

    a. *Mind reading.* You arbitrarily conclude that someone is reacting negatively to you, and you don't bother to check this out.

    b. *The Fortune Teller Error.* You anticipate that things will turn out badly, and you feel convinced that your prediction is an already-established fact.

6. MAGNIFICATION (CATASTROPHIZING) OR MINIMIZATION: You exaggerate the importance of things (such as your goof-up or someone else's achievement), or you inappropriately shrink things until they appear tiny (your own desirable qualities or the other fellow's imperfections). This is also called the "binocular trick."

7. EMOTIONAL REASONING: You assume that your negative emotions necessarily reflect the way things really are: "I feel it, therefore it must be true."

8. SHOULD STATEMENTS: You try to motivate yourself with shoulds and shouldn'ts, as if you had to be whipped and punished before you could be expected to do anything. "Musts" and "oughts" are also offenders. The emotional consequence is guilt. When you direct should statements toward others, you feel anger, frustration, and resentment.

9. LABELING AND MISLABELING: This is an extreme form of overgeneralization. Instead of decribing your error, you attach a negative label to yourself: "I'm a *loser.*" When someone else's behavior rubs you the wrong way, you attach a negative label to him: "He's a goddam louse." Mislabeling involves describing an event with language that is highly colored and emotionally loaded.

10. PERSONALIZATION: You see yourself as the cause of some negative external event which in fact you were not primarily responsible for.

The Goals of Cognitive Therapy

Cognitive therapy can enable depressed clients to see themselves realistically, with strengths and weaknesses, rather than as only inadequate, undesirable, or unworthy; as capable of mastery rather than totally helpless. Shaw and Beck (1977) assert that "the immediate goals of cognitive therapy center on the systematic modification of the depressed patient's arbitrary, distorted interpretations of reality" (p. 311).

The negative concepts of the cognitive triad are best shown by how depressed individuals *systematically* misconstrue experiences and related content. Specifically, depressed persons regard themselves as "losers." Their thinking is distorted, thus errors such as all-or-nothing thinking, overgeneralization, mental filter and the like lead them to totally denigrate themselves. The depressed client, for example, who believes he or she has lost something of substantial value, such as a personal relationship, or that he or she has failed to achieve an important objective, will take personal blame for the loss or failure, no matter what the reality of the situation. Moreover, they expect anything they do to have negative consequences and therefore are not motivated to set goals and tend to avoid engaging in constructive activities. In addition, they expect their future to be unsatisfying and filled with despair (Shaw & Beck, 1977).

Thus, cognitive therapy aims at clients' developing an objective view of the "cognitive triad": a realistic view of self, the world, and the future.

The New Mood Therapy

Burns (1980) describes cognitive therapy in the treatment of depression as *The New Mood Therapy*. By identifying distorted cognitions and subjecting them to logical analysis and empirical testing, the therapist and client work together to realign the client's thinking with reality, thereby creating a "new mood" for the depressed person.

Cognitive therapy has been proposed as a short-term approach, and time limits are frequently employed; for example, a maximum of 20 sessions in a period of 12 weeks (Shaw & Beck, 1977). Specifying a defined therapy period requires that the therapist and client use time judiciously. Shaw and Beck (1977) note especially the importance of preciseness:

> This means that every question or statement posed by the therapist should have a definite rationale or purpose. Thus, questions should be conceptually relevant to cognitive therapy and should be phrased to elicit concrete information. (Requests such as "Please give me a specific example," are frequently used.) Questioning is a major tool not only to elicit reliable information regarding specific cognitions, definitions, and meanings, but also

> to expose inner contradictions, inconsistencies, and logical flaws in the patient's conclusions. A well-timed, properly phrased question may serve to open a closed belief system. (p. 311)

In dealing with a severe case of depression, the initial focus, perhaps for the first several sessions, would appear to the untrained observer as largely behavioral. The "behavioral" interventions used in cognitive therapy, however, have a direct cognitively-oriented purpose: to change clients' passivity, avoidance, and lack of gratification in order to give them data with which to disconfirm overgeneralized beliefs of inadequacy and incompetence.

One such strategy, the *graded task assignment,* is based on the assumption that it is hard for depressed clients to complete tasks that were relatively easy before their depression. As they grow increasingly inactive, severely depressed individuals begin to think, "I can't do anything," or "It's useless to try." This cognitive reaction seems to logically follow the generalized belief that because an activity is no longer simple, it is impossible. The cognitive therapist does not try to counter this belief by contradicting it, (e.g., "Yes, you can do it if you try."), for that strategy may alienate the client. Rather, the therapist takes an empirical viewpoint ("Would you be willing to test your belief?") and divides the goal-directed activity into mini-tasks that are within the client's capability (Shaw & Beck, 1977).

Beck (1976) illustrated the use of graded task assignments with a fifty-two-year-old man who had spent over a year in a hospital without moving away from his bed. Antidepressant medications had been used to no avail. Beck spent only one session with the man and devoted it exclusively to encouraging him to walk away from his bed, first five yards, then twenty yards, and so on. Within 45 minutes, the man was able to walk about the ward; soon he was able to reward himself for his increased activity by being able to obtain a soda from a vending machine. Later, he was able to walk about the hospital grounds, play ping-pong, and go to the hospital snack bar. One month later, he was discharged. Initially, this man was convinced he hadn't the strength to walk at all! Beck was able to persuade him to test his hypothesis, offering to catch him if he fell. Obviously, the man's hypothesis proved incorrect.

Two similar "behavioral" strategies were used early in therapy:

Activity Scheduling. Since depressed clients see themselves as ineffective, the therapist and client collaborate to schedule specific daily activities that enable the client to observe himself or herself as more effective.

Mastery and Pleasure Therapy. The client keeps a running account of daily activities and marks an *M* next to each mastery experience and a *P* next to each pleasure experience. Depressed clients, who characteristically report that they can master nothing and enjoy nothing, are thus confronted with information to the contrary.

As therapy progresses, clients are trained to observe their cognitions that are associated with unpleasant affect. Clients are taught to analyze their automatic thoughts. Typically, the thoughts are negative self-evaluations—"I'm worthless," "I'll never amount to anything"—, and initially the therapist points out their unreasonable and self-defeating nature. With practice, clients learn "distancing," that is, dealing with such thoughts objectively, evaluating them rather than blindly accepting them. Homework assignments are given to facilitate distancing; a primary one is the *triple column technique*. Figure 4–2 illustrates an example of the triple column technique as used by a client of Burns (1980).

Such strategies illuminate basic self-defeating themes that clients tend to persevere in using. Cognitive distortions such as overgeneralization soon become evident and can be identified and categorized. Clients'

Excerpts from Gail's daily written homework using the "triple-column technique." In the left column she recorded the negative thoughts that automatically flowed through her mind when her roommate asked her to clean up the apartment. In the middle column she identified her distortions, and in the right-hand column she wrote down more realistic interpretations. This daily written exercise greatly accelerated her personal growth and resulted in substantial emotional relief.

Automatic Thoughts (SELF-CRITICISM)	*Cognitive Distortion*	*Rational Response* (SELF-DEFENSE)
1. Everyone knows how disorganized and selfish I am.	Jumping to conclusions (mind reading); overgeneralization	1. I'm disorganized at times and I'm organized at times. Everybody doesn't think the same way about me.
2. I'm completely self-centered and thoughtless. I'm just no good.	All-or-nothing thinking	2. I'm thoughtless at times, and at times I can be quite thoughtful. I probably do act overly self-centered at times. I can work on this. I may be imperfect but I'm not "no good!"
3. My roommate probably hates me. I have no real friends.	Jumping to conclusions (mind reading); all-or-nothing thinking	3. My friendships are just as real as anyone's. At times I take criticism as rejection of *me*, Gail, the person. But others are usually not rejecting *me*. They're just expressing dislike for what I *did* (or said)—and they still accept me afterward.

FIGURE 4–2

Three Column Technique. From FEELING GOOD: The New Mood Therapy by David D. Burns, M.D. Copyright © 1980 by David D. Burns, M.D. By permission of William Morrow & Company.

closed systems of logic and reasoning open as they distance themselves from their cognitions, analyze them with concrete evidence, and identify their patterns of thinking. Problems previously perceived as insoluble are reanalyzed as clients systematically test their cognitions, helping them approach their problems realistically. There is no attempt to deny or invalidate realistic difficulties that arise from external events. However, clients who can recognize and correct their distortions of reality are better able to attack any problems, which, in fact, do exist in their environment (Shaw & Beck, 1977).

Cognitive Therapy: A Case

Cognitive therapy's counterpart to rational-emotive therapy's "disputation" is called *alternative therapy*. Depressed persons show a systematic negative bias in their interpretations of events in their lives. In alternative therapy, the therapist teaches clients to consider alternative explanations for their experiences. By having to think of other explanations, clients are enabled to recognize their biases and substitute more accurate interpretations. Furthermore, by discussing different ways of dealing with their problems, clients are able to find solutions to problems that they had considered insoluble. They also realize that options they may have previously discarded might lead them out of their dilemmas.

Beck (1976) illustrates the use of alternative therapy with a woman who had made a recent suicide attempt and still wanted to commit suicide. She thought that she had nothing to look forward to since her husband was unfaithful. Their dialogue and a brief summary by Beck of what occurred follows:

THERAPIST: Why do you want to end your life?

PATIENT: Without Raymond, I am nothing . . . I can't be happy without Raymond . . . But I can't save our marriage.

THERAPIST: What has your marriage been like?

PATIENT: It has been miserable from the very beginning . . . Raymond has always been unfaithful . . . I have hardly seen him in the past five years.

THERAPIST: You say that you can't be happy without Raymond . . . Have you found yourself happy when you are with Raymond?

PATIENT: No, we fight all the time and I feel worse.

THERAPIST: You say you are nothing without Raymond. Before you met Raymond, did you feel you were nothing?

PATIENT: No, I felt I was somebody.

THERAPIST: If you were somebody before you knew Raymond, why do you need him to be somebody now?

PATIENT: (Puzzled) Hmmm . . .

THERAPIST: Did you have male friends before you knew Raymond?

PATIENT: I was pretty popular then.

THERAPIST: Why do you think you will be unpopular without Raymond now?

PATIENT: Because I will not be able to attract any other man.

THERAPIST: Have any men shown an interest in you since you have been married?

PATIENT: A lot of men have made passes at me, but I ignore them.

THERAPIST: If you were free of the marriage, do you think that men might be interested in you—knowing that you were available?

PATIENT: I guess that maybe they would be.

THERAPIST: Is it possible that you might find a man who would be more constant than Raymond?

PATIENT: I don't know . . . I guess it's possible.

THERAPIST: You say that you can't stand the idea of losing the marriage. Is it correct that you have hardly seen your husband in the past five years?

PATIENT: That's right, I only see him a couple of times a year.

THERAPIST: Is there any chance of your getting back together with him?

PATIENT: No . . . He has another woman. He doesn't want me.

THERAPIST: Then what have you actually lost if you break up the marriage?

PATIENT: I don't know.

THERAPIST: Is it possible that you'll get along better if you end the marriage?

PATIENT: There is no guarantee of that.

THERAPIST: Do you have a *real marriage*?

PATIENT: I guess not.

THERAPIST: If you don't have a real marriage, what do you actually lose if you decide to end the marriage?

PATIENT: (Long pause) Nothing, I guess.

> Following this interview, the patient was more cheerful and appeared to be over the suicide crisis. In a subsequent interview, she stated that the point that really struck home was: How could she be "nothing" without Raymond—when she had lived happily and was an adequate person before she ever knew him? She eventually was divorced and settled down to a more stable life.
>
> In this case, the alternative therapy was based on questioning the patient's faulty beliefs that (a) she needed her husband in order to be happy, to function, or to have an identity; (b) that, somehow, the end of the marriage would be the end of the road for her, that it would be a devastating loss; and (c) she could have no future life without her husband [the cognitive triad]. The patient was able to see the fallacy of her beliefs and consequently realized she had options besides either trying to preserve a dead marriage or committing suicide. (pp. 289–292)

TRANSACTIONAL ANALYSIS

Transactional analysis (TA) has the distinction of being the only counseling approach that had its two seminal books on the national best-seller list for longer than a year. The landmark works *Games People Play* by Eric Berne and *I'm OK—You're OK* by Thomas Harris are only two of the many books on TA that have achieved wide public recognition and popularity, making TA one of the best known and frequently used therapies.

TA stresses clients' ability to rationally recognize specific components of individual and interpersonal functioning and to make affective and behavioral changes based on this recognition. It focuses on the decisions that persons make early in their lives and posits that all humans have the cognitive capacity to reevaluate and remake decisions. TA is set apart from most other psychotherapeutic approaches by its active attempts to demystify the counseling process. A special strength of TA is its language, which communicates in common terms what most other orientations try to convey with vague theoretical concepts. James and Jongeward (1971) emphasize these points:

> The worldview of TA could perhaps be best summarized by the following: Transactional analysis is a rational approach to understanding behavior and is based on the assumption that all individuals can learn to trust themselves, think for themselves, make their own decisions, and express their feelings. Its principles can be applied on the job, in the home, in the classroom, in the neighborhood—wherever people deal with people. (p. 12)

In interpreting the basic nature of humans and how they function, TA theory posits four primary forms of analysis: structural analysis, transactional analysis, script analysis, and the analysis of games. We will address the TA perspective on human functioning through these four TA conceptual schema.

An important TA attitude advocates expressing concepts both verbally *and* visually. Explanations are accompanied by symbols—circles, arrows, triangles, and bar graphs—that increase clarity and comprehension (Dusay & Dusay, 1979).

Structural Analysis

Structural analysis provides a means of answering the questions: Who am I? Why do I act the way I do? How did I get this way? It explains intrapersonal functioning through the key TA concept called "ego states." Berne (1964) defines an ego state as "a consistent pattern of feeling and experience directly related to a corresponding consistent pattern of behavior" (p. 364). Each person has three ego states that are distinct sources of behavior: the Parent ego state, the Adult ego state, and the Child ego state.

The Parent ego state contains attitudes and behavior incorporated from external sources, primarily parents and parent-like figures of childhood (e.g., teachers, grandparents). This ego state contains the *shoulds* and *oughts* that stress responsibility and how to behave to gain recognition and approval. The parent's primary function is control of the child. As such, it can take two forms, critical and controlling, or nurturing. The Critical Parent admonishes and disapproves; the Nurturing Parent comforts and praises. The Parent ego state is very important as it provides a set of values and standards of behavior for the individual.

The Adult ego state is not related to a person's age, but rather is oriented to current reality and the objective gathering of information. The Adult ego state processes available information and produces the best solution based on it. The function of the Adult ego state is to deal with situations in a factual, precise, and organized manner. Its function is clear: rational appraising and evaluating.

The Child ego state contains all the impulses that come naturally to an infant. The Child ego state does not refer to childishness, but *childlikeness*; it is an individual's spontaneous, fun-loving part. Like the Parent ego state, the Child consists of two distinct forms: the Free Child and the Adapted Child. The Free Child represents spontaneity, curiosity, playfulness, eagerness, and intuitiveness. The Adapted Child is conforming, compromising, easy to get along with, and compliant. The Adapted Child represents adaptations of those natural inclinations of the Free Child that occur in response to traumas, experiences, and training. For example, a child is naturally programmed to eat whenever hungry. Shortly after birth, however, this natural urge may be adapted, so that the child's eating schedule is determined by his or her parents (James & Jongeward, 1971). The Adapted Child may also be manifested, however, as a pseudorebel who does the opposite of everything that is expected (Dusay & Dusay, 1979).

When individuals are acting, thinking, and feeling as they observed their parents and parent figures act, think, and feel, they are in their Parent ego state. When they are dealing with current reality, gathering facts, and objectively making decisions, they are in their Adult ego state. When feeling and acting as they did as children, they are in their Child ego state. Figure 4–3 represents these three ego states graphically.

James and Jongeward (1971) offer a case illustrating how the different ego states might be reflected in an individual's behavior.

> A client was advised to investigate a private school for his son. When he reported his findings about the school where the teaching was informal and creativity encouraged, three distinct reactions were easily observable. First, he scowled and said, "I can't see how anyone could learn anything at that school. There's

FIGURE 4–3

Ego States. From Muriel James & Dorothy Jonge-ward, BORN TO WIN, © 1971, Addison-Wesley, Reading, Massachusetts. Adapted figures from pgs. 18, 25, 27, 29, 38, 228 and 231. Reprinted with permission.

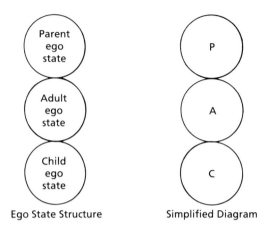

Ego State Structure   Simplified Diagram

dirt on the floor!" Leaning back in his chair, his forehead smoothed out as he reflected, "Before I decide, I think I should check on the school's scholastic rating and talk to some of the parents." The next minute, a broad grin crossed his face, and he said, "Gee, I'd love to have gone to a school like that!"

When queried about his responses, the client readily analyzed that his first was the way his father would have responded. His second was his Adult looking for more data. His third was his Child rcalling his own unhappy school experience and imagining the fun he might have had at a school such as the one he visited. (pp. 18–19)

TA does not favor any single ego state. However, determining the dominant ego state of clients is critical in understanding them and their concerns. To be a successful and comfortable human being requires parental behavior at times, adult behavior at other times, and the free creative expression of the child at still other points (Ivey & Simek-Downing, 1980).

Two types of people's problems are explained by structural analysis: contamination and exclusion. Contamination is the intrusion of the Parent ego state and/or the Child ego state into the boundary of the Adult ego state; it interferes with the clear thinking and functioning of the Adult. Contamination occurs when the Adult accepts as "true" some unfounded Parent beliefs or Child distortions and justifies them. These intrusions are problems of ego boundaries and can be diagrammed as in Figure 4–4 (James & Jongeward, 1971):

Exclusion exists when one ego state restricts the free functioning of the other two. Clients with this problem appear to behave very rigidly because they tend to respond to all situations from only one of their ego states. The client constantly responds as a Parent, as an Adult, or as a

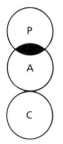 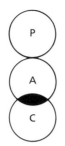 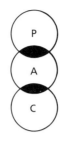

The Adult, contaminated by the Parent

The Adult, contaminated by the Child

The Adult, contaminated by the Parent and Child

FIGURE 4–4
Contamination. From Muriel James & Dorothy Jongeward, BORN TO WIN, © 1971, Addison-Wesley, Reading, Massachusetts. Adapted figures from pgs. 18, 25, 27, 29, 38, 228 and 231. Reprinted with permission.

Child. The Constant Parent excludes the Adult and Child and is typically observed in persons who are so duty-bound and work-oriented that they cannot play. The Constant Parent is usually judgmental, moralistic, and demanding of others. He or she knows all the answers and acts domineering and authoritarian. The Constant Adult who excludes the Parent and Child is overly objective. This individual appears robot-like, with little feeling and little spontaneity. The Constant Child, at the other extreme, is the sociopath without a conscience. These individuals are perpetually childlike and refuse to grow up. They don't think or decide for themselves but attempt to remain dependent in order to escape the responsibility for their own behavior. Exclusions by the three ego states are illustrated in Figure 4–5.

Dusay and Dusay (1979) point out that the structural description of ego states with circles and boundaries indicates the "what and where" of individuals' functioning; the concept of "how much" of the five potential ego states (Critical Parent, Nurturing Parent, Adult, Free Child, and Adapted Child) is answered by the use of the *egogram*. They describe the value of the egogram in stating:

A person's egogram reflects the type of person one is, the probable types of problems, and the strengths and weaknesses

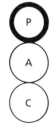 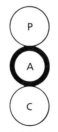 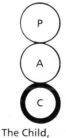

The Parent, excluding the Adult and Child

The Adult, excluding the Parent and Child

The Child, excluding the Parent and Adult

FIGURE 4–5
Exclusion. From Muriel James & Dorothy Jongeward, BORN TO WIN, © 1971, Addison-Wesley, Reading, Massachusetts. Adapted figures from pgs. 18, 25, 27, 29, 38, 228 and 231. Reprinted with permission.

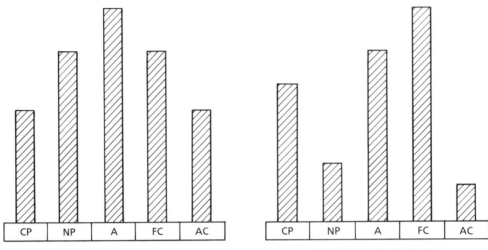

"BELL-SHAPED CURVE" EGOGRAM   "DON JUAN" EGOGRAM

FIGURE 4–6
Examples of Egograms. Adapted from Dusay, J., & Dusay, K. M. "Transactional Analysis." In R. J. Corsini (Ed.), *Current Psychotherapies.* Copyright 1979 by F. E. Peacock Publishers, Itasca, Ill. Reprinted by permission.

within one's personality. The egogram also provides a personal map for growth and change. Although there is no ideal egogram, people experience difficulties when one ego state is extremely low and another is disportionately high. Relative to that, a harmonious egogram becomes a matter of balance in the relationship between ego states. A creative artist needs a high FC; a successful district attorney needs a high CP; an accountant needs a strong A; a diplomat needs lots of AC; and a therapist needs a well-developed NP. (pp. 391, 393)

Figure 4–6 illustrates two sample egogram balances. The bell-shaped egogram implies that the individual's functioning is fairly well-balanced. The "Don Juan" by contrast has a high Free Child (interested in fun and sexual conquests), a high Critical Parent (knows how to tell partners to get lost), a low Nurturing Parent (does not care about others' feelings), a medium high Adult (logically knows how to find partners), and a low Adapted Child (feels little guilt and will not compromise).

Transactional Analysis

Whatever happens between individuals involves a transaction between their ego states. When a message is sent, a response is expected. Transactional analysis is a description of this interaction. There are three types of transactions: complementary, crossed, and ulterior. Complementary transactions occur when both parties function from the same ego state

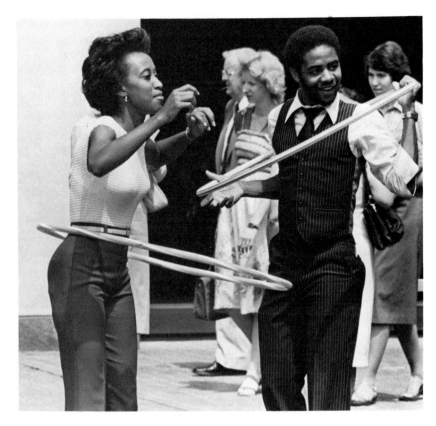

Child–child interaction is a complementary transaction

(Child to Child, Parent to Parent, Adult to Adult), or when the vectors are parallel (Parent to Child, Child to Parent, Adult to Child, Parent to Adult, etc.). The key to complementary transactions is that the response is appropriate and expected; it follows the natural order of healthy human relationships and enables persons to communicate. These transactions occur when two persons are engaged in critical gossip (Parent to Parent), solving a problem (Adult to Adult), or play (Child to Child). Examples of complementary transactions are illustrated in Figure 4–7.

Crossed transactions occur when the vectors are crossed, not parallel, and an unexpected response is made to a sent message. An inappropriate ego state is activated. At this point, persons tend to withdraw and turn away from each other or switch the conversation's direction. Examples of crossed transactions are illustrated in Figure 4–8.

Ulterior transactions are complex. They differ from complementary and crossed transactions in that they always involve more than two ego states simultaneously. When an ulterior message is sent, it is disguised

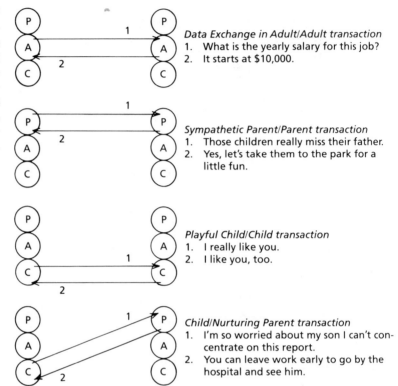

Data Exchange in Adult/Adult transaction
1. What is the yearly salary for this job?
2. It starts at $10,000.

Sympathetic Parent/Parent transaction
1. Those children really miss their father.
2. Yes, let's take them to the park for a little fun.

Playful Child/Child transaction
1. I really like you.
2. I like you, too.

Child/Nurturing Parent transaction
1. I'm so worried about my son I can't concentrate on this report.
2. You can leave work early to go by the hospital and see him.

under a socially acceptable transaction. An example of an ulterior transaction is illustrated and described in Figure 4–9.

Strokes, Scripts and Games

On its most superficial level, a stroke is a form of recognition. Strokes (human recognition) are the basic motivation for any human social interaction (Dusay & Dusay, 1979). Although positive strokes ("I like you": expressed by warm physical touches, accepting words, friendly gestures) feel better than negative strokes ("I don't like you": expressed verbally and nonverbally), people prefer negative strokes to no strokes at all. Specific patterns of giving and receiving strokes are learned early in life, and the ways in which "stroking" is learned serve to shape individuals' personalities.

Through one's early interactions with parents and significant others, a pattern of stroking usually develops that may be either supportive or attacking (Berne, 1972). From this stroking pattern, a child makes some

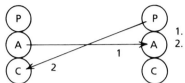

1. Boss: What time is it?
2. Secretary: You're always in such a
               hurry!

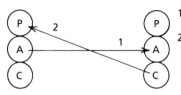

1. Husband: Can you take the car to be
              serviced this afternoon?
2. Wife: Today I iron. Johnny ex-
              pects a birthday cake. The
              cat has to go to the vet,
              and now you want me to
              take the car in!

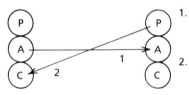

1. Boss: I need 25 copies of this re-
               port for the board meeting
               this afternoon. Can you
               get them for me?
2. Secretary: Aren't you lucky you've
               got me around to take care
               of you?

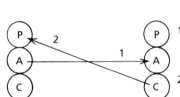

1. Scientist A: There may be some
                 variables we haven't
                 considered for this ex-
                 periment.
2. Scientist B: So what, who cares
                 around here?

FIGURE 4–8

Crossed Transactions. From Muriel James & Dorothy Jongeward, BORN TO WIN, © 1971, Addison-Wesley, Reading, Massachusetts. Adapted figures from pgs. 18, 25, 27, 29, 38, 228 and 231. Reprinted with permission.

If a car salesman says with a leer to his customer, "This is our finest sports car, but it may be too racy for you," he is sending a message that can be heard by either the customer's Adult or Child ego state. If the customer's Adult hears, the response may be, "Yes, you're right, considering the requirements of my job." If the customer's Child hears, the response may be, "I'll take it. It's just what I want."

FIGURE 4–9

An Ulterior Transaction. From Muriel James & Dorothy Jongeward, BORN TO WIN, © 1971, Addison-Wesley, Reading, Massachusetts. Adapted figures from pgs. 18, 25, 27, 29, 38, 228 and 231. Reprinted with permission.

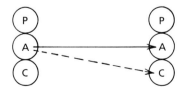

FIGURE 4–10
Development of a Life Position. From Muriel James & Dorothy Jongeward, BORN TO WIN, © 1971, Addison-Wesley, Reading, Massachusetts. Adapted figures from pgs. 18, 25, 27, 29, 38, 228 and 231. Reprinted with permission.

Experiences $\longrightarrow$ Decisions $\longrightarrow$ Psychological Positions $\longrightarrow$ Script Reinforcing Behavior

basic decisions about self and also about others. Harris (1967) identifies four general positions individuals can take:

1. *I'm OK, You're OK* is a mentally healthy position. Persons taking it have a positive self-identity and a positive image of others as well.
2. *I'm OK, You're not OK* is the position of persons who feel victimized or persecuted. They blame others for their miseries. Persons taking this position often drift into criminal behavior.
3. *I'm not OK, You're OK* is a common position of persons who feel powerless when they compare themselves to others. This position leads them to be deferential to everyone. The constant need to please others often leads to a productive but unhappy life.
4. *I'm not Ok, You're not OK* is the position of individuals who see life as hopeless and live only day-to-day.

From these basic positions children decide what life will be like. Once they take a position, they seek to keep their world predictable by reinforcing it. It becomes a life position from which games are played and scripts are acted out. This process is diagrammed in Figure 4–10 (James & Jongeward, 1971).

Scripts can be viewed as life plans that individuals feel compelled to act out (Jongeward & James, 1973). A script or "lifescript," represents "an ongoing program, developed in early childhood under parental influence, which directs the individual's behavior in the most important aspects of his life" (Berne, 1972, p. 418). Scripts are related to the early decisions and the positions of a child. Games are played as part of a lifescript. Games are "ongoing series of complementary ulterior transactions progressing to a well-defined, predictable outcome" (Berne, 1964, p. 48). When seeking positive strokes and unable to receive them in a straightforward manner, persons employ ulterior methods and use games to receive strokes. More simply stated, a game is an ulterior transaction; a way of cooperatively interacting on a superficial level for the purpose of concealing the real meaning of the interaction on a deeper level (Belkin, 1980).

Dusay and Dusay (1979) provide the following further explanation and example of a game:

> A *game* is defined as an orderly series of ulterior transactions (with both an overt and a covert level), which results in "payoffs"

with specific bad feelings for both game players. The overt series of transactions is straightforward and in this particular example is an Adult-to-Adult transaction: The boss asks his secretary, "What time is it?" She answers, "3 o'clock." However, his covert nonverbal message emanating from his Parent to her Child is, "You're always late." Her hidden nonverbal response from her Child to his Parent is, "You're always criticizing me." Even though neither the boss nor his secretary express these hidden sentiments out loud, each is fully aware of the hidden messages and each will receive a personal payoff of bad feelings. The boss is playing his part in the game colloquially known as *Now I Got You, You SOB*, and he feels angry and powerful; his secretary is playing *Kick Me* and feels bad and picked on. . . . After several repeated episodes of these games with themselves and perhaps with other players, the secretary will entitle herself to a "free" depression while the boss will entitle himself to a "free" rampage and rage. (pp. 376–377)

Redecision: The Emphasis for Therapeutic Efforts

The basic therapeutic goal of transactional analysis is to help clients in making new decisions about their present behavior and the direction of their life. TA seeks to help clients become more aware of how they restrict their choices by following early decisions about their life positions. In doing so, it offers options for attaining alternative, more satisfying ways of living. The essence of therapy is to substitute an autonomous lifestyle characterized by awareness, spontaneity, and intimacy for a lifestyle characterized by manipulative game playing and self-defeating scripts (Corey, 1982).

Harris (1967) asserts the therapeutic emphasis of TA as enabling individuals "to have freedom of choice, the freedom to change at will, to change the responses to recurring and new stimuli" (p. 58). Individuals who seek therapy for one reason or another are unable to redecide; to break through impasses that stem from early injunctions and decisions. Consistent with this goal, Goulding and Goulding (1979) label their use of TA principles redecision therapy. According to the Gouldings, when the therapeutic goal of redecision has been attained, persons tend to think, behave, and feel in different ways. They can be autonomous, and they experience a sense of freedom, excitement, and energy.

Berne (1966) set forth four general objectives that allow redecisions to be better realized:

1. Help the client decontaminate any damaged ego state.
2. Assist the client in developing the capacity to use all ego states when appropriate.

3. Help the client in developing full use of the Adult; in effect, to facilitate the establishment of a thoughtful, reasoning person with the capacity to govern his or her own life.

4. Assist the client in replacing the inappropriately chosen life position and life script with an *I'm OK* position and a new, more productive life script.

The Therapeutic Process as Contractual

Harris (1967) sees the TA therapist's role as a "teacher, trainer, and resource person with heavy emphasis on involvement" (p. 206). As a teacher, the therapist explains principles such as structural analysis, transactional analysis, script analysis, and game analysis to clients. The therapist helps clients discover the disadvantageous conditions of the past in which they made certain early decisions, adopted life positions, and developed strategies for dealing with people that they might now wish to reconsider. Although the therapist has the TA knowledge base, he or she does not function as a detached, aloof, superior expert who is there to cure the "sick client" (Corey, 1982). Rather, the therapeutic process is viewed as an equal relationship. The importance of the therapeutic contract highlights this equality.

Dusay and Dusay (1979) describe the primary process of client change in TA therapy as being defined by a *treatment contract*. Both therapist and client address the question, central to contractual therapy: "How will both you and I know when you get what you came for?" Therapist and client are allies working together to accomplish mutually agreed-upon goals. During therapy, both therapist and client define their responsibilities in achieving their goals. Contracts must be specific and concretely delineate the ways of actually working to fulfill the agreed-to terms.

Dusay and Duasy (1979) identify four major components of the TA treatment contract:

1. *Mutual Assent.* Both therapist and client, through Adult-to-Adult transactions, agree on the objectives for therapy.

2. *Competency.* The competencies of both parties are defined. The therapist agrees to provide only those services he or she can competently deliver. The client realistically assesses his or her potential for achieving contractual objectives.

3. *Consideration.* Consideration is addressed: from the therapist, professional skill and time; from the client, the therapist's fee as well as time and effort in working toward positive change.

4. *Legal Object.* The contract must have a legal aim and be within the ethical limits of the therapist. For example, " 'Provide me with mind-

altering drugs, Doctor, so I can become more aware of myself' is not a legal contract. 'I want to graduate from college with a B average,' may be an acceptable contract" (Dusay & Dusay, 1979, p. 401).

Goulding and Goulding (1979) similarly posit the contract as the basis for therapy in TA. They advocate that clients choose the aspects of their functioning that they want to change in order to attain their goals. Clients then work with the therapist to create the contract, with the therapist serving as both witness and facilitator. The Gouldings propose that the therapist work with a contract as long as it is therapeutic for the client.

A Case: Redeciding to be a Winner

The following case illustrates how a TA therapist might act as a teacher or trainer and advocate client responsibility for learning TA terminology. The client is asked to compare relevant concepts to his or her own situation and then redecide about his or her life based on all the information available.

In counseling, Fred reported, "If I heard it once, I heard it a hundred times, 'What a stupid thing to do, Fred. Can't you do anything right?' I couldn't even talk fast enough for my folks, and I still stutter sometimes. When I went to school, I just couldn't seem to do anything right. I was always at the bottom of the class, and I can remember teachers saying, 'Fred, that was a stupid question.' Teachers were just like my mom. When they read the grades out loud, my name was last, and the kids laughed at me. Then I got to high school, and the counselor said I could do better. That I wasn't dumb, just lazy. I don't get it."

In subsequent counseling sessions, Fred learned that early in life he had taken the position, "I'm stupid. I'm not OK." He thought of himself as a failure and acted out the role. Though he did poorly, Fred remained in school, played the game of *Stupid*, and evoked negative comments, low grades, and nagging from his teachers. This reinforced his basic psychological position.

Fred discovered his script was that of a loser. In his Child ego state he felt stupid and played the part of *Stupid*. He also discovered that his Parent ego state agreed with this position and thus encouraged him to fail. Fred's analysis of his ego states gave to his Adult the objective data about who he was, how he got that way, and where he was going with his life. It took Fred a while to decide which ego state would control his life. Finally, his Adult won out. He enrolled in college and maintained good grades.

After discovering his loser script, Fred decided that he didn't have to be a loser. He could become a winner if he chose to. (James & Jongeward, 1971, pp. 38–39)

COGNITIVE APPROACHES: THEORETICAL ANALYSES

Cognitive approaches to counseling and psychotherapy focus first and foremost on the types of thoughts clients have and their impact on emotional and behavioral difficulties. Counselors operating from this perspective consider cognitive change the primary goal of therapy. The emphasis is on changing how one thinks in order to change the way one feels and acts.

Rational-emotive therapy and Beck's cognitive therapy agree in that emotional disturbance results from mistaken, distorted, and dysfunctional beliefs with which individuals tend to keep indoctrinating themselves. While their terminology differs, RET looking at rational versus irrational and cognitive therapy considering clients' rules, their actual therapeutic differences are more in emphasis than content. Transactional analysis places primary importance on understanding three distinct patterns of intrapersonal functioning called ego states: Parent, Adult, Child. It too posits that emotional disturbance is a result of faulty thinking; thus its therapeutic efforts focus on "freeing up the Adult so that the individual may experience freedom of choice and the creation of new options above and beyond the limiting influences of the past" (Harris, 1967, p. 199).

All three approaches advocate a therapeutic alliance between counselor and client, especially TA, with its treatment contract. Although lacking a formal contract, cognitive therapy similarly seeks sharing of responsibility in client-counselor interchanges. The therapist does not attempt to directly counter clients' beliefs but rather asks, "Would you be willing to test that belief?" Wessler and Wessler (1980) describe how cognitively-oriented therapists must create and maintain collaborative counselor-client relationships.

> Keep in mind that RET, and presumably all therapies if they are to be effective, is a collaborative venture. Clients need information to decide whether or not to collaborate in their therapy. One explanation, however, is rarely sufficient to keep the client focused on cognitive change. For one reason or another, including years of conceiving the emotional problems differently, many clients easily stray to attributing the cause of their emotional problems to the situations they are in or to past events. At these times it is important to *continue* to set the stage, which may mean going back to the beginning and explaining again the ABC theory . . . In short, setting the stage may occur throughout therapy and not just during the first session. (pp. 80–81)

While displays of warmth and affection facilitate good counselor-client relationships, as Wessler and Wessler emphasize, giving clients appropriate information and communicating a respect for their ability to make their own decisions conveys confidence and creates collaboration. Harris (1967) wrote that humans have choices: "What was once decided can be undecided." All three orientations in this chapter consider the therapist as a teacher, trainer, and resource person who offers information to help clients gain the understanding and awareness needed to make new decisions that enable them to live more satisfying lives.

A common criticism of cognitive approaches is that the focus remains too much *in the head*. All three approaches we discussed, however, emphasize putting newly acquired understanding and insights into action. They all stress the value of homework in order that clients can experience situations in which they are able to practice new ways of thinking and thus confirm their efficacy.

The power of cognitively-oriented approaches is increasingly being recognized by practitioners who were previously more affectively or behaviorally oriented. When cognitive emphases are used by practitioners of other approaches, there is evidence that therapeutic power is increased (Ivey & Simek-Downing, 1980). For example, Corey (1982) writes in this regard:

> A trend in contemporary behavior therapy is the increased emphasis on the role of thinking and "self-talk" as a factor in behavior. One of the most interesting areas of this approach is cognitive behavior modification, which consists of teaching people to change what they are thinking in order to change how they are acting. (p. 155–156)

Likewise, Corey similarly stated in reference to TA:

> In my opinion one of the shortcomings of the Gestalt approach is that it deemphasizes intellectual factors. In Gestalt therapy, one is frequently called to task if one thinks and is told that one is "bullshitting" or, even worse "elephantshitting!". . . . Thus, it is the marriage of many of the concepts and techniques of Gestalt with those of TA that is most useful. (p. 137)

The next chapter will provide a closer look at how the various approaches to counseling and psychotherapy compare and contrast. Should you desire to explore the cognitive approaches presented here further, consider the suggested readings that follow.

SUGGESTED READINGS

Rational-Emotive Therapy

Ellis, A. (1962). *Reason and emotion in psychotherapy.* New York: Lyle Stuart.
Ellis's initial assertions forming the foundation for RET are found in this

volume. He describes RET's origins, major concepts, and differences from other psychotherapeutic approaches.

Ellis, A. (1973). *Humanistic psychotherapy.* New York: McGraw-Hill. This book presents most of the key components of RET, elaborating on Ellis' philosophy of the means by which individuals achieve personal growth and self-acceptance.

Ellis, A., & Harper, R. (1975). *A new guide to rational living.* Hollywood, CA: Wilshire. A bibliotherapeutic reference for the layperson, this easy-to-read book applies the principles of RET to everyday living.

Walen, S. R., DiGiuseppe, R., & Wessler, R. L. (1980). *A practitioner's guide to rational-emotive therapy.* New York: Oxford University Press. This book offers step-by-step instructions on how to practice RET.

Wessler, R. A., & Wessler, R. L. (1980). *The principles and practice of rational-emotive therapy.* San Francisco: Jossey-Bass. This work contains a wealth of contributions to the theory and practice of RET, particularly the authors' expansion of Ellis's ABC model.

Cognitive Therapy

Beck, A. T. (1967). *Depression: Clinical, experimental, and theoretical aspects.* New York: Harper & Row. In this book, Beck emphasizes the dominance of certain cognitive schema creating depression, which he labels the "cognitive triad of depression."

Beck, A. T. (1976). *Cognitive therapy and the emotional disorders.* New York: International Universities Press. In this book Beck expounds on his theory to consider emotional disorders other than depression: anxiety, phobias, obsessions, and psychosomatic disorders.

Beck, A. T., Rusch, A. J., Shaw, B. F., & Emery, G. (1979). *Cognitive therapy of depression.* New York: Guilford Press. A total volume illustrating the application of cognitive therapy for overcoming this disabling emotional disorder.

Burns, D. D. (1980). *Feeling good: The new mood therapy.* New York: The New American Library. Written as a bibliotherapeutic resource for the layperson, this book outlines a systematic program to control cognitive distortions that lead to pessimism, lethargy, procrastination, low self-esteem, and other "black holes" of depression.

Ellis, A., & Greiger, R. (Eds.) (1977). *Handbook of rational-emotive therapy.* New York: Springer. Although focusing generally on the theory and practice of RET, this book contains chapters written by Beck in which he presents basic concepts and research relating to his cognitive therapy.

Transactional Analysis

Berne, E. (1964). *Games people play.* New York: Grove Press. Berne's initial book that launched the TA movement remains current in relevant content. It is particularly valuable for understanding basic life scripts and parent–adult–child transactions.

Berne, E. (1972). *What do you say after you say hello?* New York: Grove Press. In this book, Berne covers the entirety of TA and its development. The concept of scripts is given special attention.

Goulding, M., & Goulding, R. L. (1979). *Changing lives through redecision therapy.* New York: Bruner/Mazel. The authors clearly address both the theory and practice of TA, focusing on basic TA concepts, pragmatic topics such as contracts, and the importance of working on redecisions as a major part of therapy efforts.

Graham, B. (Ed.) (1977). *Transactional analysis after Eric Berne.* New York: Harper's College Press. Different authors address TA and its applications. This book offers similarities and subtle differences in the application of the approach providing comprehensive examples of TA in actual practice.

Woolams, S., & Brown, M. (1979). *TA: The total handbook of transactional analysis.* Englewood Cliffs, NJ: Prentice-Hall. This book provides a description of the theory and practice of TA. Redecision therapy is included as a predominant part of this presentation.

5

Comparing and Contrasting: Clarifying a Pragmatic Therapeutic Position

All counseling approaches and techniques are ultimately
concerned with freeing people from immobility.

(Ivey & Simek-Downing, 1980, p. 413)

Although each approach in the preceding chapters places a different degree of emphasis on the three domains of human functioning, the ultimate goal of each of them is to free clients from their immobility. Persons seeking therapeutic help find themselves in some way powerless to change the actions, thoughts, or feelings that prevent them achieving their immediate and longer-range life goals. One individual stays socially isolated, not knowing how to meet people; another person cannot stop thinking certain thoughts that make life miserable; a third individual is always too depressed to function in a personally satisfying way. In all cases, these people are unable to break free from their present maladaptive functioning.

Counseling and psychotherapy attempt to help people become better at pursuing their immediate and long-range goals. Therapy is aimed at stimulating mastery over the thoughts, feelings, and actions that hinder this competence (Watson & Morse, 1977). Other than sharing this very general assumption, however, each major approach differs in its view of human nature, its goals of therapy rooted in that view, and its assumptions about how therapy is ideally experienced.

This chapter reviews the major approaches to counseling and psychotherapy by comparing and contrasting these differences. We then present a case that illustrates how the various approaches might be used with the same client to help you clarify and thus more completely comprehend the value of a pragmatic therapeutic position.

As we point out in chapter 1, developing a pragmatic therapeutic position is a two-step process:

1. Primary assessment, goal setting, and intervention according to one dominant theoretical orientation in which you have developed expertise. For example, if you have assumed a cognitive stance, you initially help your client modify the way he or she thinks. THEN:

2. Secondary assessment and direct intervention focusing on the remaining two domains.

Accurately comprehending how the different affective, behavioral, and cognitively-oriented approaches differ is vital to effectively assuming a pragmatic therapeutic position. Concise, crisp assessment, goal setting, and intervention in each domain of a client's functioning must be different, not overlapping and thus overdone. Distinguishing the essentials of one's primary approach and the secondary orientations is critical for this to occur.

One of the most difficult questions that must be addressed by every therapeutic approach is on the nature of the human being. Therapists must clarify their conceptions of persons' role in the world before they can hope to help them. Yet, human beings are likely the most complex organisms known, and this complexity is reflected in the diversity of opinions that have been considered.

Affective approaches' understanding of human nature is characterized by existential therapy's view that human beings possess awareness and the freedom to make choices that shape their lives. Human life is construed as having infinite possibilities. Person-centered therapy also takes a positive view of humans; individuals are naturally inclined to move in a self-enhancing direction. Inherent in each client is worth, dignity, and self-direction towards greater growth and health. Affective approaches view every individual as unique and able construe the world differently. One's view of self is seen as the way one establishes a view of the world. Thus, problems arise when there is a discrepancy between what one wants to be and what one is. Congruence between the real self and the ideal self, by contrast, is considered the definition of mental health.

Gestalt therapy perhaps best typifies the affective approaches on congruence. People are viewed as wholes, not parts, seeking to find completeness in themselves. The person divided into parts experiences difficulties. Thus, it is the whole person who takes responsibility, completes unfinished business, experiences, and is aware who is fully functioning.

By contrast, behavior therapy posits that humans are shaped primarily by sociocultural conditioning. Human development is basically determined by what an individual is exposed to and thus able to learn or not learn. Human behavior is seen as following laws and can be explained through systematic study of learning principles. Problems in living are viewed as resulting from lack of or faulty learning experiences.

Reality therapy, although a behaviorally-oriented perspective, is middle ground between behavior therapy and the affectively-oriented positions. Reality therapy is directional in proposing that all persons are motivated by their need for identity and can develop either a success identity or a failure identity. Individuals must act in the context of reality, however, to attain identity. The emphasis is clearly on the actions and consequences that occur in person–environment interactions.

Cognitive approaches recognize dual possibilities for human beings. Humans are born with equal potential for adaptive, rational thinking and maladaptive, irrational thinking. Although persons may be shaped by early maladaptive decisions and learning experiences, they tend to maintain their faulty thinking by consistently reindoctrinating themselves with ineffective and dysfunctional assumptions from the past. Thus, people's beliefs are at the root of their problems. Examining the validity of present beliefs and finding alternatives enables persons to remake decisions with greater awareness.

The major approaches to counseling and psychotherapy have basic differences in the principles they emphasize in their conceptualizations of human nature. It is important, however, to note one overriding commonality among them that is not directly stated, but rather implied: All these approaches advocate the possibility of human change. A related belief is that certain events in persons' lives are causes of concern and are serious enough to warrant some kind of change. Thus, all of the approaches agree that sometimes individuals are in situations that cause them to need help, and that help can be offered with the expectation that changes can occur (Hansen, Stevic, & Warner, 1982). The goals in offering therapeutic assistance again distinguish the approaches.

THERAPEUTIC GOALS

In comparing the goals of the various approaches, one finds diverse objectives which are derived from the different views of human nature proposed by the particular orientations. Corey (1982) considered the question of a common denominator or point of integration among these various therapeutic goals. He proposed that the issues raised by diverse goals could be simplified by viewing them in terms of their degree of generality or specificity. "Goals can be seen as existing on a continuum from general, global, and long-term objectives to specific, concrete, and short-term objectives" (Corey, 1982, p. 221). Affectively-oriented approaches tend towards the general; behaviorally-oriented and cognitive approaches stress specific goals. The goals are not necessarily contradictory, they merely differ in specificity.

Existential therapy takes a positive, trusting, optimistic view of human nature. Persons can do for themselves. Thus, its goals of therapy allow for more leeway. The existential therapist seeks to create conditions in which clients can know themselves better and remove the blocks that prevent them from fulfilling their human potential. Clients are therefore able to feel free to take responsibility for the direction of their own lives. Person-centered therapy similarly seeks to help clients unlock their potential to be open to new experience, to trust themselves more completely, to possess an internal locus of evaluation, and to be willing to be a process, not static. Gestalt therapy too has a more general goal, focusing on clients becoming more aware of their moment-to-moment experiences and accepting responsibility for the direction of their lifes.

Behavior therapy specifies concrete, observable, and measurable therapeutic objectives, in stark contrast to the broad affective goals just described. The behavior therapist is not opposed to general global goals, but broad goals should be defined through subgoals that can be evaluated. Krumboltz (1966), a noted behavior therapist, admitted that he himself was not opposed to a relatively vague goal like self-actualization, but rather:

> All of these ways of stating goals suffer from being so global and general that they provide no guidelines for what is to be accomplished. . . . In order to make such generalities useful they must be translated into specific kinds of behavior appropriate to each client's problem so that everyone concerned with the counseling relationship knows exactly what is to be accomplished. (pp. 9–10)

Like any good teacher, the behavior therapist needs to accurately assess what a client knows and what he or she needs to learn. Reality therapy helps clients make clear and concise value judgments about their behavior and decide on a concrete plan of action for change. Clients learn more realistic and responsible behavior in order to develop a success identity. Clients experience difficulties because of prior faulty learning. Without new learning, they will not be able to change.

Cognitive approaches have precise, short-term goals similar to behaviorally-oriented approaches. They focus, however, on a different domain of human functioning: thought. Beck's cognitive therapy is especially diagnostically-oriented and explicitly relates particular patterns of thought to specific categories of psychopathology. Transactional analysis's use of structural, transactional, script, and game analyses and its emphasis on contractual therapy similarly emphasize concrete short-term goals. Rational-emotive therapy seeks to eliminate clients' dysfunctional, self-defeating beliefs and replace them with more functional, adaptive ideas. While specific irrational and rational beliefs are explicated to help the client practice this skill, the overriding goal is more general in terms of a more tolerant and rational outlook on life. Like Krumboltz, Ellis advocates subgoals (although cognitive) in order to make a general goal such as changing one's outlook on life workable and thus attainable.

THE THERAPEUTIC PROCESS

All the major approaches to counseling and psychotherapy accept the importance of a positive working relationship as a foundation for the therapeutic process. All stress the value of clients feeling accepted and understood, of feeling that the therapist is concerned and competent, and feeling the therapist to be genuine and honest. In effect, the therapist must be perceived as a real person, deserving of trust and able to help.

Patterson (1973) discusses the importance of the therapeutic relationship, maintaining that research indicated that the most meaningful element within therapy is the relationship. He asserts that the therapist serves as a reinforcer, for the therapist's respect and concern for clients

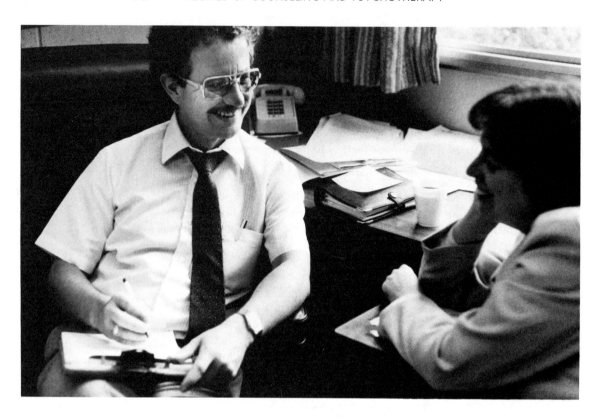

A positive working relationship is the foundation of therapy

become very powerful influences on their behavior. The therapist also can model a good personal relationship that clients can use for their own growth. Patterson clearly stresses the value of a sound therapeutic relationship in stating:

> The evidence seems to point to the establishment of a particular kind of relationship as the crucial element in counseling or psychotherapy. It is a relationship characterized not so much by what techniques the therapist uses as by what he is, not so much by what he does as by the way he does it. (pp. 535–536)

Given that therapeutic efforts are directed at change on the part of the client, this change occurs as a result of what transpires in the therapy setting. Affective approaches, for example, believe that awareness gained through affective experiencing will lead to client change. The affectively-oriented approaches tend to emphasize most the conditions of the therapeutic relationship. Person-centered therapy highlights this in considering these conditions as "necessary and sufficient" for clients to improve. The relationship that exists between counselor and client is vital to successful therapy. The ability of the therapist to be congruent and empathic, to have positive regard for the client, and communicate these qualities to the client is stressed. If these conditions are communicated, clients can enter into a real relationship with the therapist that will lead to self-exploration, learnings, and subsequent goal attainment.

Similarly, the existential position sees the therapist's main task as establishing a personal and authentic encounter with clients. Clients are helped to discover their own uniqueness in the relationship they have with the therapist. A human-to-human encounter is sought wherein clients can grasp their being-in-the-world. As opposed to this almost exclusive emphasis on therapeutic conditions, Gestalt therapy offers a set of powerful procedures to facilitate their presence. The therapist does not interpret and do for clients, but rather helps them develop the means to make their own interpretations and attain greater awareness. Clients gain experience in the present where they can identify and work on past unfinished business or potential impasses that will interfere with their functioning.

While traditionally, behavior therapists have generally been less concerned about relationship variables, a good working rapport is seen as an important groundwork for implementing behavioral intervention strategies. The behavior therapist is an active and directive teacher who functions as a trainer and resource person in helping clients learn more effective and adaptive ways of behaving. Clients themselves must be active in the process and willing to experiment with their new learning. Reality therapy, on the other hand, does emphasize strongly an involvement of counselor and client as an essential part of therapy. The aim of this therapeutic relationship, however, is not to establish a warm and positive rapport with clients but to have them assume responsibility for their own behavior. The learning process is still considered paramount, with the therapist teaching clients how to be autonomous and responsible for who they are and who they want to become by developing realistic plans of action to fulfill their goals.

Like the reality therapist, the cognitively-oriented therapist seeks to teach clients specific ideas they can use to get more satisfaction from life. As it is in behavior therapy, a good working relationship between the counselor and client is important in creating collaborative situations where clients can learn new ways of thinking. All three cognitively-oriented approaches presented in this book advocate teaching clients the basic concepts of the approach, be it RET, TA, or cognitive therapy. While the specific concepts differ, clients are helped to use their new knowledge to acquire more enhancing rather than self-defeating belief systems.

What therapists are and what they do is a result of missing their therapeutic position, that integration of an internalized personal philosophy of helping and an externally accepted model of what constitutes a mature, well-functioning human being. Counselors can use such understandings to develop therapeutic goals and select existing therapeutic techniques. They can then match intervention strategies with identified goals to help their clients.

JANET: DEPRESSED AND IN DANGER OF LOSING HER JOB

After being told by her employer that she had to "get some help or find another job," Janet, 27 years old, arranged for a counseling appointment. During the initial interview she relates the following information:

I just don't know what to do anymore. I feel like everything's just falling down around me. I don't even know why I came here. It's not going to help. The only reason I did come is because my boss said if I didn't I was out of a job. It won't be the first time though and probably not the last either.

My own father took off before I was even born. My mother said that he didn't want to be burdened with a child. Mom never remarried and had to support the two of us by herself. She was always working. I hardly ever saw her and the different sitters I was left with never seemed to like me.

Maybe because I was always sick and missing school, I never got along well there either. But my jobs all seem to end up like school. I'm afraid to go half the time. My doctor told me that most of my illness must be psychological because she can never find anything physically wrong with me. She thinks I might make myself sick so that I have an excuse to stay home from work.

I don't have any social life to speak of. I just don't know how to act around people. I try to please but it seems like I just don't have what it takes to make it in life.

The following discussion outlines how therapists operating from the different theoretical perspectives presented in the previous chapters would work with Janet.

Before reading further, we ask that you briefly refer to our introduction, in which we discuss the functions of theoretical models. Three functions in particular are vital to successful therapy: 1) organizing information into hypotheses that can guide therapy, 2) understanding adaptive and maladaptive functioning, and 3) developing and evaluating specific therapeutic strategies. Note how each of the following therapist's perspectives uses a particular theoretical approach to serve these essential functions.

THE AFFECTIVE APPROACHES

An Existential Therapist's Perspective

"My approach to therapy has evolved from my philosophy about life. I believe that Janet has the capacity to expand her awareness, and in doing so, decide for herself the future direction of her life. I view the process that Janet and I will enter to be a human encounter, a dialogue in the deepest and most genuine sense—an exchange wherein I will be as authentic and open as I am able. I hope that through the trusting and honest relationship Janet and I develop, she will understand herself more fully. She will come to realize more than anything else that she does not have to continue as a victim of past misfortune but can design her destiny.

As an existential therapist, I do not stress specific therapeutic procedures, but rather focus on certain themes that I consider to be part of the human condition. I will work to be my true self with Janet by challenging her and by reacting to her. My challenges might include:

- ☐ Are you living as fully as you want to or are you merely existing?
- ☐ Are you living your life according to your own choices or according to the desires of others?
- ☐ What are some choices you are currently faced with? How do you deal with the anxiety that is a part of making choices for yourself and accepting the freedom to choose your own way?
- ☐ What are you doing to provide yourself with a sense of purpose that will make you feel more significant and alive?

In my relationship with Janet, I will be genuinely honest and open, inviting her to respond in a similar manner. I expect that we will both be affected by this encounter. She may touch off emotions and reactions within me. I will try to understand her world from her subjective viewpoint and at the same time communicate what I am feeling in our relationship. In summary, I hope to create a climate in which Janet can evaluate her past choices and come to freely choose for herself and take responsibility for her choices. As she learns how she has limited her existence, I hope she will take steps toward freeing herself and creating her being-in-the-world anew."

A Person-Centered Perspective: Janet Finds Personal Power

"It is difficult to predict how therapy with Janet may proceed, but in general, when clients begin therapy, there is a discrepancy between the way they see themselves and the way they would like to be. This seems to be true for Janet. She will likely look to me for direction and magic answers for solving the problems in her life. Janet appears to mistrust herself and tends to externalize the cause of her difficulties. She also seems very reluctant to try new things.

I believe that Janet has within herself the necessary resources for pursuing her own personal growth. Therapy will be aimed at helping Janet to tap her inner resources so she can deal better with her problems. I think that this is best accomplished by creating a climate in which Janet feels free to express her feelings and be fully accepted by me. I would not judge or criticize her for what she expresses, but rather try to fully experience in the present what it must be like to live in Janet's world.

By my being congruent, showing positive regard, and communicating empathic understanding, Janet should begin to grow personally in our relationship. Eventually, Janet will learn to be more open to all of her experiences. She will use our relationship to learn to accept herself as a person with strengths, not just limitations. She will realize within herself a personal power to make her own decisions and guide her own future."

Gestalt Therapy: Gaining a Fuller Sense of Self

"My goal with Janet is to foster her ability to take responsibility for herself. Although philosophically I hold an existential view of the human condition, I will draw heavily on experiential exercises that will enable Janet to gain a fuller sense of herself in the present. The exercises will help Janet focus on how she obstructs her present functioning.

Janet appears to have significant "unfinished business" in her resentment towards her parents, which she has turned inward toward herself. While we will emphasize Janet's present situation, she may also need to reexperience past feelings (toward her parents especially) that keep her from developing intimacy with others. Janet will not merely talk about past experiences; rather, she will be asked to imagine herself in earlier scenes with her mother or, more creatively, her unknown father, as though the painful situation were actually happening. She will relive the situation, perhaps by using the empty chair exercise to talk directly to her father, telling him of her resentment toward him for leaving her and the hurt she has felt without a father, eventually completing her unfinished business with him.

Janet will find that she will not necessarily get rid of any of her feelings but that she can learn to live with them, especially those that seem contradictory, for example, both love and hate toward her parents. In therapy sessions, we will work with these polarities that Janet does not generally express. Janet in particular appears to be most critical and judgmental of herself. We would thus work to increase Janet's self-acceptance, which she does not recognize or express. In this manner, Janet will explore aspects of herself that can be further developed and integrated. Along this line, I will ask Janet to try different experiments, such as expressing previously repressed body movements or gestures. I want to invite Janet to try out new behaviors and see what she can learn from experimenting with them. As Janet learns to pay greater attention to whatever it is she is experiencing at any given moment, this awareness itself can lead to positive change. The more aware she is, the greater her opportunity to find her own center and live for her own purposes."

Behavior Therapy: A Learning Perspective

"I would begin therapy with Janet by assessing her present behaviors (or lack of certain behaviors). We will identify Janet's strengths and weaknesses and then determine those behaviors she wants to increase or decrease in frequency. Our goals will therefore be concrete and measurable. Together we will work out a treatment plan with strategies that are designed to meet those goals.

We will choose the procedures that seem most appropriate to achieving the stated goals. I believe that Janet's present difficulties result from a lack of skills or from using skills inappropriately. She needs to learn new behaviors and new ways of using previously learned behaviors. Be it classical conditioning, instrumental conditioning, or observational learning, we will focus on Janet's behavior.

For example, Janet is afraid to go to work. While this fear was likely learned while she was going to school, we would not emphasize the past unless it is necessary in modifying her faulty learning. We may choose systematic desensitization to work with this aspect of Janet's present functioning. First she would learn relaxation procedures, then she would develop a hierarchy of her specific fears of her job. We would then use imagery, pairing relaxation with lesser fears and working our way up the hierarchy to her greatest fear. Janet could thus learn to be less anxious and more relaxed at work. Instrumental principles might then be considered for building a better behavioral repertoire to help her function better at work.

Janet also lacks social skills. Modeling procedures might be used to teach her more assertive social amenities. As a behavior therapist, I will continually keep track of her progress and evaluate the results of therapy to determine how well Janet is proceeding toward her goals, as well as the efficacy of the procedures we are using. For lasting behavioral change to take place, Janet will need to be active in and outside of our sessions. She will be asked to keep records of relevant daily behaviors and put the skills she will be learning into action everyday."

Reality Therapy With Janet

"As a reality therapist, I believe that evading reality and living irresponsibly are the major causes of human problems. Therefore, I want to help Janet take a critical look at what she is doing with her life and judge how effective her behavior is in attaining her life goals. Once she is able to make this assessment, we can begin therapy by deciding upon specific ways in which she wants to change.

I will focus on what Janet can and will do in the present to change her behavior. I will challenge her to look at her current behavior and to make value judgments about the way she is now living with questions such as "Are your needs being met by your current behavior?" "If not, what can you do to change?" "Are you willing to commit to changing some of those behaviors that prevent you from meeting your needs?" Therapy will emphasize behavioral change, not feelings or attitudes. What Janet can do right *now* to start living in a responsible manner and thus achieve a success identity will be of foremost importance.

To this end, I will help Janet develop plans to change her present failure-oriented behavior into success behavior. She will make a commitment to carry out these plans, for if change is to occur, then action is necessary. It will be critical that she accept responsibility for changing and not blame outside forces for the way she is or give excuses why she doesn't meet her commitments. We may develop a therapeutic contract that spells out goals, the means to achieve them, and commitments to carry them out.

One final point: the importance of client responsibility cannot be overstressed. It is critical to reality therapy. For example, when Janet says that she is depressed, I don't ask why she is depressed, nor do I dwell on feelings of depression. Instead, I ask her what *she has done* that day to contribute to her depression. Through my caring, concerned involvement with Janet, I hope to show her the benefits of responsibly facing reality and actively living in it."

THE COGNITIVE APPROACHES

Rational-Emotive Therapy: Janet's ABCs

"My major goal with Janet will be to help her gain a more rational and realistic outlook on life. Within that general goal, however, my subgoals will be to consider Janet's specific patterns of irrational thinking that lead to her emotional and behavioral difficulties. I will function as a teacher, focusing on what Janet needs to learn to change her thinking. To begin, Janet will learn that she is maintaining her present irrational beliefs by reindoctrinating herself with them without examining their validity or functionality. She will accomplish this by analyzing her thinking using an ABC framework.

She will first learn that, like most persons, she probably believes that activating experiences (A) cause the emotional and behavioral consequences (C). She will learn that it is actually her beliefs (B) about A that cause C. This will lead to us examining the demands, devastation, and self-denigration that Janet has blindly accepted. Her major irrational beliefs appear to be devastation and self-denigration, for example, "It's utterly horrible that my father deserted my mother and me before I was even born!" and "Because I have been seemingly rejected by so many persons, I must be no good."

Janet will then learn to evaluate and dispute (D) her irrational beliefs by challenging their validity and functional value with questions such as, "How is it the end of *your* world that your father was disturbed?" "Because some persons reject you, how does that define you as a person as 'no good'?" "How does maintaining these beliefs help you in any way?" By challenging her present beliefs, Janet can discard them as much as is realistically possible and substitute more rational, logical thinking. While she might be disappointed that her father was the way he was and feel somewhat sad about it, she does not have to be miserable over something that happened before she was born and over which she had no control whatsoever. "Some persons may reject me; however, I don't have to reject myself and the fact is that 'some' is not 'all'."

Thus, therapy will be a reeducation process. As in any educational endeavor, Janet will be asked to practice what she is learning. Homework assignments are a critical component of therapy, and Janet will complete cognitive, emotive, and behavioral tasks to more firmly establish her new belief system. Janet will experience more functional and satisfying emotional and behavioral effects (E) as a result of her new beliefs and develop a more rational view of life so that her future will be proactive rather than reactive."

Cognitive Therapy's Triad of Depression

"As a therapist trained in Beck's cognitive therapy, I am well prepared to deal with Janet's depression. While Janet may have overt emotional and behavioral symptoms, I believe that specific distorted cognitive conceptualizations about herself, her present circumstances, and her future potential that are the basis for her developing and maintaining her depressive symptoms. Janet clearly seems to distort her life experiences. For example, her father leaving before her birth she misinterprets as a *personal* failure. Janet is maintaining a systematic bias against herself.

Therapy with Janet will consist of identifying her cognitive distortions and subjecting them to logical and empirical testing. My goal is to help Janet realign her thinking with reality. Therapy will be relatively short so that we both see the need for judicious use of our time. Initially I will ask Janet to complete graded task assignments. I won't try to counter her "I can't" and "It's no use" beliefs by taking an opposing stance. Rather, I will simply ask Janet to test her present beliefs. She says that she makes herself ill and can't go to work. I might ask that she go to work the next time she isn't feeling well and test her belief that she "can't."

As therapy progresses, I will help Janet recognize and collect her automatic thoughts and learn "distancing," dealing objectively with such thoughts rather than blindly accepting them. She will complete homework such as the triple column technique to facilitate distancing. Basic self-defeating themes will emerge and her commonly employed cognitive distortions will be identified and categorized. Through alternative therapy Janet will then learn to consider alternative interpretations of her experiences. By having to think of other explanations, Janet will learn to recognize her biases and substitute more accurate interpretations. I won't attempt to invalidate the real difficulties that Janet may experience as a result of external events in her life. But by discussing with me and herself different ways of dealing with obstacles, Janet will find solutions to problems that she previously considered hopeless and insoluble."

Janet from a TA Perspective

"Since an important part of Transactional Analysis is the counselor and client working on mutually agreed-upon goals, Janet and I will first develop a therapeutic contract to guide what we will do during our sessions. This contract will be a clear set of statements of what she wants from therapy, what she wants to change, and what she is willing to do to make those changes. One important aspect of Janet's life is that she feels "not OK" much of the time. She wants to learn to feel "OK" about herself and others.

Therapy will primarily focus on present behavior and transactions with others as well as the attitudes Janet has about herself. Janet and I will explore her past to learn what decisions she made as a child. I will teach her the fundamental vocabulary of TA: the Parent, Adult, and Child ego states, scripts, and games. Janet will learn that her decisions about how to survive as a child may no longer be appropriate and that she can change these decisions. For Janet, one major decision appears to have been "I'm not OK. I'm a loser."

In addition to making this early decision, Janet appears to have accepted a list of early parental messages such as "You're not worthwhile." Janet's inability to garner positive strokes from those around her led her to seek negative strokes. Now she finds it difficult to accept positive strokes and develop intimate relationships with others. She invests considerable time and energy in collecting bad feelings and these will need to be explored. I will confront Janet with the games she plays, the ulterior transactions between her and others that prevent intimacy and result in the bad feelings. "Poor Me" and "Helpless" seem appropriate games to analyze with Janet.

As our therapy sessions proceed, Janet will be taught to analyze her life scripts. She will come to understand that she bases her present life on a series of decisions. We will explore in depth the ways in which she has particularly programmed herself and how she acts and feels as a result of her early decisions. Through script analysis, Janet will learn to actively do something about changing her programming. Through this increased understanding, she should be able to break free of her early scripting."

You have just read how different therapists would work with Janet from each of the therapeutic perspectives we have discussed. However, the basic theoretical theme of this book is the systematic and direct consideration of all three domains of client functioning for the most effective and efficient clinical practice. A pragmatic therapeutic position fully and directly deals with all three domains of human functioning: affective, behavioral, and cognitive. The order in which they are addressed is a function of one's personal philosophy of helping and preferred theory in which one has developed expertise. If you assume a primary cognitive stance, your initial concern will be directed toward changing Janet's thinking. In operating from a pragmatic therapeutic perspective, however, it is not always enough, nor is it realistic to focus on only one sphere. Affective and behavioral change *is* likely to occur as a result of cognitive change; nevertheless, in order to *maximize* therapeutic effectiveness and efficiency, a focus on one single domain may be less than optimal. Direct assessment, goal setting, and intervention addressing all three areas of Janet's functioning will surely increase the likelihood of therapeutic success.

The following perspective is that of a therapist using the pragmatic therapeutic position from an affective/cognitive-behavioral stance:

"I believe that awareness can be curative in and of itself. I also feel strongly that the goals that person-centered therapy advocates are the ultimate road to self-actualization: openness to experience, trust in oneself, an internal locus of evaluation, and the willingness to be a process. I find these concepts, the positive and forward moving view of human nature, and the idea of communicating core conditions in therapy to be most closely aligned with my own personal philosophy of helping. I very much feel a comradery with the idea of using myself and my relationship with clients as the major force for change. Person-centered therapy thus constitutes my primary theoretical orientation when working with clients.

I see the development of a trusting relationship as critical to therapeutic progress. I will try to build this trust with Janet by being fully genuine with her in our sessions. I will encourage her to talk openly about the feelings that she has felt must be kept hidden. I will try to model the behaviors and attitudes that I want Janet to acquire. If I am open and honest during our sessions and don't try to hide behind pretenses and professional roles, then Janet will be able to drop her masks and be

A PRAGMATIC THERAPEUTIC PERSPECTIVE TOWARD WORKING WITH JANET

genuine with me. If I can really listen to her nonjudgmentally, then I have a basis of coming to know her world as she sees it. I will seek to communicate my empathic understanding to her. If I am able to be truly sensitive and open with Janet, she will probably begin to be sensitive and open to herself. She will have less need to deny or distort her feelings and therefore her ability to clearly know what she is feeling at any given moment will increase.

I am confident that with this awareness, Janet will be freed from her need to draw her self-image from things outside herself. She will learn to trust her own ideas and to act in healthy, self-actualizing ways. One concern I have is that while Janet will be aware of her feelings, cognitive and behavioral changes may come more slowly. I do believe that these changes in the latter two domains can come without additional intervention. However, I want to give Janet every advantage in facilitating this growth. For this reason, I will also directly address the cognitive and behavioral areas, primarily by helping Janet learn more adaptive thinking and acting skills.

In considering the cognitive domain, I would draw heavily from Beck's cognitive therapy, especially its cognitive conceptualization of depression. By helping Janet understand her specific beliefs that create and maintain depression, she will be better prepared to cope with her present or future depressive symptoms. With this increased understanding, Janet will learn to distance herself from her negative attitudes and see the cognitive distortions that prevent her from living a more satisfying life. Through alternative therapy, we will work on how Janet can consider different explanations for her experiences. She will see that she has alternatives in the ways she thinks as well as feels.

Janet can spend countless hours expressing the feelings she has hidden for so many years. She can learn to think about the things she tells herself that lead to an unsatisfactory existence. Yet without acting upon this new awareness and these cognitive constructions, Janet's success in therapy is incomplete. I would stress that now having addressed both her affective and cognitive domains, Janet is likely to function much better and be happier. Again, however, I want to help this growth process in every way. Therefore, I will work with her to change her behavior as well.

Through modeling, for example, Janet can be taught specific social skills that she now lacks. Assertiveness might be the goal of observational learning, which may comprise attention, retention, motor reproduction, and motivation. Janet could also practice her new assertive behaviors in our sessions through role rehearsals. I could play the role of a social acquaintance, and Janet could practice the way she'd like to act assertively with me. This exercise lets her experiment and receive corrective and supportive feedback on the effects of her new social skills. Practice will be essential, and homework assignments of going out between sessions and *doing* will be equally emphasized.

In summary, like a nutritionist, I realize that while one food may be sufficient to sustain life, a balanced diet from each of the major food groups is best for optimal physical well-being. Nourishing counseling and psychotherapy likewise is composed of "foods" for each of the three areas of human functioning: the affective, the behavioral, and the cognitive.

Ponzo (1976) recounts his mother's early advice in writing:

EPILOGUE

> When she was annoyed with me, my mother would say, "Zander, there is a time and place for everything." I did not appreciate the depth of her wisdom then but saw the statement only as a precursor to more physical means if I did not stop inappropriate "time and place" behavior. However, maturity has enabled me to appreciate and utilize the wisdom of my mother's words in many areas of life.
>
> I have lived through an era of proliferating therapies, each of which asserts that there is a time and place for its system—and it is always. . . . Fortunately, I sensed that dogmatism and deification contradicted Mother's wisdom, and I resisted the demands. Instead, I worked to become a wise, time-and-place-for-everything counselor/therapist, a person who sought to integrate the wisdoms of the gurus into a system in which the different teachings worked together rather than against each other. (p. 415)

Ponzo's time-and-place philosophy is quite apt in concluding our discussion of theoretical approaches. We partially dispute his contention; we believe that each major approach is actually *always* appropriate in every situation. Our concern, however, is with the degree of appropriateness, and the therapeutic efficiency and effectiveness of a singular focus. For these reasons, we advocate our pragmatic therapeutic position. The previous cases have shown how each approach we have presented can be used to help Janet achieve therapeutic successes.

We present Janet's therapy from a pragmatic therapeutic perspective to show its increased efficacy as a systematic and integrated approach, a *more* effective and efficient approach. From that therapist's perspective, a person-centered orientation was the primary focus, followed by a cognitive therapy, then a behavior therapy, which addressed directly the other major domains of Janet's human functioning. They were addressed not because affective intervention alone was insufficient, but because their addition made the total therapy process more effective. The selection of those orientations was purely a matter of personal and professional preference. As long as the three domains are each given attention, the choice of particular orientation is discretionary.

We stress that your choice of a primary theory of expertise should be the one that most closely aligns with your own personal philosophy of helping. The choice of secondary theories are best selected similarly. We propose that our modification of Ponzo's time-and-place perspective (a pragmatic therapeutic position) is the most effective and efficient therapeutic approach one can pursue, because clients and their concerns, and counselors, are all unique.

SUGGESTED READINGS

Belkin, G. S. (Ed.). (1980). *Contemporary psychotherapies*. Chicago: Rand McNally. This book offers clinical case studies to illustrate realistic examples of how various theories of counseling and psychotherapy are translated into practice.

Corey, G. (1982). *Case approach to counseling and psychotherapy*. Monterey, CA: Brooks/Cole. In this book, the author creates a client (Ruth) and demonstrates how therapists using the different major theoretical orientations might work with her.

Corey, G. (1982). *Theory and practice of counseling and psychotherapy* (2nd ed.). Monterey, CA: Brooks/Cole. The author provides an excellent introductory overview of the major approaches to counseling and psychotherapy, particularly the later chapters, which contrast major concepts through description and a comparative single case study.

Corsini, R. (Ed.). (1979). *Current psychotherapies* (2nd ed.). Itasca, IL: Peacock. The editor has compiled contributions from major exponents of a number of popular approaches to counseling and psychotherapy. Each contribution contains detailed case study material to illustrate primarily points.

Wedding, D., & Corsini, R. (1979). *Great cases in psychotherapy*. Itasca, IL: Peacock. This book is intended as a companion reader to *Current psychotherapies* cited above. It offers further examples of case reports illustrating applications of the major psychotherapeutic approaches.

Part Three

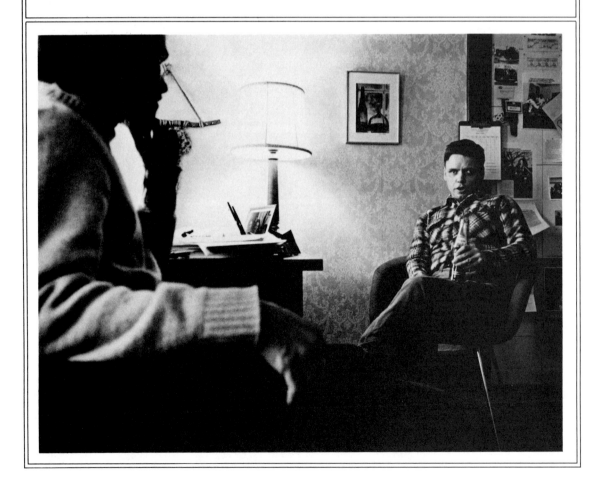

Putting Theory into Practice: A Skills Approach

In this section we present a systematic skills model of the therapeutic process. We don't claim to have reinvented the wheel; rather, we have synthesized and integrated the established models that have been reported as most effective in clinical and research literature with models we have found work best with our own clients and in training future practitioners. We keep theory clearly in focus and use it as a basis for specific skills and phases of the therapeutic process throughout these chapters. Our many cases and illustrations should enhance your understanding of the skills and overall process.

Chapter 6 is an overview of our systematic skills model of counseling and psychotherapy. Four distinct phases with relevant therapist skills constitute this presentation of the therapeutic process. Chapter 7 presents therapist skills for creating a positive therapeutic climate. Chapter 8 delineates therapist skills to help clients discriminate and define their problems. Chapter 9 investigates goal setting, and chapter 10 discusses proactive problem intervention.

We again note that there is much literature devoted to systematic skills models of the therapeutic process as well as each of the associated therapist skills characteristic of a model's specific phases. At the end of each chapter we list recommended resources to direct you to additional information.

The Course of Counseling and Psychotherapy

Research data and clinical experience strongly suggest that certain key dimensions of interviewing underlie all counseling and therapeutic approaches.

(Evans, Hearn, Uhlemann, & Ivey, 1979, p. 5)

Clients are both unique and predictable. They are unique in that therapists can rarely anticipate the specific concerns a particular client will present. Experienced therapists often admit that they are frequently surprised by the variety of topics different clients introduce. At the same time, however, clients are predictable in that they share many similar problems and distressing situations to some degree. Everyone has felt angry, confused, indecisive, or overwhelmed. They have had depressing, destructive, self-denigrating thoughts and have acted in dissatisfying and inappropriate ways. Expressing these concerns *and* doing something constructive about them is often quite difficult for many persons. Thus, they need trained professional help.

As clients are both unique and predictable, so too are the theoretical approaches therapists use to help them cope with their problems and develop more satisfying lives. The discussion of affective, behavioral, and cognitive approaches in the preceding chapters illustrates that each orientation has unique aspects. All have commonalities as well. The different theoretical approaches emphasize different elements of the therapeutic process as well as different therapist skills. The particular skills a therapist uses most often are thus determined by personal experience and primary theoretical orientation. Research has clearly shown that therapists of different theoretical orientations use different skills in differing degrees (Ivey & Simek-Downing, 1980). Research has also suggested, however, that certain key dimensions and skills underlie all counseling and therapeutic approaches (Evans et al., 1979).

We have been using the term *process* when we discuss what happens between a therapist and client—the therapeutic process. This term aptly communicates the essence of this interaction. Process refers to an identifiable sequence of events taking place over time (Patterson & Eisenberg, 1983). Process usually implies progressive stages. For example, there are certain identifiable stages in the healing process of a serious physical injury such as a broken arm. Similarly, the generally predictable stages of human development from birth to death have been well-documented (Erikson, 1963; Gould, 1972; Kimmel, 1974; Neugarten, 1977).

This second parallel also applies to the process of counseling and psychotherapy. While therapists' primary theoretical approaches may differ and the specific circumstances and concerns of every client may vary, the stages of the therapeutic process generally are the same. It is in implementing these components in therapeutic process that divergence may occur; the basic components themselves remain constant. Although they differ by terminology, most all major writers have conceptualized the counseling process as distinct phases (Brammer & Shostrom, 1982; Carkhuff & Berenson, 1977; Egan, 1982; Ivey & Simek-Downing, 1980; Patterson & Eisenberg, 1983). We too see the process as proceding through identifiable phases:

☐ Phase I: Creating a Therapeutic Climate
☐ Phase II: Problem Discrimination and Definition
☐ Phase III: Goal Setting
☐ Phase IV: Proactive Problem Intervention

This therapeutic process is developmental; that is, it is systematic and cumulative. The success of Phase II depends on the quality of the therapeutic climate that is created in Phase I. Similarly, the success of Phase III depends on the work conducted during Phase II, and so on. Each phase has specific tasks as well as identifiable therapist skills for completing tasks. For example, if the therapist does not possess those skills that facilitate the establishment of a working relationship in Phase I, problems cannot be accurately discriminated nor defined in Phase II. Thus, assisting the client to establish meaningful goals (Phase III) without knowing what the problem was would be virtually impossible! No matter the theoretical orientation, understanding the therapeutic process in general and possessing the therapist skills to implement the process are obvious essentials which will now be considered.

Most clients voluntarily seek therapeutic help. They become aware of problems in their lives and realize that they need assistance. Other clients are reluctant to present themselves for therapy. Although they are experiencing difficulties, they either do not acknowledge they need help or do not recognize that their present life is less than adequate. With all clients, however, caution and some anxiety are inevitable; they must be made to feel comfortable and confident that therapy will help them. As students must be prepared to learn a new subject, so too clients must be ready to enter and benefit from therapy. This readiness to enter Phase II of the therapeutic process is the goal of Phase I; it is accomplished by therapists creating a set of conditions through using specific skills.

CREATING A THERAPEUTIC CLIMATE

Core Conditions

Certain core conditions underlie the entire process of counseling and psychotherapy. They are actually attitudes that must be expressed in a variety of ways during therapy. Studies show that therapists' skills in conveying these attitudes affect the success of therapy and play a central role in establishing and maintaining an effective therapeutic climate. They include:

☐ Empathic Understanding: therapists' ability to convey to clients that they can understand the client's world from the client's frame of reference.

☐ Respect: therapists' conveying to clients that they have a positive regard for the client as a person of worth and value and for the client's potential to improve his or her life situation.

☐ Genuineness: therapists' being themselves with clients and not hiding behind any professional role, but showing interest in a human being–to–human being exchange.

☐ Concreteness: concentrating on specific feelings, thoughts, and behaviors and encouraging clients to similarly concentrate on identifiable and thus changeable aspects of their intrapersonal functioning and relationships with others.

Research has indicated that effective therapists, regardless of their theoretical orientation or training, convey these core conditions to their clients (Berenson & Carkhuff, 1967; Carkhuff, 1969a, 1969b; Rogers, Gendlin, Kiessler, & Truax, 1967; Truax & Carkhuff, 1967; Truax & Mitchell, 1971).

Social Influencers

Another important set of elements critical in creating an effective therapeutic climate are social influencers. Clients must be confident that their therapist can actually help them. Research supports the idea that how a client perceives a counselor in terms of *expertness, attractiveness,* and *trustworthiness* determines the counselor's ability to help (Barak & La Crosse, 1975; Corrigan, Dell, Lewis, & Schmidt, 1980; Schmidt & Strong, 1971; Strong & Schmidt, 1970a, 1970b).

Social influencers are:

☐ Expertness: the client believes that the therapist has the training and background to help him or her in terms of information, understanding, and skills.

☐ Attractiveness: the client likes and respects the therapist, feels compatible with him or her, and wants to emulate some of the therapist's behaviors.

☐ Trustworthiness: the client feels secure in the therapist's ability and willingness to maintain confidentiality and respond to him or her with care, respect, and professional competence.

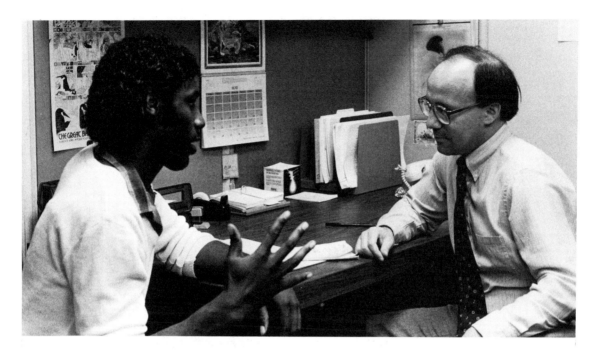

Structuring and Attending Skills

Attending is a vital therapist skill

Although core conditions and social influencers must be established before problem discrimination and definition (Phase II) can begin, therapists
must possess still more skills to create the best possible therapeutic environment. These skills are structuring and attending.

Structuring. Structuring refers to statements by therapists that let clients
know what to expect from the therapeutic process. Structuring gives
therapy a common meaning for client and counselor and helps keep it on
track. If therapy is to be of any value, clients must begin with an accurate
understanding of *where* they are, *who* they are with, and *why* they are
there (Brammer & Shostrom, 1982).

Attending. A client must know that the therapist is truly listening, and
that during the time they are together the therapist is available to work
with the client. Attending is done both psychologically, by listening atten-
tively to and considering what the client says, and physically, by displaying
a posture of interest.

Examinations of sessions conducted by ineffective counselors have revealed that they are frequently unable to help clients rank their many
problems and thus choose and clearly define the best way to deal with

**PROBLEM
DISCRIMINATION
AND DEFINITION**

them. These counselors seem to wander aimlessly from topic to topic, discussing much but accomplishing little (Ivey & Simek-Downing, 1980). In Phase II of the therapeutic process, the client must be helped to articulate personal concerns and put them in context so that something can be done about them.

Counseling is primarily a verbal process that involves a great deal of dialogue. Therapists need to respond to clients in ways that help them explore and clarify their concerns and that show clients that the therapists understand what they are experiencing. Understanding alone is not enough; it must be communicated. In addition, therapists must help clients to articulate their concerns specifically and concretely so that they can be actively dealt with.

Therapist skills in Phase II can be categorized by its two predominant tasks; organization and focusing.

Organizational Understandings

A therapist's organizational skill is the ability to distinguish variations in and correlate aspects of a client's total functioning. This therapist skill is prerequisite to problem definition. From the presentation on human functioning and counseling theory, we know that clients' affective, behavioral, and cognitive functioning are affected by any concerns they experience. Therapists' ability to distinguish among the explicit and implicit aspects of clients' affective, behavioral, and cognitive modes of functioning is therefore critical.

The environmental *context* in which clients function is another vital component for therapists to recognize and respond to. At all times, what exists around clients will play a dominant role in how clients choose to react. Often the best of intentions and most enthusiastic efforts are thwarted by a hostile, unbending environment. In comparison, a supportive, encouraging environment dramatically enhances clients' potential for solving problems.

Focusing Skills

Focusing skills enable therapists to direct clients' attention to therapeutically appropriate areas of affective, behavioral, and/or cognitive functioning and relevant environmental contexts. Observations of skilled therapists reveal that they selectively focus on and selectively ignore certain client communications (Ivey & Simek-Downing, 1980). Since different theories stress the importance of different information, therapists must be able to focus on the client communications that are the most relevant in their primary theoretical approach. Three such therapist-focusing skills that are very useful are reflection, inquiry, and summarization.

Reflection. Reflection seeks to accomplish precisely what it implies: a mirroring of feeling, thought, and behavior in their context as presented by a client. Responding with reflections enables therapists first to communicate empathic understanding, showing the client the therapist's comprehension of his or her internal frame of reference. Reflection also helps clients focus on what the therapist has reflected back to them, setting the stage for discrimination and definition in the addressed area.

Inquiry. Inquiries are questions that help clients discriminate and define their problems more clearly. Inquiries that are open-ended, unlikely to be answered with a simple *yes* or *no*, are invitations to explore and elaborate. Closed inquiries, by contrast, likely to be answered *yes* or *no*, are used to get more specific information.

Summarization. Summarization is the gathering together of the major points of a client's communications and presenting them back to the client in a more pointed, outline form. Summarizations serve as a bridging response to help clients converge and organize the essentials of their concerns.

Clients' Responsibilities in Phases I and II

Clients' major responsibility in Phases I and II is to explain their problems, how they feel and think about them, how they have acted, and the context in which problems are occurring. With the therapist's assistance— first in creating a conducive therapeutic climate, then in helping clients explore their difficulties in a concrete, focused manner—clients can rank and define specific issues of primary concern and commit to pursuing them.

Reconsidering Phases I and II in the Therapeutic Process

Core conditions, social influencers, structuring and attending of Phase I, and the therapist skills of Phase II will be developed in upcoming chapters. It is valuable to again emphasize the developmental nature of the therapeutic process. Phase I and Phase II variables are critical not only in beginning the process, but throughout it as well. Therapists who fail to create a conducive therapeutic climate or to actively exhibit organizational and focusing skills will not be able to successfully accomplish Phase III and Phase IV tasks, as those tasks build upon the accomplishments of Phase I and II tasks. While the way in which initial skills are expressed in later phases may change, therapists' need to use them is constant. A conducive therapeutic climate, for example, can be readily reduced to chaos if therapists lose sight of its vital importance *throughout* the entire therapeutic process.

Harold came to therapy after being referred by his family doctor. He had gone to see the doctor complaining of a variety of physical ailments including constant nervousness, headaches, and stomach upset. His physician was unable to determine any physical basis for Harold's complaints and suggested they had a psychological source. In their initial session, the therapist provided Harold sufficient structure so that he immediately knew what his responsibilities were and, similarly, what the therapist wanted to accomplish with him. Harold was impressed by the therapist's self-assurance and the generally professional manner in which he conducted himself. He also was confident because this particular therapist, whom his physician suggested, had an excellent reputation.

Harold first felt anxious about sharing his concerns with the therapist, but became more comfortable and trusting as the session proceeded. He could see that this person was intently listening to him and seemed to fully understand what he was going through by the responses he gave to Harold's expressed concerns. Harold's initial concerns were about his physical ailments and his physician's belief that they had a psychological basis. To help Harold concretely analyze this problem, the therapist asked him to remember some specific situations in which his physical symptoms seemed to worsen. Of the four situations Harold shared, three were at home and appeared to result from his wife's behavior toward him, which he described as pushy and hostile. The therapist summarized this observation, also telling Harold that his general physical symptoms might be more easily termed anxiety. Harold agreed with the therapist. They both then committed themselves to looking more intensively at Harold's relationship with his wife and the anxiety it produced.

Problem discrimination and definition, while absolutely necessary, are not ends in themselves. Clients cannot work on their problems without setting specific goals that point out how their lives might be made more satisfying. This goal setting constitutes Phase III.

GOAL SETTING   Once a therapeutic climate has been created and problems ranked, the next task is for the client to gain a greater level of self-understanding; in doing so, setting specific goals. In Phase III of the therapeutic process, clients should begin to formulate a new sense of direction. Patterson and Eisenberg (1983) suggest that emerging goals be thought of as the "flip side" of problems—"so that, as problems are more clearly understood, the direction in which the client wishes to move also becomes clearer" (p. 33). In Phase III, the means for reaching new goals may not be clear to clients, but the goals themselves begin to take shape.

Therapeutic goals are of two types: outcome goals and process goals. Outcome goals are the results clients expect to attain from therapy.

Outcome goals normally result automatically from the problem definition that takes place during Phase II. For example, in the previous case illustration, Harold and the therapist defined and tentatively committed themselves to concentrating on Harold's anxiety from his interactions with his wife. Thus, Harold's immediate outcome goal is implied: lessening the anxiety caused by his relationship with his wife.

By contrast, process goals are the objectives the therapist considers necessary to accomplish if clients are to realize their outcome goals. The different theoretical orientations' process goals come from the domain of human functioning on which they are primarily based. During Phase III, therapists' theoretical grounding is most critical for it is here that *theory* provides direction to the process. Assume that Harold's therapist uses rational-emotive therapy, and remember that RET emphasizes cognitive change and cognitive causation of clients' problems. Harold's thoughts are the primary consideration in Phase III. Part of a session during this phase might appear as follows:

THERAPIST: Harold, you've mentioned that you feel highly anxious when your wife is hostile towards you or when you think about her acting angrily with you. Where do you think that anxiety comes from?

HAROLD: From the way my wife is, of course. If she would be nicer, then I wouldn't feel so anxious around her.

THERAPIST: It would seem that way; however, if your wife acted angrily towards me, I wouldn't necessarily feel anxious. Why wouldn't I feel anxious and you would?

HAROLD: Because she's not your wife.

THERAPIST: Well, let's assume that she was my wife. I still wouldn't have to feel anxious. Now what might be the difference?

HAROLD: Maybe she just doesn't mean as much to you as she does to me.

THERAPIST: That's very true. The word *meaning* is a key. It's the meaning we put on situations, in this case your wife's behavior, that leads to how we feel. What meaning do you put on your wife's behavior?

HAROLD: (pause) I'm not sure what you're getting at.

THERAPIST: Well you're obviously not thinking to yourself, "Oh, I really love it when she acts in such a hostile manner." Are you?

HAROLD: No, of course not.

THERAPIST: What might you be thinking?

HAROLD: It's terrible the way she acts! And for no good reason at all.

THERAPIST: Right! You're thinking to yourself how horrible and unfair it is that she acts that way. And if you think that, how will you feel? Wonderful?

HAROLD: No, anxious as I always do feel.

In this brief interchange the therapist helps Harold attain a new perspective on his anxiety from his wife's behavior. It is not necessarily his wife's actions but rather the meaning Harold attaches to her actions that creates his anxiety. Once Harold can see the implications of this new perspective, goals can be set to be pursued in Phase IV. Returning to a later portion of the same session:

THERAPIST: Harold, we seem to agree that it's primarily the meaning that you give to your wife's behavior that creates your anxiety. If lessening the intensity of the anxiety you feel around her is your goal, then we have to look at how we might work to change your thoughts about her behavior.
HAROLD: That sounds reasonable. How do we begin?

Now both an outcome goal and a process goal are present. The therapist and client can move on to Phase IV, selecting and implementing strategies for attaining goals.

Promoting a New Perspective

The specific process goals different therapists choose are largely determined by therapists' theoretical orientations. The therapist skills that help clients recognize the value of specific goals suggest diagnostic understandings but let clients diagnose themselves. Therapists thus seek to give clients new perspectives. The skills necessary to accomplish this task are both integrative and challenging.

- ☐ Information Giving. Clients often have problems because they lack information. Information giving means providing new information as well as correcting misinformation. It includes pointing out the consequences that potential actions may have in clients' lives and offering specific suggestions. With additional information, clients can often see their problems in a new light.

- ☐ Interpretation. Though interpretations may vary in content depending upon the theoretical orientation on which they are based, the therapist trys to explain connections among seemingly isolated information (in the client's view) from the client. In doing so, the client is offered a different perspective on his or her concerns.

- ☐ Confrontation. Confrontation involves finding and pointing out mixed messages, conflicts, and incongruities that clients express or that exist in their lives. Clients are challenged to explain discrepancies and thus clear up any distortions that they have.

- ☐ Self-disclosure. Effective self-disclosure entails therapists sharing experiences with their clients that will help clients understand themselves better and find appropriate goals for their own betterment.

- ☐ Immediacy. Immediacy is communicated when therapists convey what they themselves are experiencing in their relationship with clients in the here-and-now. The goal is to spontaneously challenge clients to consider their interpersonal style and the quality of their cooperation in the therapeutic process.

Specifying Goals

All that has gone on up to this point has largely been preparatory. A therapeutic climate has been created to help clients discriminate and define their primary problems so that they can commit to outcome goals. The therapist has challenged the client to promote a new perspective from which to perceive the primary problems. This new perspective enables clients to better understand what needs to be done to alleviate the discomfort caused by their problems. Setting process goals completes this

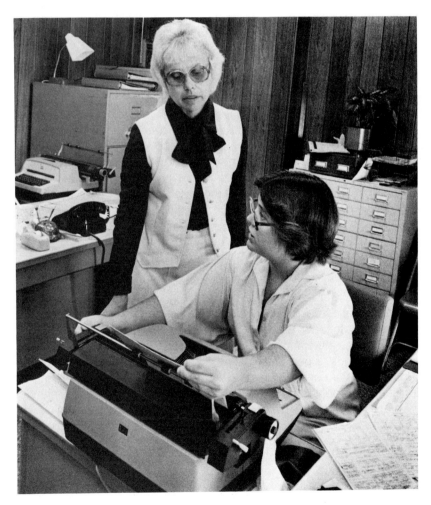

Improved job performance can be an outcome goal of therapy

preparatory portion of the overall therapeutic process. All that takes place subsequent to goal setting is done to see that the goals established are achieved.

Outcome goals differ by clients' definitions of their problems. These goals, however, directly relate to what clients seek in counseling. As clients more clearly comprehend their concerns via the therapist's primary theoretical perspective, process goals come to be recognized as the means by which their difficulties are dealt with. Process goals are the therapist's responsibility. They come from a carefully considered theoretical position; clients cannot be expected to spontaneously recognize their therapeutic importance without introduction.

Clients' Responsibilities in Phase III

Ideally, in Phase II clients will collaborate with the therapist in a variety of ways. They will carefully consider the therapist's challenges, new information, and alternative points of view about their problems. They will gain and invest more in therapy. They won't simply develop some kind of theoretical understanding of themselves and their difficulties. Rather, they will develop what Egan (1982) calls *dynamic understanding,* "the kind of understanding that sits on the edge of action. It has a flavor of 'Now I see what I am doing and how self-destructive it is, and I've got to do something about it' " (p. 41).

Together with the therapist, clients will then clarify, specify, and commit to pursuing stated process goals. The aim of the theoretically-oriented process goals is to achieve the stated outcome goals. That, however, is the work of Phase IV.

Reconsidering Phase III and Its Place in the Therapeutic Process

In Phase III clients must be helped to expound on the explanations offered in Phase II so that they can see the bigger picture and view problems in their total context. Clients' perceptions of their problems are often too narrow or somehow distorted. In Phase III, therapists must help their clients develop new and more objective points of view about their concerns, the kinds of perspectives that help clients set process goals. These process goals are best promoted when the therapist challenges clients to look at their problems through the therapist's eyes using his or her primary theoretical orientation. That orientation gives direction to what would otherwise be a directionless process. Finally, therapists help their clients to further clarify, specify, and commit to stated goals based on the clients' increased awareness and understanding of both outcome goals and process goals.

The skills of Phase III will be more fully explored in upcoming chapters. These skills are best suggested to clients, not forced on them. Clients must be responsible for considering their problems from new perspectives. If the therapist is too dogmatic and domineering, clients can be put off and become overly resistant. Egan (1982) dramatically notes in this regard:

> Confrontation can become a club; helper self-disclosure can become exhibitionistic; immediacy and the offering of alternative frames of reference can lead to a power struggle. (p. 41)

Here, the importance of creating a therapeutic climate in Phase I again becomes evident. In Phase III, the social influence aspect of the therapeutic process must be firmly established if clients are to accept the therapist's challenges. In Phase I therapists create a power base by being perceived as attractive, expert, and trustworthy. In Phases II and III, therapists can use this social influence to help clients develop more accurate and useful perceptions of themselves, their environment and the interactions between the two.

The skills of Phase III are, like the skills of Phases I and II, tools to achieve certain goals. Phase III is successful only if it completes the process of setting goals. In Phase II, information was gathered and problems ranked. Initially, Phase III promotes new perspectives in clients so they can perceive their problems in a more goal-oriented manner. If this new view is facilitated by a counselor well versed in a primary theory and focused on identifiable process goals, the client can come to realize that pursuing process goals will help them attain outcome goals.

Ideally, as Phase III progresses, clients realize more succinctly that they must change, be it an affective, behavioral, or cognitive adjustment. Clients may well be reluctant to change and doubt their ability to do so. These fears and doubts need to be dealt with before moving on in therapy, as the client experiencing them is likely still not ready for more proactive problem interventions: Phase IV.

PROACTIVE PROBLEM INTERVENTION

Counseling and psychotherapy are not just talking and planning. Clients must ultimately do something differently—*change*—if they are to live a more satisfying life. This is what is meant by the term *proactive*: actively and assertively seeking to change how one feels, thinks, and acts. Clients' intending to change and specifying goals that will have the desired effects culminates Phase III. Selecting appropriate intervention strategies, implementing them, and then evaluating the results is the work of Phase IV.

Selection Skills

There is almost an infinite number of intervention strategies that can be used with clients. Each theoretical orientation has its own set. Affective intervention strategies, which seek emotional change, include imagery, sensory awareness, and verbal and nonverbal expressions of feeling. Cognitive interventions change thinking. Didactic (instructional) strategies that focus on step-by-step verbal processing of decision making, analyzing, and problem solving are the primary forms of cognitive intervention. Cognitive Restructuring, identifying dysfunctional thinking and replacing it with more functional ideas, is a notable example. Behavioral interventions focus on learning and/or reinforcing functional behaviors and developing different contingencies for dysfunctional behaviors to increase positive behaviors.

Given that a therapist has a primary theoretical orientation, there are still likely several intervention strategies that could be equally effective in achieving a specific goal. Different interventions will work differently with different clients for different problems and for different goals. For example, if a client's goal is to develop a greater sense of self-worth, and the therapist's approach is cognitive, various strategies such as cognitive restructuring, self-monitoring, and thought stopping could all be potentially effective in reducing negative thoughts about self (Hackney & Cormier, 1979). An extensive knowledge of research and case history documentation can be invaluable in such situations, pointing to methods, clients, and types of problems with which specific interventions have been more or less effective.

When more than one intervention appears viable, they can all be explained to the client. Okun (1982) proposes the following be shared with clients in such cases:

1. An explanation of the intervention strategies applicable to the client's situation
2. A rationale for each strategy
3. The time and activities involved in each strategy
4. The possible consequences of each strategy, including the advantages and disadvantages

Client input regarding intervention strategies will facilitate their implementation, if not be vital to them. Alone, a therapist might choose a strategy a client cannot or will not take part in. For example, some interventions call for clients to imagine or fantasize; a client who has difficulty generating vivid images is not likely to gain from such a procedure (Hackney & Cormier, 1979).

Similarly, interventions should be consonant with clients' values. Consider the case of a college student unable to stay in school without accepting financial help from relatives. For a person seeking to be as independent as possible, however, such assistance may be more of a burden than dropping out of college temporarily to earn the needed money. Without the client's investment in the intervention plan, or with only minimal investment, the use of a particular strategy could create more problems than existed before.

Finally, intervention strategies should be considered in terms of clients' environment. One sure way to lose weight would be to be locked in a room without food until the weight was lost. While this obviously is unrealistic for most individuals, clients could consider not keeping fattening foods in their home.

Implementation Skills

Once a specific strategy has been decided upon, its effective implementation is the next consideration. It is tempting to conclude that clients who have moved successfully through Phases I, II, III, and strategy selection in Phase IV will have little difficulty in implementing interventions they have helped to choose. This conclusion is often erroneous for two reasons (Patterson & Eisenberg, 1983):

1. Any new way of thinking, acting, or feeling will be unfamiliar and always includes the risk of failure, no matter how logically it has been derived.
2. Old familiar ways of functioning frequently have their own rewards along with the problems they create. Even though change may reduce or diminish the problem situation, it may also reduce the old familiar rewards.

Because it is hard for many clients to change in ways that will ultimately improve their lives, therapists must have skills for helping clients implement change strategies. Cormier and Cormier (1979) propose that complete intervention implementation involves presenting interventions in positive terms, then therapist modeling, client rehearsal in the session, and help in transferring in-session experiences to clients' daily lives. Egan's (1982) "provision of support and continued challenge during strategy implementation" warrants emphasis as well.

The effective therapist will preface interventions with rationales; the positive benefits the client will derive from changing, such as achieving goals, feeling more in control of one's life, or eliminating an unwanted hassle. The therapist also tries to reduce the client's apprehension by summarizing the intervention strategy and reviewing potential difficulties.

The therapist helps the client to perceive such problems as not too difficult. For example, if a person is trying to stop smoking, difficulties might be the longing that comes from giving up a pleasurable habit, or the envy the client could feel in the company of smokers. Clients may need to learn certain coping skills to make it easier for them to overcome these difficulties and concentrate on changing. Motivation could be enhanced by identifying the feeling of better health or the thought of how much money the client is saving and the other things it can buy, such as finer clothes or entertainment. It is important to note that this is not blind encouragement, but rather part of intervention implementation in preparing for contingencies that may occur.

Therapist modeling, client rehearsal in the therapy session, and helping clients generalize their changes to outside the session constitute the balance of intervention. Along with these therapies, in providing support and continuous challenge, therapists make the success of an intervention strategy more likely. While the probability that a strategy will succeed is increased if it is reasonably planned, clients often need continuing help during implementation as well. The focus is not *doing for* clients, but rather helping them mobilize potential resources to increase the strength of their motivation and capabilities and decrease the impact of difficulties.

For example, should a client feel inadequate and discouraged as he or she attempts to change, the therapist can provide empathic understanding. The therapist can further challenge the client to mobilize whatever resources are necessary to persevere.

Jane and Harry were experiencing a great deal of marital discord. Harry refused to seek any form of assistance, either with Jane or alone. Jane decided that she still wanted to see what she could do to save their relationship. Together with the therapist, she decided to try, alone, a strategy of "positive focusing" with Harry. She had an especially difficult time in the beginning. It was extremely discouraging to her when Harry not only did not appreciate her efforts to compliment him and give him more positive attention, but also actually denigrated her for "wanting something from him." The therapist's explaining to Jane that with unilateral interventions "it usually gets worse before it gets better" and constantly reminding Jane of this fact through confrontation, enabled her to be patient and tolerate frustration until Harry began to respond positively.

Evaluation Skills

One of the primary problems most counselors have during Phase IV is failing to effectively monitor and evaluate the effects of an intervention strategy. As Gottman and Leiblum (1974) sadly report, "Too often, evaluation is done by consensus among professionals involved with the case when treatment terminates" (p. 2). Many counselors seem to regard data gathering for evaluation as something that is unnecessary, therapeutic results being obvious, or something that is aversive and therefore easily ignored (Hackney & Cormier, 1979). Egan (1975) pointedly notes the importance of concrete evaluation efforts, however, in stating:

> Tangible results form the backbone of the reinforcement process in counseling. If the client is to be encouraged to move forward, he must see results. Therefore, both counselor and client should be able to judge whether the action program is or is not being implemented, and to what degree, and the results of this implementation. (p. 225)

Egan (1982) proposes three principal questions to guide therapy evaluation.

1. **Quality of participation.** Is the client actually carrying out the intervention strategies? What is the client's quality of participation? If clients are not investing themselves in a selected strategy or strategies, or do so only halfheartedly, this needs to be assessed and appropriately dealt with.

2. **Quality of intervention strategies.** If the client is actively invested in the intervention strategies, are the goals toward which the strategies are directed being achieved? Wholly? Partially? If the client is implementing a strategy as it has been designed and not achieving the goal, then it is likely that the strategy needs to be redesigned.

3. **Quality of problem resolution.** Are the problems that were originally defined actually being dealt with? Are the client's needs being met? If the client's problems persist, if the problem situation is not becoming more manageable, then new goals likely should be considered and new strategies devised. If the problem situation is becoming more manageable and the quality of the client's life is improving, then this is a signal that termination will be forthcoming.

Evaluation is a critical part not only of Phase IV, but also of the entire therapeutic process. It is presented here as a final portion of the process for ease of explanation. In practice, however, evaluation is effective only if it is *ongoing*. The questions above should be considered throughout the entire process, at all phases, not just at the end.

Client's Responsibilities in Phase IV

Clients must be motivated and cooperative if proactive problem intervention is to take place. Although initial reluctance and resistance is a natural client response to the inconvenience and discomfort of change, lasting results are achieved only if implementation of intervention strategies is a collaborative effort with the therapist. Clients must actively involve themselves in Phase IV activities.

By providing adequate preparation, support, and challenge, therapists help clients assume a greater willingness to take risks. While risk is inherent throughout the entire therapeutic process, in Phase IV clients risk the most. They face new ways of functioning and the consequences that this incurs. Risk taking is not simply leaping into a void, however. It is the therapist's role to help clients take reasonable risks (Egan, 1982).

Finally, clients are ultimately responsible for carrying out the agreed-upon intervention strategies in their own lives. Clients can accomplish this in many ways, but in general therapists must be sure that clients are fully prepared to effectively implement strategies. No client should be expected to do the impossible.

Reconsidering Phase IV and Its Place in the Therapeutic Process

It is not uncommon for many therapists to ignore or ineffectively implement all or aspects of Phase IV. Some therapists never get to this phase. They assume proactive problem intervention to be the sole responsibility of the client. Some clients, once they can set specific goals, do possess the power to change on their own. Many, however, need the planning, information, practice, support, and challenges of a skilled therapist to change. Some therapists *begin* with Phase IV. They might listen briefly to a client's concerns, tell the client what to do, and then rather blindly send him or her out to do it. All too often such failures are blamed on "unmotivated" clients (Egan, 1982). The more likely cause is an incomplete therapeutic process.

THERAPISTS' SKILLS VERSUS THERAPISTS' THEORY In our view, it is a mistake to equate effectiveness in counseling and psychotherapy with either skills or theory. Therapists' skills should not be isolated from their primary theoretical approach nor the approach isolated from the skills. However, as Kagen (1973) asserts, the basic issue confronting the field of counseling and psychotherapy is not its validity, but rather reliability. He stated:

> Not, can counseling and psychotherapy work, but does it work consistently? Not, can we educate people who are able to help others, but can we develop methods which will increase the likelihood that *most* of our graduates will become as effective mental health workers as only a rare few do? It is my basic premise that attempts to validate therapy derived from

personality theories have failed, not because of the inadequacy of the theories, but because the average practitioner has not been adequately educated to implement the theory. This is not to deny that better theories are needed but rather to assert that there is enough truth in extant ones to ameliorate the critical mental health problems of our world if only we could translate their implications into effective action with greater consistency. (p. 44)

Thus, we need a skills model with which to implement theoretical concepts of counseling and psychotherapy consistently and sytematically. The rest of this section expands on the general therapeutic model and specific therapist skills of this chapter. We will apply specific skills to specific theoretical approaches in an attempt to integrate, not exclude, theory and technique.

SUGGESTED READINGS

Brammer, L. M., & Shostrom, E. L. (1982). *Therapeutic psychology: Fundamentals of counseling and psychotherapy.* (4th ed.). Englewood Cliffs, NJ: Prentice-Hall. The authors outline a detailed seven-step process of counseling and psychotherapy in chapter 4.

Carkhuff, R. R. (1969). *Helping and human relations.* (Vols. 1–2). New York: Holt, Rinehart and Winston. These two books detail Carkhuff's framework for the helping process. Volume 2 includes what have come to be his well-known and influential five-point scales for evaluating counselor effectiveness.

Egan, G. (1982). *The skilled helper: Model, skills, and methods for effective helping.* (2nd ed.). Monterey, CA: Brooks/Cole. Egan presents an atheoretical three-stage model of helping focused on "problem-management." The skills and methods that make the model work are spelled out in detail.

Ivey, A. E., & Simek-Downing, L. (1980). *Counseling and psychotherapy: Skills, theories and practice.* Englewood Cliffs, NJ: Prentice-Hall. The authors devote Part I of this book to their view of counseling and psychotherapy as a decision and problem-solving process wherein therapists and clients first define the problem, then generate alternatives, and last, take action.

Patterson, L. E., & Eisenberg, S. (1983). *The counseling process.* (3rd ed.). Boston: Houghton Mifflin. Although a short, compact introduction to the counseling process, this book still offers a careful analysis of the counselor/client experience in a three-stage framework.

7

Phase One: Creating a Therapeutic Climate

THE QUESTION . . . But what are the characteristics of those relationships which do help, which do facilitate growth? And at the other end of the scale, is it possible to discern those characteristics which make a relationship unhelpful, even though it was the sincere intent to promote growth and development?

(Rogers, 1961, p. 41)

The average client enters therapy with certain misgivings, and for understandable reasons (Brammer, 1973):

1. It is not easy for many persons to accept assistance.
2. Many persons find it difficult to commit themselves to changing.
3. Some individuals find it very awkward to submit to the influence of a therapist; their esteem, integrity, and independence is threatened.
4. Most people cannot readily trust and be open at an intimate level with a stranger.
5. It is often difficult to see one's problems clearly at first.
6. Sometimes problems appear too large, too overwhelming, or too unique to share easily.

Readiness for learning is a well-recognized educational requirement. For example, children are not ready to study a new subject until they have a certain level of maturation, motivation, and skill development. Readiness for counseling and psychotherapy is similar. Certain conditions must be created before clients can fully participate in and gain from therapy (Brammer & Shostrom, 1982). This readiness is the goal of the skills therapists use in Phase I of therapy, illustrated in Figure 7–1.

FIGURE 7–1
Phase I of therapy

```
┌─────────────────────────────────────────────┐
│                  Phase I                      │
│        client presents self for therapy       │
└─────────────────────────────────────────────┘


┌─────────────────────────────────────────────┐
│ client readiness for upcoming phases of the   │
│ therapeutic process is created:               │
│       • core conditions communicated          │
│       • social influence established          │
│       • structuring provided                  │
│       • therapist attending evidenced         │
└─────────────────────────────────────────────┘
```

Similarly, clients will have to be prepared to enter Phase II, problem discrimination and definition, which we will discuss in the next chapter.

Certain core conditions form the foundation for establishing and maintaining an effective therapeutic climate. Although different numbers, specificities, and names for these conditions appear in professional literature, we believe four primary conditions comprise the prerequisite components. These conditions are empathic understanding, respect, genuineness, and concreteness. The ability to communicate these characteristics to clients is an essential therapist skill.

CORE CONDITIONS: ESSENTIAL ELEMENTS FOR A THERAPEUTIC CLIMATE

Empathic Understanding

Carl Rogers (1942, 1951, 1961) introduced empathic understanding as a core condition of therapy, describing it as the therapist's ability to "enter the client's phenomenal world—to experience the client's world as if it were your own without ever losing the 'as if' quality" (Rogers, 1961, p. 284). Empathic understanding means that therapists respond sensitively and accurately to clients' thoughts, feelings, and actions as if they were their own, while maintaining a sense of separateness and objectivity.

George and Christiani (1981) refer to a therapist's empathic understanding as "trial identification," comparing it to the relationship that a reader establishes with the main character of a novel. They quote Truax and Carkhuff (1971) in this regard, who note:

> As we come to know some of *his* wants, some of *his* needs, some of *his* achievements, and some of *his* failures, we find ourselves living with the other person much as we do the hero or heroine of a novel . . . we come to know the person from his own internal viewpoint and thus gain some understanding and flavor of his moment-by-moment experiences. (p. 315)

In adopting a client's internal frame of reference, the therapist comes to better understand a client's private world and the meanings he or she attaches to aspects of it. The therapist is thus able to help the client comprehend more clearly these meanings by reflecting them back to him or her. Empathic understanding also means considering the client's frame of reference without judging it. As clients share their feelings, thoughts, and actions, the therapist tries to understand without labeling anything good or bad, right or wrong. This nonevaluative attitude allows clients to become more accepting of themselves.

While recognizing the importance of empathic understanding as described by Rogers, subsequent authors have expounded upon the concept, proposing different levels of empathy. For example, Egan (1982) speaks of two distinct degrees of empathic understanding: (1) primary-level accurate empathy, and (2) advanced accurate empathy. Primary-level empathy is the early focus in therapy and advanced empathy is used later. In this chapter, we will look at primary-level empathy. Advanced empathy will be examined in chapter 9 with the therapist skill of interpretation.

Empathic understanding as a therapist skill involves "communicating *initial basic* understanding of what the client is feeling and of the experiences and behaviors underlying these feelings" (Egan, 1982, p. 87). Egan (1975) describes a therapist as using empathic understanding when he or she (1) *discriminates:* "gets inside" the client, looks at the world from the client's perspective or frame of reference, and tries to understand what the client's world is like; and (2) *communicates* to the client this understanding in such a way that the client believes the therapist knows both his or her *feelings* and their *apparent basis.*

If a client begins a session by sharing how a family illness and the associated expenses and grief seem overwhelming, the therapist using empathic understanding might say:

THERAPIST: You're really depressed by all of the heartache and hardship your parent's illness has created.

The therapist discriminates the client's feelings ("depression") and their basis ("heartache and hardship"), and then communicates this understanding to the client, how the therapist perceives the client's world.

In communicating empathic understanding, the therapist's task is to directly tell clients what they have explicitly said verbally and/or nonverbally about themselves. Empathic understanding is not an attempt to derive implications from only parts of what the client says, or indirectly alludes to. That kind of advanced-level empathy, à la Egan (1982), belongs under the rubric of interpretation, a therapist skill primarily used later in the total process to help clients develop new perspectives from which to set goals. Empathic understanding, although presented as a critical component of Phase I, should be continuously used throughout therapy. The following are some further examples of therapists' communication of empathic understanding:

CLIENT: Home has been more of a hassle everyday. I just can't seem to keep up with all the chores that have to be done and with the kids wanting so much attention. Wow!

THERAPIST: You're frustrated seeing yourself so overwhelmed with household responsibilities and the children's demands as well.

CLIENT: Things are really looking up. With graduation only 2 weeks away and a job waiting for me, I'm feeling really great.

THERAPIST: It's a joy to have things falling into place.

For cognitively-oriented therapists in particular, Walen, DiGiuseppe, and Wessler (1980) add the importance of letting clients know that not only what they are feeling, but also what they are *thinking* is being understood. For example,

CLIENT: I don't know what I'll do if I don't get this job. My savings are almost gone.

THERAPIST: You sound very worried about what will happen if you don't get *this* job, almost as if you're thinking it's your last chance.

When the therapist points out both the client's thought and emotion, along with relevant actions and circumstances, the client has the option of dealing with either of them; identifying and reflecting an emotion alone, however, precludes this option. Often clients are startled by such multiple identifications and seem amazed that the therapist can virtually read their mind.

With most clients, empathic understanding immediately helps build rapport. It also aids clients to more clearly consider their thoughts, feelings, and behaviors and their problems. In a sense, empathic understanding serves both as a relationship-building skill and a problem discrimination and definition skill. Therapists therefore have criteria for evaluating how well their empathic understanding is creating a therapeutic climate. Do their responses help develop or maintain a positive working relationship with clients? Do they help clients consider their problems more fully in terms of relevant thoughts, feelings, and behaviors? Consider the following interchange:

CLIENT: I'm not sure I'll ever develop any closer friendships with the people I work with. I just don't seem to be able to say the right things. I always seem to come across as either shy or clumsy.

THERAPIST: You're feeling kind of hopeless; like, what's the use of trying cause I'll just mess up again.

CLIENT: Exactly, and the worst part is that I know that's much of my problem. I know what to say, yet my pessimistic attitude prevents me from feeling free to just say, hey did you hear about . . .

When the therapist "hits the mark," the client can gain by more accurately discriminating and defining the problem. When therapists are able to consistently communicate empathic understanding, clients often respond with a "yes set." A client repeatedly says "Yes, that's how I feel and that's what's been going on in my life," then often further explores and clarifies his or her concerns. It should be remembered, however, that empathic understanding is never sufficient in and of itself; it is only effective to the degree that clients perceive it as such.

Respect

Respect as we define it is not some vague attitude but a specific therapist action essential to creating an effective therapeutic climate. If therapists want to help clients change, they must believe that clients have the potential to do so. Respect is evident when therapists exhibit a deep, sincere acceptance of clients' inherent worth, separate from their problems. The fact that clients exist justifies this respect. Therapists also show respect when they let clients make their own decisions, even if they are in error, for much can be learned from mistakes. The respectful therapist is neither rejecting nor overprotective. Rather he or she fosters client independence and self-confidence.

Carl Rogers uses the term *positive regard* in stressing respect as critical to the counseling process. He regards individuals as forward mov-

Carl Rogers

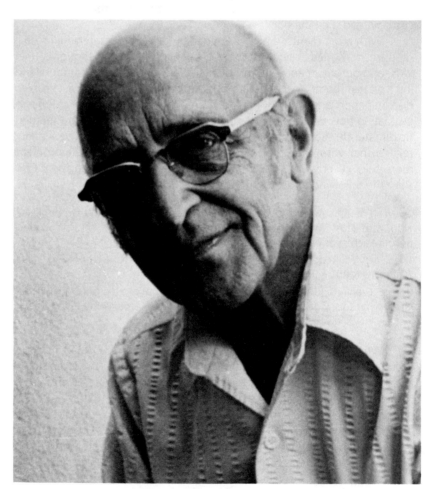

ing, positive, and capable of growth. His work demonstrates this emphasis on exhibiting respect in therapy:

> From a first glance, one would think the helpee has no assets, no hope. But, out of a dark morass of discouragement, Carl Rogers always seems to find something positive in an individual and highlights that positive dimension. (Ivey & Gluckstern, 1976, p. i)

Other counseling theories similarly emphasize communicating respect for clients. Behavioral therapists believe that virtually all clients can cope more effectively with problems if they are appropriately reinforced for any movement toward greater personal development. While the terminology and procedures may differ, respect in the sense of having positive regard for clients is a part of all effective therapeutic approaches.

It should be noted, however, that respect is not simply optimistically focusing on clients' positive aspects. Respect is optimistic, but it must also be realistic. While therapists should constantly search for assets in their clients, they should simultaneously deal frankly with their very real life issues. Therapy does not exist to smooth things over, but rather to help individuals cope with the world as it is (Ivey & Simek-Downing, 1980). Respect thus also involves challenging clients to make use of the resources they possess.

In such challenges, therapists do not act for clients unless absolutely necessary and then only as a means to help the client act on his or her own. Consider the following therapist's responses:

CLIENT: I just can't think of any alternatives open to me. I'm sure with your experience you could tell me what I should do.

THERAPIST A: Your situation does sound to be awfully difficult. I have advised others in similar situations to begin by . . .

THERAPIST B: You sound quite frustrated and at a loss as to what to do next. I could offer you some suggestions from my experience, but they might only solve your immediate discomfort. We might better spend our session considering *together* how *you* can identify possible alternatives so that similar situations in the future won't present such a problem.

Therapist A simply offers the client advice, possibly changing the immediate situation but offering little insight to help the client deal with similar occurrences in the future. Therapist B challenges the client. Therapist B assumes that the client does have, somewhere, the necessary resources to begin to deal with the problem presented. Therapist B recognizes that experiencing discomfort in the short term is worth the long-term gains that a client can achieve by learning to cope with problems on one's own.

Respect is showing positive regard for clients in a down-to-earth, nonsentimental manner. Respect also ultimately involves placing demands on clients as well. Respecting clients then, refers to clients' basic humanity *and* to their potential for being *more* than they may be at present. Respect is therefore both gracious and tough-minded (Egan, 1975).

Genuineness

Genuineness, like respect, can be viewed as some vague attitude or quality. However, like respect, genuineness can be expressed through the actions therapists exhibit. Genuineness refers to the ability of therapists to be themselves in their interactions with clients. They do not need to present a professional "front" or facade. They express their personal thoughts and feelings when appropriate. Therapists must always, however, keep in mind what will benefit their clients; this sometimes calls for withholding genuine expressions (Carkhuff, 1971).

Egan (1982) proposes that being genuine means doing some things and not doing others.

☐ *Refusing to overemphasize role.* The genuine therapist does not take refuge in a professional role. He or she avoids being contrived or planned, but rather is personal and responds to clients as people, not objects.

☐ *Being spontaneous.* Genuine therapists, while tactful (as part of their respect for clients), do not constantly weigh what they are going to say. Genuineness does not call for expressing *every* thought to clients. Rather, as Rogers (1957) suggests, therapists should express negative feelings to clients only if these feelings persist or if they interfere with therapists' ability to progress with clients. Whether a response will benefit the client is the deciding factor. For example:

CLIENT: What do you think are my chances for improvement?

THERAPIST A: You've told me you're willing to change, but you just won't do anything, and nothing will happen until you put forth the actual effort.

THERAPIST B: You're curious as to my prognosis. Maybe it's time for us to evaluate where we are and what the future looks like.

Therapist A takes the client literally and replies somewhat bluntly. Therapist B realizes the importance of direct feedback, but also recognizes the client's inquiry as an opportunity to mutually evaluate therapeutic progress as well as allow the client to learn important self-evaluation skills.

☐ *Avoiding defensiveness.* Genuine therapists recognize they possess strengths and limitations. When clients express negative attitudes toward them, they seek to understand what they are saying and then work with them to clarify and correct the situation. Consider the following therapists' reactions:

CLIENT: You're no help at all. Week after week and nothing has changed for me!

THERAPIST A: Well, you might want to look more carefully at YOUR role in any lack of progress. How much effort have you exerted?

THERAPIST B: It has been tough sledding so far. Let's review what we've done and what we might have to do differently.

Therapist A reacts negatively. Therapist B recognizes that lack of progress can emanate from the therapist, the client, or both. Therapist B is open to examining the situation and trying to improve future performance. Therapist A sees only one possible block to progress—the client.

☐ *Being consistent.* Genuine therapists practice what they preach. The values they share with clients are the same ones that they practice in their everyday living. This genuineness is most evident in therapists' ability to talk openly and honestly about themselves and their experiences. The essence of counseling and psychotherapy is clients' ability to adequately share themselves with the therapist in a real, personal way. Genuine self-disclosure on the part of therapists will produce further self-disclosure on the part of their clients.

Concreteness

Clients often begin therapy with ambiguous complaints. A major task of therapy is to help clients move from confusion to clarity about the issues they are struggling with. This change requires that the therapist and client speak clearly and specifically with each other. Vagueness, abstractness, and obscurity are opposites of concreteness. They prevent therapeutic progress (Patterson and Eisenberg, 1982). For example, consider the following client problem and proposed solution:

PROBLEM: The client is dissatisfied with a low-paying job.
SOLUTION: The client must find a better-paying job.

Vague solutions to vague problems cannot lead to effective action. In this example neither the problem nor the solution is sufficiently concrete to lead to any form of realistic goal setting and thus positive client change. Concreteness is paramount in creating a progressive therapeutic climate and cannot be overstated. This condition, perhaps more than empathic and understanding, respect, and genuineness, moves clients through the therapeutic process by encouraging exploration of specific problem areas (George & Christiani, 1981). And yet, of the core conditions presented here, concreteness is perhaps the easiest to implement. Ask clients to recount specific events in their lives. Follow up any descriptions that are still unclear with more questions or empathic understanding so that the full, rich sequence of their lives becomes clearer not only to you but also to them as well. The following example illustrates this.

CLIENT: Things have been going real poorly. (vague)

THERAPIST: What might be a specific example of that thing going most poorly? (concrete)

CLIENT: Well, I was down in bed with the flu all weekend (concrete) and I couldn't get anything done. (vague)

THERAPIST: The flu was surely an unpleasant experience for you. (concrete). You said that you couldn't get anything done. What specifically is of such immediate concern that it had to be done? (concrete)

Often, clients will not readily express themselves in concrete and specific terms. It is the therapist's responsibility to help them to do so. Egan (1975) summarizes the essence of concreteness in stating:

> If the counselor is as concrete as possible in his responses to the client, the client will learn to be concrete in the exploration of his behavior. . . . Concreteness is extremely important in counseling. Without it, counseling loses that intensity or density that marshals the energies of the client and channels them into constructive action. Low-level helpers often prefer to have clients talk in generalities. They seem to think that mere talking is enough, whatever the focus. Concreteness means that the client must risk more in the counseling interactions, but little happens without risks and without facing the crises precipitated by reasonable risk taking. (pp. 101, 105–106)

ENHANCING THERAPY WITH SOCIAL INFLUENCERS

In almost all human relationships, individuals try to influence each other. Although many influencing attempts are indirect and inadvertent, deliberate and direct influence is common when persons seek to do things with, for, or to each other. History has provided ample evidence that people suffering from a variety of emotional disturbances and physical ailments, of psychogenic origin in particular, have been "cured" by their belief in a helper's curing powers (Frank, 1973). Counseling and psychotherapy try to help clients change how they act, feel, and think. These attempts can be construed as purposeful influence whether or not therapists or clients conceptualize them as such (Corrigan, Dell, Lewis, & Schmidt, 1980).

In 1968, Stanley Strong wrote what has become a landmark paper on counseling as an interpersonal influence process. His propositions stimulated much research, which was intensively reviewed by Corrigan, et al., 1980. In abstracting the major points from Strong's article, they report:

> Based on cognitive dissonance theory (Festinger, 1957), Strong hypothesized that counselors' attempts to change clients' behavior or opinions would precipitate dissonance in clients. Clients could reduce dissonance by one of five means: (a) change in the direction advocated by the counselor, (b) discredit the counselor, (c) discredit the issue, (d) change the counselor's opinion, or (e) seek others who agree with the client. Strong suggested that counselors could increase the likelihood that the first alternative would occur by reducing the likelihood of the second and third. Extrapolating from research in social psychology, Strong postulated that the extent to which counselors are perceived as expert, attractive, and trustworthy would reduce the likelihood of their being discredited. By increasing clients' involvement in counseling, the likelihood of discrediting the issue would be reduced. From these hypotheses, Strong suggested a two-stage model of counseling. In the first stage, counselors enhance their perceived expertness, attractiveness, trustworthiness, and clients' involvement in counseling. In the second state, counselors use their influence to precipitate opinion and/or behavior change in clients. (pp. 395–96)

Corrigan, et al., (1980) cautions that Strong's position and the work that emanated from it rest on one basic assumption: it is a client's *perception* of a therapist's expertness, attractiveness, and trustworthiness that determines the therapist's ability to exert influence. Strong and Matross (1973) elaborate this point in defining a therapist's ability to influence a client as dependent upon the client's judgment of the correspondence between his or her needs and the therapist's resources appropriate to those needs *as perceived by the client*. Thus, upon gathering information about a therapist, the inferences a client draws from that information, not the information itself, determine how effective the therapist can be with that client. Research suggests that therapists' actual experience and clients' ratings of therapists' experience may be unrelated (Dell & Schmidt, 1976).

Communicating Expertness

Hoveland, Janis, and Kelly (1953) define expertness as "the extent to which a communicator is perceived to be a source of valid assertions" (p. 21). Using this definition, Strong (1968) proposed that clients' perceptions of therapists as experts is influenced by: "(a) objective evidence of specialized training such as diplomas, certificates, and titles, (b) behavioral evidence of expertness such as rational and knowledgeable arguments and confidence in presentation, and (c) reputation as an expert" (p. 216).

Corrigan, et al. (1980) reports that research on therapists' perceived expertness has focused on three primary points: visible evidence, reputation, and interview behavior.

Visible Evidence. Visible evidence of therapists' expertness is demonstrated when therapists are identified as professionals (therapist, counselor, social worker, etc.), and as possessing credentials (diplomas, certificates, and the like) attesting to their expertise. Kerr and Dell (1976) found that therapists in casual dress were viewed as less expert than those dressed more professionally. Other visible evidence found to suggest therapist expertness include office decor, name plates, and titles.

Reputation. Reputation is direct or indirect testimony that therapists are experts, of which clients are aware. The testimony may come from various sources, such as former clients or professional colleagues. Therapists may also derive status from their association with a prestigious institution. Egan (1982) notes that therapists' reputations may or may not be deserved and are not absolute indications of actual competency. Nevertheless, therapists' attributed experience and status clearly affects their perceived expertness (Corrigan, et al., 1980).

Interview Behavior. Interview behaviors that contribute to clients' perceptions of therapists as experts include the judicial use of abstract psychological terminology (Atkinson & Carskadden, 1975), therapists' directiveness (Atkinson, Maruyama, & Matsui, 1978), effectively communicated core therapeutic conditions (Scheid, 1976), an attentive, confident, and reassuring manner (Sprafkin, 1970), and fluent, spontaneous speech manner denoting preparation and the asking of relevant, thought-provoking questions (Strong & Schmidt, 1970).

Strong (1968) in particular proposes that an important source of expertness is therapists' confidence in the theoretical approach or model they employ. This confidence is communicated not by blind adherence but by therapists' speaking and acting with authority and enthusiasm. Strong (1968) also emphasizes the value of therapists' formal structuring efforts during initial sessions in particular. He states:

> Most counselors pay considerable attention to structuring the interview. They point out the roles and requirements of the client and the counselor in the interview, the sequences of the process, and events likely to occur as they work toward problem solution. Such structuring, whether explicit or implicit, gives evidence of

the counselor's expertness. Since the client must perceive that the counselor knows what he is doing, explicit structuring may be more effective than implicit structuring. . . . The client is provided a "rational" framework to view his problem, the means of problem solution, and the importance of his own efforts and further information. He is thus more able to guide his own efforts toward problem solution. (p. 221)

Accentuating Attractiveness

Strong (1968) suggests that clients' perceptions of therapists' attractiveness are based on "perceived similarity to, compatibility with, and liking for" (p. 216). For example, group similarity or dissimilarity such as race and sex may have an effect on clients perceptions of therapists (Merluzzi, Banikiotes, & Missbach, 1978; Merluzzi, Merluzzi, & Kaul, 1977). Likewise, the presence or lack of similar attitudes and experiences can affect whether a therapist is perceived as attractive.

Other factors affecting perceived attractiveness seem much like those affecting expertness. Egan (1982) proposes that therapists may appear attractive to clients because of visible evidence such as physical characteristics, because of professional role or reputation, and as a result of therapists' actions within the counseling interview. He suggests that interview behavior is most important, however, stating:

> I emphasize behavior because there is little that can be done about the other categories, even though you know they are affecting a client. For instance, some clients might find ministers more attractive helpers than psychologists, but if you are a psychologist, you would hardly become a minister for that reason. (p. 135)

Corrigan, et al., (1980) reports that research has found the most reliable indicators of clients' perceptions of therapist attractiveness come from interview behaviors. These behaviors include a moderate level of self-disclosure (Mann & Murphy, 1975), therapist disclosure that conveys similarly-held attitudes (Daher & Banikiotes, 1976), and the display of a number of nonverbal behaviors indicating interest in clients, including eye contact, forward body orientation and body lean toward the client (Hasse & Tepper, 1972; LaCrosse, 1975), less distance between therapist and client (Hasse & Tepper, 1972), and smiling and head nodding by the therapist (LaCrosse, 1975).

Trustworthiness

Strong (1968) asserts that therapists' perceived trustworthiness is based on their "(a) reputation for honesty, (b) social role, such as physician,

(c) sincerity and openness, and (d) lack of motivation for personal gain" (p. 217). Corrigan et al., (1980) reports that therapists' perceived trustworthiness has received relatively little research attention and thus the factors that might enhance trustworthiness are not well verified.

Common sense and the little research that has been conducted suggests, however, that trustworthiness is communicated similar to expertness and attractiveness. Clients judge trustworthiness based on visible evidence such as physical appearance ("He has an honest face," or "She reminds me of an old rival who would go to any length to win."), professional role or reputation ("My doctor referred me to you saying your integrity was without question in these types of situations," "I just feel most comfortable speaking with my minister."), and interview behavior. In emphasizing the overriding importance of therapists' interview behavior in increasing their trustworthiness in the eyes of clients, Egan (1982) recommends the following therapist actions:

- ☐ Make agreements with clients and live up to the provisions
- ☐ Maintain confidentiality
- ☐ Be optimistic about clients' abilities to face their problems, but always realistic as well
- ☐ Be willing to give clients information or feedback that may help them
- ☐ Use your social influence power carefully and for clients' best interests
- ☐ Be open to clients' feedback and attempts to exert social influence themselves
- ☐ Avoid behavior that might indicate the presence of ulterior motives as voyeurism, selfishness, superficial curiosity, personal gain, or deviousness

Actual Accomplishment

Egan (1982) states accomplishment is the "bottom line" of social influence. He maintains that if a therapist is perceived as an expert (in the sense that he or she engages in behaviors that *appear* competent to the client), as attractive, and as trustworthy, but in the long run *is of no actual help*, the client is worse off than before therapy began. If clients possess reasonable expectations for therapy and these expectations are not met, then they lose any faith in the process itself. Consider the client who says,

CLIENT: I give up. I sought therapy like you suggested. The therapist was an OK person and by the looks of all the degrees on the wall, a qualified professional. I felt comfortable during our sessions. But nothing changed in my life. In fact, things got worse.

One cannot automatically assume that the therapist was at fault. However, even though the client perceived the therapist as expert, attractive, and trustworthy, opening the client to potential social influence, the client wasn't helped by therapy. It is therefore critical that therapists *deliver* what is promised in the therapeutic agreement, whether that agreement is implicit or explicit (Egan, 1982). Strong (1968) sees an ingredient of effective therapy in addition to clients' perception of expertness, attractiveness, and trustworthiness in the initial stages: Clients must be involved in therapy to reduce the likelihood that they will try to discredit it.

Increasing Client Involvement

Clients' ability to change is greatly increased when they are intrinsically involved in the influence process. Gilbert (1978) proposes that individuals tend to do things when there are enough *incentives* to motivate them. Individuals tend not to be motivated if there are no incentives or if the incentives are of little value to them. People also tend to avoid behaviors for which they are punished. Egan (1982), in applying these basic principles to client motivation in therapy, identifies three means by which therapists can involve clients more actively:

1. *Reducing Psychological Pain.* Clients will be generally motivated if they are in psychological pain. The disorganization in their lives makes them susceptible to therapists' influence. They view therapy as a potential source of relief and are even willing to pay a price to find relief, which is to change the way they feel, think, and act. By contrasting past and present psychological pain with potential immediate and future relief, therapists can motivate clients to become more actively involved in seeking therapeutic gains.

2. *Maintaining a Client Focus.* Clients will involve themselves in therapy more fully if they are dealing with issues they think are of intrinsic importance to them. Communicating the core condition of empathic understanding is of critical value in this step. The more therapists understand clients' internal frames of reference and their perceived world, the more likely it is that they will deal with issues that are important to clients and that clients will be personally cognizant of this relevance.

3. *Properly Pacing Therapy.* The amount of physical and psychological effort that therapy demands of clients affects their motivation to actively and consistently involve themselves in it. If too many demands are placed upon clients too soon, they may terminate therapy prematurely. If too little is asked of them and little progress is evident,

again, premature termination is likely. Watson and Tharp (1981) describe effective therapy as greatly affected by "shaping," in which therapists guide clients step by *gradual* step toward more constructive patterns of thinking, feeling, and acting. They identify the loss of client motivation and involvement during therapy as due to inadequate shaping, too much or too little effort demanded of the client.

STRUCTURING SKILLS

Many clients come to counseling having little idea of what to expect, and others arrive with unreasonable or inappropriate expectations. If therapy is to be of any value, clients must begin by knowing *where* they are, *who* they are with, and *why* they are there (Brammer & Shostrom, 1982). To state this another way, therapists should explain to clients what constitutes a "good client" (Eisenberg & Delaney, 1977) so that they are best prepared to begin therapy.

Structuring skills tell clients what to expect from the therapeutic process. The therapist must decide how much structuring to use and when to use it. Too little structuring reduces the potential of productive sessions; too much structuring sounds "preachy" and may make clients reluctant to participate fully, fearing that they will not be behaving "properly" (Patterson & Eisenberg, 1982). Relatively short and to-the-point statements that describe the working agenda are ideal. Long-winded speeches about the therapeutic process and its intricacies only detract unnecessarily from valuable session time. Structuring statements should be initially used to set a working agenda for therapy and later used to maintain clients' momentum toward achieving therapeutic gains.

Therapists differ in their primary theoretical orientation and the techniques they employ; institutions and agencies differ in policies and regulations; and clients differ in issues they present, needs, and background. Consequently, the structure of therapy will differ among therapists, institutions and agencies, and clients. Day and Sparacio (1980) reviewed structuring procedures in counseling and identify three themes that regularly recur across them all: practical structuring, consumer structuring, and process structuring. We will also address session termination skills, a part of all three.

Practical Structuring

Practical structuring is "the procedure by which a joint understanding and agreement is reached between counselor and client on the logistical, pragmatic, and procedural aspects of the counseling situation" (Day & Sparacio, 1980, p. 248). Practical structuring includes specifying names and titles of participants, the length of sessions, scheduling sessions, making up missed sessions, cancellations, crises and emergency contacts, and fees and fee payment procedures.

The structuring of practicalities should be concrete, brief, and matter-of-fact. Practical structuring is often performed by secretarial or other support staff or with literature that the client and therapist can discuss. Because these issues can directly effect whether an effective therapeutic relationship is established and maintained, it is the therapist's responsibility to see that the client knows the essentials.

An example offered by Benjamin (1974) illustrates practical structuring by a therapist:

> So we have agreed, Carol, to meet for the time being every Monday at four in the afternoon. We'll have about forty-five minutes each session to talk over whatever is on your mind. (p. 17)

Consumer Structuring

Consumer structuring is "the procedure by which a joint understanding and agreement is reached between the counselor and client on consumer-oriented concerns relating to the counseling encounter" (Day & Sparacio, 1980, p. 248). Consumer issues include confidentiality, taping sessions, record keeping, therapist qualifications (and sometimes limitations), client rights and responsibilities, and the potential for client success given the problem presented.

The following statement suggested by Pietrofesa, Hoffman, Splete, and Pinto (1978) depicts the use of consumer structuring.

> I'm Mrs..........You are probably not familiar with our counseling procedures here. From your application, you know our session is being taped. What is said is still private and confidential between us. (p. 226)

Process Structuring

Process structuring is "the procedure by which a joint understanding and agreement is reached between counselor and client regarding the dynamics and methodology of the counseling encounter" (Day & Sparacio, 1980, p. 248). Process structuring issues entail definitions of what counseling and psychotherapy are, how the therapeutic process begins and ends, how sessions begin and end, goals to pursue, therapist and client roles and responsibilities in the therapeutic framework being used, and information regarding referral, consultation, and follow-up.

Stewart, Winborn, Johnson, Burks, and Engelkes (1978) provide a fine illustration of process structuring:

> My job as a counselor is to listen and try to understand how you feel and think about things. I won't make decisions for you, but together we may come up with some things for you to consider in making a decision. If you make a decision, I will help you find ways to carry it out. Your part in counseling is to help me understand how you feel and think. You also have to make decisions and carry out tasks that need doing before you can reach your goals. (p. 99)

Termination Skills

There is a minimum of time required for a counseling session. Sessions that continue for no more than ten to fifteen minutes make effective interchange between client and therapist difficult. In fact, many therapists normally require five to ten minutes just to re-orient themselves and to change their focus from a preceding activity to the present moment with the client (Hackney & Cormier, 1979). Compounding this reorientation, research has indicated that clients tend to postpone addressing their most distressing concerns as long as possible. Sessions that are not time limited exacerbate this tendency to postpone. Thus, time limits help clients focus on primary problems early in therapy sessions.

Effective termination skills greatly enhance counselor–client interaction. Benjamin (1974) suggests two considerations as basic to terminating a counseling session:

1. Both therapist and client should know that the session is ending, the therapist in particular.
2. Termination concerns that which has already taken place; therefore, no new topics should be introduced. If a client tries to introduce new material at the end of a session, it is generally best to postpone addressing it until the next meeting. The therapist might simply suggest, "That seems like a good place for us to begin our next session."

Usually a brief, to-the-point reference to time limits is the simplest way to end a session.

Summarizations are another, more detailed and concrete, method of ending a session. They provide a specific focus that the client can consider until the next session. A summarization can come from the therapist, be requested of the client, or be a combination in which mutual feedback is offered.

ATTENDING SKILLS Counseling and psychotherapy are interpersonal transactions that demand a certain intensity of presence. Therapists' presence, or "being with" clients, is what is meant by *attending*. In working with clients, therapists should look at them and maintain natural eye contact. A therapist's body should also communicate interest. Although it was once believed that counseling was solely a verbal interchange, increased study of videotapes and films have shown that nonverbal communications are vital to any therapeutic relationship's success. Thus, eye contact and body language are the physical fundamentals of attending.

If therapists are to fully attend to clients, more than their physical presence is needed; they must also listen. Listening, however, is not an overtly observable behavior. It must be made so with therapist responses that communicate true and active listening to their clients. For example:

CLIENT: I had just the most miserable day. Everything that could have gone wrong did.
THERAPIST: Every darn thing!

Restating a portion of the client's concerns shows that the therapist is truly listening, not just physically appearing to.

Finally, passive listening, allowing silence to occur, is also an important attending skill. Clients often need time to think. Patiently giving them this opportunity (although not to excess) communicates that what they have to say is important and worth waiting for.

Physical Attending

Egan (1982) proposes an acronym, SOLER, to represent five major appropriate physical attending skills.

- [ ] *Face the client SQUARELY:* This communicates to the client, "I'm available to you; I'm with you." Turning one's body away, either to the side or opposite, suggests a lessened degree of interest and involvement.
- [ ] *Provide an OPEN posture.* Crossing one's arms or legs can be perceived as signals of standoffishness or defensiveness. An open posture suggests an openness to what the client has to say. It communicates that there are no blocks preventing direct access to the counselor.
- [ ] *At times, LEAN toward the client.* In observing individuals intensely involved in conversation, their attraction for each other as if drawn by a magnet is evidenced in their tendency to lean toward one another. A slight forward trunk lean communicates, "I'm interested." A reclining or slouchy upper body says "I want to back off" or "I'm bored."
- [ ] *Maintain EYE contact.* By maintaining eye contact with clients, therapists show that they are trying to hear what is being said. A natural

style of eye contact with clients is best. Frequent breaks in eye contact suggest discomfort with what is being said. Avoiding eye contact is self-explanatory, and rigid staring is not natural. Again, observe two individuals in serious conversation. They very likely have uninterrupted eye contact. What is being said is so interesting that they don't even take a moment to look up to stop and reflect.

☐ *RELAX:* If the therapist appears rigid, the client will probably find it difficult to relax. A natural, relaxed position on the part of the therapist makes it easier for both to feel more comfortable. Facing the client squarely, an open posture, leaning toward the client, and maintaining eye contact all can be taken literally or metaphorically. Effective counselors are not overly self-conscious about their physical presence. They use SOLER as a general guide, not as an absolute set of rules to be applied in all cases. Using this guide, they ask themselves, "To what degree am I physically attending to my client?"

Active Listening

Active listening by therapists consistently tells clients that they are being paid attention to. It reassures them that what they have to say is important and encourages them to explore, and thus discriminate and define, their concerns. Less therapist "talk time" and prompting is required and more time is available for client self-exploration and elaboration. Minimal encouragers and restatements are counselor skills that facilitate active listening.

Minimal encouragers are brief one- or two-word prompts that punctuate a therapy session. "Uh-huh," "and so," "mmm," "yes," "ah," and similar utterances keep clients talking once started and let therapists show their involvement with little intrusion into a client's conversational flow (Ivey & Simek-Downing, 1980). Minimal encouragers also act as reinforcement to clients to continue. The client speaks and the therapist gives a minimal encourager, suggesting the client continue and thereby enhancing self-exploration.

CLIENT: What a bummer today was. First, I got a flat tire on the way to work and then when I finally got there, the downhill slide continued.
THERAPIST: Oh, wow.
CLIENT: Yea, my boss started on me about . . .

Minimal encouragers can be nonverbal as well as verbal. Nonverbal encouragers are a valuable adjunct to verbal encouragement.

CLIENT: I never get my way. My parents seem to think that they can just order me around with their bossy "no you can't."

THERAPIST: (Shakes head from side to side)
CLIENT: It's really bad. I'm to the point that I'm ready just to take off.

Restatements are "repetitions of all or a selected portion of the client's previous communication, and neither add nor detract from the basic communication" (Hackney & Cormier, 1979, p. 68). Restatements confirm for clients that the therapist has heard what they have just said. Restatements should be used judiciously. To be most effective, they should be interspersed with other types of responses. Otherwise, they can create a "parroting" effect that puts off some clients. Examples of restatements illustrate the value of this skill:

CLIENT: I'm looking forward to summer vacation.
THERAPIST: Can't wait for vacation to come.

CLIENT: I get along with most of the persons I work with, but my boss, that's a different story.
THERAPIST: Your boss is a different story.

Passive Listening

The most basic, yet overlooked, therapist skill is passive listening, or effectively using silence in a counseling session. Clients frequently need opportunities to pause and internally explore their thoughts, feelings, and behaviors. They need someone to simply wait, listen, and allow them to prepare to share their story. New therapists typically are uncomfortable with time lapses during counseling sessions and tend to interrupt them unnecessarily. They are not yet sensitive to the various meanings of silence, nor are they skillful in handling these pauses. Silences, however, can prove important in terms of attending to clients.

First, silence lets clients know that they have a responsibility for providing independent input into the session. Too often, therapists rush in to fill up space, thus taking on an inappropriate amount of responsibility for session content. Second, silence allows clients to delve further into their thoughts, feelings, and actions and to ponder their implications as well as what has just happened during the session with the therapist. Clients need this time to reflect without feeling pressured to maintain constant overt communication (George & Christiani, 1981).

Brammer and Shostrom (1982) suggest that silence has a number of significant meanings, and counselors must try to identify the correct meaning in order to respond appropriately. Silence can mean that the client feels uncomfortable and is anxious or embarrassed in having to present himself or herself, or a specific idea or concern, in therapy. It can also indicate client resistance, particularly when the client has been coerced into coming for counseling. Silence can be a sign that the client has reached the end of an idea and is merely wondering what to say next. Silence can also be considered "anticipatory," wherein a client pauses expecting something from the therapist—some type of reassurance, information, or other reaction. In each of these instances, the question that therapists must consider is whether or not to interrupt the silence.

Brammer and Shostrom (1982) advocate that clients be allowed to assume responsibility for going onward when they are responsible for initiating the original silence. They see this as avoiding interfering with a forward-moving activity. Yet, it is important that therapists recognize situations in which clients should be supported over rough places rather than forced to face them before they are ready. George and Cristiana (1981) propose that statements communicating empathic understanding combined with tentative inquiries are a positive method of interrupting client-initiated silences.

CLIENT: (Silence)

THERAPIST: You appear somewhat apprehensive about being here. I'm wondering if you might share what you're thinking at the moment?

In summary, the therapeutic use of passive listening as an attending skill cannot be overstated. Silence can communicate to clients a sincere and deep acceptance. It demonstrates the therapist's concern and willingness to let the client assume control of their part in the therapeutic process. As an intentional response, properly implemented, passive listening can be an important facet of the experience clients gain from a therapy session: they can say to themselves, "Here I was really listened to" (Benjamin, 1974).

THERAPIST SKILLS I: THEORETICAL APPLICATIONS

This chapter addressed creating a therapeutic climate. We initially considered four core conditions therapists can help create by displaying certain skills. We then examined ways to further enhance the counseling environment with social influencers. Finally, we examined the essential elements of structuring and attending skills as means for preparing clients to begin discriminating and defining their major concerns.

All of the theoretical approaches to counseling and psychotherapy postulate similar common conditions for creating an appropriate therapeutic climate. Most also agree that therapists' skills crucially influence the kind of environment that ultimately evolves when therapist and client meet. Variations do exist though in the manner and degree with which each approach attempts to apply these therapist skills and thus provide specific prerequisite conditions.

Core Conditions

With the exception of concreteness, which is emphasized by all the major approaches, the diverse skills that facilitate core conditions of empathic understanding, respect, and genuineness are well illustrated by the opposing views of Carl Rogers and Albert Ellis. For Rogers (1961), communicating qualities such as empathic understanding, genuineness, and respect are of primary importance if positive client change is to occur. In the person-centered perspective, how therapists display themselves as persons is far more important than any challenging skills and intervention strategies they might use.

By contrast, Ellis (1973) maintains that clients can make positive changes even if therapists don't create these core conditions. He wrote in this regard:

> Actually, quite effectual therapy, leading to a basic personality change, can be done without any relationship whatever between client and therapist. It can be accomplished by correspondence, by readings, and by tape recordings and other audiovisual aids, without the client having any contact with, or knowing practically anything about, the person who is treating him. (p. 140)

While Ellis does not view core conditions as essential for client change, he also does not ignore them. The more conducive the therapeutic climate, the more likely efficient and effective therapy will occur. Ellis posits that these conditions are secondary, not prerequisite, elements for positive client change.

Between the opposing views of Rogers and Ellis, various emphases are placed on therapists' skills at creating core conditions. Existential therapists emphasize the person-to-person encounter in therapy. Therapy is seen as a shared journey in which both the therapist and client strive for authenticity, and the client is a partner. Thus, empathic understanding, and especially genuineness and respect are key ingredients. By contrast, Gestalt therapists do not consider these core conditions as critical to therapy. Their view is quite similar to that of behavior therapists.

Stereotypically, behavior therapists have been viewed as mechanical, manipulative, and highly impersonal. This misconception seems to have been an overreaction to how many behavioral therapists' view therapists' facilitation of core conditions compared to those of person-centered and existential therapists. Although they don't place the same weight on core conditions, most behavior therapists do contend that establishing a conducive therapeutic climate is a prerequisite for positive client change, but not sufficient in itself for "maximally effective therapy" (Goldstein, 1973, p. 220). Behaviorally-oriented reality therapists place a greater emphasis on therapists' facilitation of core conditions. Glasser (1965) maintains that a relationship with clients must be established before effective therapy can occur. He proposed that clients need to know that the therapist cares about and accepts them, and believes in their capacity to succeed. In this way, clients learn that there is more to living than focusing on failures and irresponsible behavior. Reality therapists especially engender respect by refusing to accept blaming and excuses. They display respect further by viewing clients in light of what they can do if they face up to reality.

In the other two cognitive-oriented approaches, Transactional Analysis and Beck's cognitive therapy, empathic understanding, genuineness, and respect are perceived similar to behavior therapists; valuable and facilitative, but not in and of themselves curative.

Social Influencers

Research has clearly indicated the social influencing nature of counseling and psychotherapy (Corrigan, et al., 1980). All therapists by virtue of their professional position exert social influence by being perceived as expert, attractive, and trustworthy. Some theoretical approaches explicitly emphasize therapists' social influencers while others do not directly address them.

Because of their value as a teaching tool, social influencers play a critical therapeutic role for behavior therapists, rational-emotive therapists, and reality therapists. Rational-emotive therapists, in particular, actively direct clients in examining their beliefs and teaching them new ways of thinking. This influence is reflected most dramatically in Ellis's (1973) assertion that he will "persuade, cajole, and at times even command" clients to change as an integral part of the therapeutic process (p. 154).

Reality therapists likewise strongly emphasize the importance of their social influencing skills. Glasser (1965) criticizes conventional psychiatry for failing to deal with issues of right and wrong in the course of therapy. He proposed emphatically:

> Our job is to face this question, confront them with their total behavior, and *get them to judge* the quality of what they are doing. We have found that unless they judge their own behavior, they will not change. (p. 56)

While not as intense in asserting their social influence, behavior therapists actively direct intervention strategies and, more important in terms of social influence, serve as explicit reinforcers and contingency contractors for clients. As Goldstein (1973) states, "Therapy is the therapist's responsibility. It is the therapist who at the very least implicitly establishes himself as the expert, and any failure is the therapist's failure" (p. 222).

The affectively-oriented approaches all tend to downplay therapists' roles as social influencers. In some ways, these approaches posit clients' ability to see themselves, not their therapists, as social influencers as a key ingredient for therapeutic success. Beck's cognitive therapy and Transactional Analysis, although didactic, tend to deemphasize therapists' social influencing skills. Equality within the therapeutic environment is sought. Contracts are usually made between therapist and client stating the terms of their relationship. Both therapist and client possess significant social influence, which must be directed toward a common goal for effective therapy to take place.

Structuring and Attending Skills

Attending, practical, and consumer structuring skills are an obvious necessity for any therapist, regardless of therapeutic orientation. The different emphases on these skills seems a moot point. Therapists' use of process structuring skills, however, does vary widely among the various approaches.

Although Carl Rogers stresses the responsibility of therapists to display core characteristics, he views the client as responsible for structuring the sessions. Existential therapists hold a similar view on process structuring. The founder of Gestalt Therapy, Fritz Perls, went further in claiming that full responsibility for structuring therapy rests with the client. He believed that most persons seek therapy because they are unwilling to accept responsibility for their own lives. A significant quote in this regard was made at one of his workshops: "So if you want to go crazy, commit suicide, improve, get 'turned on,' or get an experience that will change your life, that's up to you" (Perls, 1969, p. 75).

Rational-emotive therapists and behavior therapists emphasize therapist structuring skills. Both view therapy as an educational endeavor in which therapists teach clients more adaptive ways of functioning. These therapists therefore assume a great share of responsibility for structuring what goes on during therapy. In between are cognitive therapy, reality therapy, and Transactional Analysis, which emphasize establishing contracts between therapist and client and thus making structuring a joint venture.

A Caveat

This discussion of theoretical applications of the various therapist skills is based on the common conceptualization of what the founder, primary spokespersons, or majority of relevant practitioners of a particular approach advocate. There is no reason not to use any of the skills presented in this chapter or upcoming chapters with any theoretical position. As we have stressed before, therapist skills and techniques are not theory; they are a way to implement theory. Using different skills to different degrees need not prevent you from adopting a specific primary theoretical orientation. Common conceptualizations are presented here to explain how a particular therapist skill is *typically* used by the *typical* therapist of one of the major orientations presented in the second section of this book.

The following annotated case summarizes the therapist skills presented in this chapter. The case continues through the upcoming chapters so that you can follow the client, Charles, as he and his counselor progress through the therapeutic process.

CHARLES: PHASE I

The client, Charles, is 25 and currently a part-time graduate student. The setting is a University Counseling Center. This is the beginning of his first session with the counselor. Key identifying data in the case have been changed and condensed to highlight key issues.

THERAPIST SKILLS I

COUNSELOR: Hello, Charles. Come on in and sit down. My name is Kay Simmons.

CHARLES: Hi.

structuring/respect/ genuineness

COUNSELOR: From the information you gave the secretary, I notice that this is the first time you've seen a professional counselor. Before we discuss what's brought you here, it might be beneficial to talk about counseling, my role, and your responsibilities.

CHARLES: Okay, sounds like a good place to begin. I would like to know a bit more about what I should expect.

structuring/social influence expertness, trustworthiness, respect/genuineness

COUNSELOR: I'm a professional counselor licensed by the state of Florida. Any specific questions you have about my credentials or the Counseling Center, feel free to ask . . . I see my job as a counselor being to set up a climate where you would feel comfortable to present your concerns. I won't make decisions for you, but rather work with you in defining your main concerns, setting goals to deal with them, and selecting strategies to achieve those goals. As you know from the release you signed that accompanied the intake sheet, I'm taping our session. I do this in case I feel a need to review what has transpired between us. I often recommend that clients listen to their session tapes and I make them available to you . . . What is said here is confidential unless there is a danger to you or someone else or unless I have your permission to consult with a colleague on a critical point that he or she might have some special expertise providing extra assistance to us. Any questions?

CHARLES: Not right now.

structuring/respect

COUNSELOR: Our session will last for 45 minutes and we can leave some time at the end so that we can decide . . . or you can decide, whether you'd like to continue and meet together again.

CHARLES: Okay.

COUNSELOR: Your intake sheet notes only that you "want to talk to someone." Why don't you explain a bit more specifically about why you decided to come see a counselor.

structuring

CHARLES: Well, I feel a little bit silly about coming. But, I've just been real restless inside. Just confused with my life.

COUNSELOR: Go on.

minimal encourager

CHARLES: It seems like I'm going through a lot of restructuring . . . I'm not sure of what to do with myself.

COUNSELOR: You're feeling uncomfortable with the changes you've been experiencing. And confused about where to go from here.

empathic understanding

CHARLES: Yeah, for sure. I guess I structured my life a couple of years a certain way . . . now all of a sudden I have to change. And I'm having a hard time dealing with that . . . I'm not sure if I want it changed but I feel like I have to.

COUNSELOR: So, you're uncertain about whether or not you really want to change the way you have been living your life.

empathic understanding

CHARLES: Exactly. I don't know . . . I'm used to being independent . . . but what happened is that I've met someone very special in my life and you know how that goes. You start falling in love . . . you're no longer thinking of yourself. You have to start thinking of another person.

COUNSELOR: Another person.

restatement

CHARLES: I don't know. It's frustrating right now because I feel like I have to do a lot of changing just so I can be with this person.

COUNSELOR: Sounds like you're unsure not only of your new role, but also about whether or not you even want to continue it at all.

empathic understanding

CHARLES: Right, yeah.

COUNSELOR: How exactly do you perceive your need to change? What is a specific example of how you must adapt to this new life situation?

concreteness

SUGGESTED READINGS

Core Conditions

Gazda, G. (1973). *Human relations development.* Boston: Allyn & Bacon. Developing his ideas from a Carkhuff framework, Gazda singles out some especially valuable points on empathic understanding and related constructs.

Ivey, A. E., & Authier, J. (1978) *Microcounseling* (2nd ed.). Springfield, IL: Charles C. Thomas. This book offers a most distinct discussion of what the authors refer to as "qualitative dimensions" of effective counseling and psychotherapy. Of particular value is the authors' analysis of how the major theoretical orientations emphasize or deemphasize specific core conditions.

Patterson, C. H. (1974). *Relationship counseling and psychotherapy.* New York: Harper & Row. Patterson suggests some particularly fine points to consider from what he terms the "response dimension" related to necessary therapeutic conditions.

Social Influencers

Egan, G. (1982). *The skilled helper: Model, skills, and methods for effective helping* (2nd ed.). Monterey, CA: Brooks/Cole. Egan offers a brief but superb overview of "helping as a social influence process" as well as other topics.

Gilbert, T. F. (1978). *Human competence: Engineering worthy performance.* New York: McGraw-Hill. Gilbert emphasizes that competence does not lie principally in behaviors but rather more so in the accomplishments toward which specific behaviors are directed.

Kanfer, F. H., & Goldstein, A. P. (Eds.) (1980). *Helping people change: A textbook of methods* (2nd ed.). New York: Pergamon. One of the editors (Goldstein) offers an exceptional contribution on "relationship-enhancement methods," describing a social influence process that is complementary to Strong's landmark conceptualization.

Structuring/Attending

Brammer, L. M., & Shostrom, E. L. (1982). *Therapeutic psychology: Fundamentals of counseling and psychotherapy* (4th ed.). Englewood Cliffs, NJ: Prentice-Hall. The authors address "client readiness" and "opening techniques" as topics in their overall discussion of the counseling process in a way that offers unique ideas for the beginning therapist to consider.

Evans, D. R., Hearn, M. T., Uhlemann, M. R., & Ivey, A. E. (1979). *Essential interviewing: A programmed approach to effective communication.* Monterey, CA: Brooks/Cole. This book offers chapters devoted directly to both specific structuring and attending skills.

Patterson, L. E., & Eisenberg, S. (1983). *The counseling process* (3rd ed.). Boston: Houghton Mifflin. The authors' discussion of "structuring and leading techniques" provide some thoughtful practices.

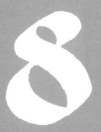

8

Phase Two: Discriminating and Defining Client Problems

A detailed and comprehensive assessment is often a sine qua non for effective therapeutic intervention. The cliche "diagnosis must usually precede treatment" points to the obvious fact that when the real problems have been identified, effective remedies (if they exist) can be administered.

(Lazarus, 1981, p. 17)

neffective counselors tend to wander with clients in therapy and fail to identify basic issues that must be resolved, or they may form a simple definition of a client's problem without considering all the factors involved. The initial task in any counseling relationship is to discriminate among diverse client concerns and define a specific problem to pursue. Therapists' discrimination skills involve the ability to "distinguish, or tell apart, two or more behaviors, concepts, events, objects, or feelings" (Cormier & Cormier, 1979). These discrimination skills are prerequisites to problem definition.

Usually, a client presents one or more concerns superficially in therapy. The counselor then helps the client create and explore all possible definitions of the client's expressed concerns. The client and therapist then select one problem and commit themselves to addressing it. This process constitutes Phase II of the therapeutic process and is illustrated in Figure 8–1.

The temptation to accept a problem as presented by a client and then immediately try to solve it can be enticing. However, the client's

FIGURE 8–1
Phase II of therapy

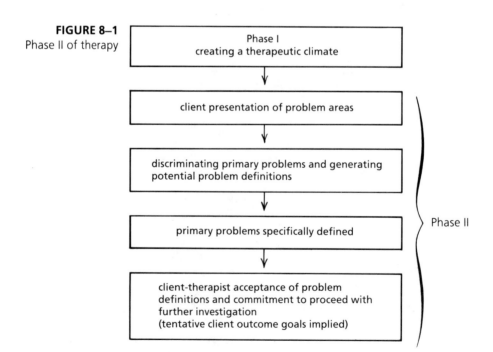

initial definition of a problem may be incomplete. Consider the following example:

Lou: I'm new in town and I'm feeling awfully lonely. I don't know anyone. I don't know where to go to meet people. I'm just feeling real down on myself too.

If Lou's key problem is immediately defined as loneliness, then therapy will be directed toward alleviating Lou's loneliness. This direction may be the most desirable to pursue, but immediately choosing it without considering alternative possibilities may severely limit the effectiveness of therapy. The therapist's choice to accept or enlarge the client's definition of the problem is one of the most critical elements of ultimate therapeutic effectiveness (Ivey & Simek-Downing, 1980).

Lou's problem may be a poor image of self, a lack of social assertiveness, an inability to maintain meaningful conversation, unrealistic expectations about meeting new people, confusion in orienting himself to a new environment, a new boss making inordinate demands on his leisure time, whatever. With limited information, there are many possible definitions of his problem. More information and a more detailed examination of the problem are needed so that many alternatives can be considered in alleviating it. One tool for conceptualizing how therapists can gain more information is the Johari Window.

The Johari Window (Luft, 1970) is a visual illustration of how exploration and elaboration of client problems can occur. As pictured in Figure 8–2, the Johari Window illustrates how in any relationship between two persons there are four types of information: four panes in a window. The first pane, Area 1, is information that both the client and the therapist know about the client. This is normally intake information that clients would readily share such as name, address, presenting problem, and the like.

STIMULATING CLIENT EXPLORATION AND ELABORATION

	Known to Therapist	Unknown to Therapist
Known to Client	1 Open Area	2 Hidden Area
Unknown to Client	3 Blind Area	4 Unknown Area

FIGURE 8–2
The Johari Window

Area 2 is information clients generally do not readily disclose: intimate fears, anxieties, sexual difficulties, first impression dislike of the therapist, and so on. Area 3 is information the therapist has about the client of which the client is not aware, such as impressions about the client and possible theoretical explanations of his or her difficulties. Area 4 is information as yet unknown to either client or therapist, such as why the client is unable to independently find a solution to his or her problem or what the ultimate direction of therapy will be.

Figure 8–2 illustrates that to explore and elaborate on their concerns, clients must be helped to feel secure and unthreatened about moving material from Area 2 (information known to self but unknown to the therapist) into Area 1 (information known to both self and the therapist). For many clients, this is very difficult; the material to be shared may never have been revealed to anyone before. Feelings of fear, anger, and certain "unacceptable" beliefs are a part of Area 2. They have not been shared because they create anxiety and discomfort for the client. Effective therapists frequently hear clients say they "have never told this to anyone before." When this happens the client often is relieved (Eisenberg & Delaney, 1977).

As the client begins to talk more about self to the therapist, the amount of information known by both the client and the therapist expands and the amount known to the client but not the therapist contracts. This change is graphically shown in Figure 8–3: Area 1 increases as Area 2 decreases.

As therapist–client interaction continues, therapists will respond to clients with empathic understanding and try to help clients concretely define their concerns, with honesty and respect. Clients will learn more of how the therapist perceives their situation from their interactions with the therapist. The therapist's sharing allows a still further increase in Area 1, in this instance decreasing Area 3. As clients receive and consider this feedback from the therapist, they learn more and more about themselves.

FIGURE 8–3
Area 1 increases as the
client shares information
with the therapist

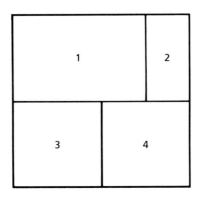

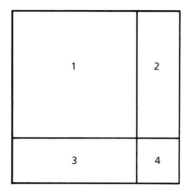

FIGURE 8–4
Both client and therapist
share information

Some of the unknowns of Area 4 begin to become more understandable as well. Over time, what occurs can be illustrated in Figure 8–4. The information available to both client and therapist has steadily expanded: problem definition gains from being better informed.

When is enough information available to adequately define a problem area? How much clarity is necessary for a client and therapist to proceed with the therapeutic process? Given our presentations on human functioning and theoretical approaches for understanding it, we believe that sufficient information exists when clients' affect, behavior, cognitions, and their contexts have been determined. Problem situations clearly conceptualized in this manner offer both beginning therapists adhering to one primary theoretical orientation and therapists sufficiently experienced to adopt a pragmatic therapeutic position all the relevant information necessary to work with a client in defining specific problem areas. Client and counselor can then commit themselves to focused change in upcoming phases of the therapeutic process.

DIAGNOSIS: ORGANIZING CLIENTS' TOTAL FUNCTIONING

Recognizing Nonverbal Client Communications

Knapp (1978) defines nonverbal behavior as all human communication events that transcend spoken or written words. All persons constantly transmit information about themselves by the manner in which they make or don't make eye contact, their body language and facial expressions, vocal qualities, and proxemic behaviors. Clients send many messages about their thoughts, feelings, and general pattern of acting without uttering a word. Mehrabian (1971), in reporting his and his associates' research on expressed like and dislike between individuals, states:

> Our experimental results show:
> Total liking equals 7% verbal liking plus 38% vocal liking plus 55% facial liking.

> Thus the impact of facial expression is greatest, then the impact of the tone of voice (or vocal expression), and finally that of the words. If the facial expression is inconsistent with the words, the degree of liking conveyed by the facial expression will dominate and determine the impact of the total message. (p. 43)

If a client says to a therapist "Everything has gone real well since our last session" in a flat, unenthusiastic voice while looking down at the floor and frowning, the true message is likely the nonverbal one. While the exact percentages stated by Mehrabian might be disputable, little question exists as to how important nonverbal communications are in fully understanding clients' total functioning.

Ivey (1983) offers a number of especially relevant therapeutic considerations when seeking to "read" specific client nonverbal communications. Two further important client signals are recognized.

Nonverbal communication

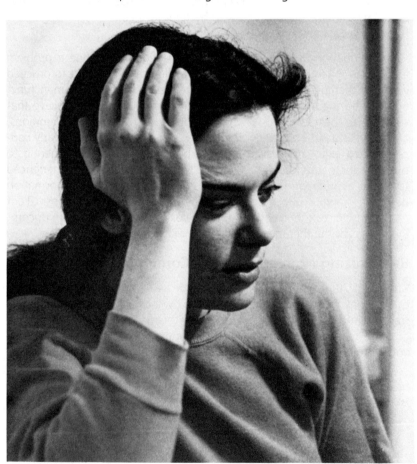

Eye Contact. When a topic is interesting to clients, their pupils tend to dilate. By contrast, when an issue is uncomfortable or boring, the pupils contract. Breaks in eye contact are also significant. Clients tend to look away when discussing issues that particularly depress or disturb them.

Cultural differences are significant in understanding eye contact. Direct eye contact is considered a sign of interest in white middle-class culture. However, even there clients will tend to offer more eye contact while listening and somewhat less while talking. Some blacks in the United States have been found to have reverse patterns; they look more directly when talking and slightly less while listening. Further, among some Hispanic groups, eye contact by the young is a sign of disrespect.

Body Language. Just as cultural differences in eye contact exist, body language patterns differ. For example, a comfortable space for conversation between North Americans is slightly more than arm's length. The British seem to prefer even larger distances. South American Spanish-speaking people frequently prefer less than half that distance, as do most continental Europeans.

Just as shifts in eye contact provide potential information about client discomfort, so do changes in body language. A client leaning forward is likely interested. Clients leaning away may be bored or frightened.

Autonomic Physiological Behaviors. Autonomic physiological responses such as blushing, commonly suggesting embarrassment, and quickened breathing, denoting nervousness, are observable and tell about clients' present functioning. They are likely the most expressive and difficult to conceal of observable behaviors.

Vocal Qualities. A client's voice communicates much about how he or she feels toward another person or situation. Changes in pitch, volume, and speech rate suggest similar true messages as changes in eye contact and body language. Timing of vocal changes may indicate comfort or discomfort. Speech hesitations and breaks suggest confusion or stress.

Verbal emphases are especially useful in understanding the essence of clients' communications. Louder volume and increased accent will be given to certain words or short phrases. The key words clients emphasize with volume and accent often denote issues of interest or special meaning.

Facial Expression. Smiles, frowns, raised eyebrows all communicate commonly recognized messages. Yet the manner in which they are expressed can communicate additional information.

> Let us consider a very simple form of facial expression—an
> ordinary smile. One of the most common instances is the "simple

smile," a mere upward and outward movement at the corners of the mouth. It indicates inner bemusement; no other person is involved. The "upper smile" is a slightly more gregarious gesture in which the upper teeth are exposed. It is usually displayed in social situations, such as when friends greet each other. Perhaps the most engaging of all is the "broad smile." The mouth is completely open; both upper and lower teeth are visible.

Yet without other facial movements, particularly around the eyes, smiles would not really mean what they seem to mean. For appropriate warmth, the upper smile is usually enhanced by slight changes around the corners of the eyes. Even the smile is not always an entirely convincing expression of broad surprise or pleasure unless it is accompanied by an elevation of the eyebrows. (Saral, 1972, p. 474)

Gazda, Asbury, Balzer, Childers, and Walters (1977) emphasize viewing nonverbal communications as clues rather than positive proof. They urge counselors to interpret nonverbal messages cautiously and remember that a given behavior can have different meanings for different individuals or even for the same individual on different occasions. Counselors must be sensitive to cultural background and context in recognizing potential variations in meaning.

It is often valuable to bring clients' attention to their nonverbal behaviors as a means of clarifying their meaning. For example:

THERAPIST: You always appear to be breathing rather hard when we begin our sessions. (suspecting possible client apprehension or nervousness in getting started)

CLIENT: I know. I've gotten caught in rush hour traffic coming here each time so far. I have to run from my car to make my appointment time.

THERAPIST: You hadn't mentioned this. Perhaps we might arrange for a later interview time.

CLIENT: That really would be better. I would have asked, but I didn't realize that was a possibility.

Even though the therapist initially interpreted the client's nonverbal message incorrectly, bringing the behavior to the client's attention helped the client share previously unknown information with the therapist. Likewise, the therapist was then able to share previously unknown (to the client) information about arranging a later session time. In terms of the Johari Window, Area 1 has thus increased with Areas 2, 3, and 4 decreasing.

This example illustrates the value of therapists' attending to clients' nonverbal communications. The ability to observe and respond to messages being sent enables therapists to project an unusual warmth, sensitivity, and perceptiveness that enhances the intimacy of the counseling relationship. This interchange may help clients perceive the therapist as clearly possessing professional expertise.

Clients' Affective Functioning

Affective functioning is the feelings clients experience in their problem situation. If a client communicates being "down all the time," the affect is some type of depression. Affective functioning can be explicitly or implicitly communicated.

Feelings are explicit if a client both experiences them and expresses them.

☐ "I just mope around all day."

☐ "I can't seem to control my temper. Every time my wife brings up my drinking, I start yelling."

Feelings and emotions are implicit if a client experiences them, but does *not* allow them to be observably expressed.

☐ "I boil inside when my boss starts ordering me around. I can't say anything to her though because I know it will mean the end of my job."

☐ "I want to tell my father how much I love him, but when we're together, I just can't seem to share my feelings with him."

Clients' Behavioral Functioning

Behavioral functioning is the actions of clients in problem situations. Like affective functioning, behavioral functioning can be both explicit and implicit; that is, actions clients observably do, or actions they can do but refrain from.

Behaviors are explicit when they can be observed by others.

☐ "When he speaks to me like that, I get up and walk away."

☐ "I was beginning to feel depressed again and decided it was time to do something about it. So I picked up the phone and made an appointment to come and see you."

Behaviors are implicit when clients are able to perform them, but refrain from doing so.

☐ "I knew exactly what to do, smile and say 'I love you,' but I just couldn't do it."

☐ "Walking away from the argument was my other option. Next time I'm going to do just that instead of responding back so negatively."

Clients' Cognitive Functioning

Cognitive functioning is the thoughts, beliefs, and expectations clients maintain about themselves, others, and the world. Cognitions are not observable, and thus are always implicit unless made explicit by clients verbalizing them.

- ☐ "When my husband and I aren't getting along, I think to myself, 'Why shouldn't I divorce him and start over?' "
- ☐ "I just start crying every time I think of my child having to suffer so much after the accident."
- ☐ "When the sun finally came out, I said to myself, 'I'm going to get out and enjoy myself.' "

The Importance of Context

Personality theorist George Kelly's position on the importance of considering the context that clients function in mirrors our own and addresses the necessity of maintaining a constant view of "client in context." Kelly (1955) states:

> It is a mistake to assume that a psychologically healthy person can immediately adjust himself happily to any kind of situation. Adjustment can only be achieved in relation to something. It makes a difference what one has to adjust to. Diagnosis is not complete until the clinician has some understanding of the milieu in which adjustment is to be sought. This position represents a departure from the common notion that diagnosis involves the analysis of the client only. From our point of view, diagnosis is the planning stage of client management. Therefore, *both* the client and his milieu must be understood. (p. 804)

In considering context, the major questions that therapists face are the degree to which environmental factors affect clients' functioning and the degree to which clients' functioning affects their environment. For example:

Harris took an early retirement from his work when he was 61. He and his wife Martha wanted to take advantage of their retirement annuity and have more free time to enjoy all they had worked so hard to attain. Suddenly Harris had a heart attack and died only six months after retiring. Martha is still distraught and refuses to go out and engage in any enjoyable activities although Harris's death was over a year ago.

In Martha's case, environmental factors, i.e., the untimely death of her husband, have heavily influenced her total functioning. However, her depressive affect, negative thoughts, and unwillingness to engage in activities without her husband a year after his death have contributed to her limiting her activities. Obviously, environmental change in the form of bringing Harris back is not possible. Martha can be helped to change her functioning and thus change her *current* environment by changing the way she feels, thinks, and/or acts.

At times, the environment can be changed, and this can be an appropriate tack to consider. For example:

John is a 17-year-old high school senior whose parents have arbitrarily imposed a 9 P.M. weekend curfew on him. John is unable to attend evening sporting events and social affairs that all of his classmates go to. He has been invited to a number of parties but always turns the invitation down, making up an excuse to hide his embarrassment over his parents' unreasonable curfew rule. Peers are beginning to ostracize him, calling him "stuck up."

John, like Martha in the previous illustration, feels depressed, has negative thoughts, and cannot engage in social activities, although this last situation is not of his own choosing. Changing his affective or cognitive functioning would do little to change his environment. He could learn to more comfortably bear his plight, at least temporarily. His parents' unreasonable rules, however, might better be addressed and his parents directly involved in the therapeutic process. Alternatives to therapy with individuals that involve significant others in a social-ecological therapeutic process will be discussed in chapter 11.

FOCUSING SKILLS

Focusing skills enable therapists to direct clients' communications toward the therapeutically appropriate areas of affective, behavioral, and cognitive functioning and their relevant contexts. In counseling and psychotherapy, clients are affected by the focus therapists choose to take. For instance, if a therapist is trying to understand what a client thinks about a problem, and focuses on the client's cognitions, the client will be influenced to talk about his or her relevant thoughts.

Therapists' choice of words in their communications reflects their primary orientation. The therapeutic focus is best implemented by the *verbs* chosen by therapists in discussing concerns with clients. For example, a therapist with an affective focus would use the verb *feeling,* as in "You are feeling quite happy today." A behavioral therapist would use the verbs *behaving, acting,* or *doing,* as in "You were acting oddly at the party last evening." A cognitive therapist would employ such verbs as *thinking, imagining, telling yourself,* as in "What might you be thinking when you're at work?"

Contextual focus accompanies an affective, behavioral, or cognitive orientation. A contextual focus is gained by the *nouns* chosen by therapists in discussing an area of concern; for instance, "You are very worried about *your job.*" Another aspect of context is time: past, present, or future. It is addressed by the verb *tense* therapists use in communicating with clients. For example, "You feel somewhat apprehensive with him" is in the present tense and reflects a current context. "You felt somewhat apprehensive with him," in the past tense, addresses a previously experience. Finally, "You will feel somewhat apprehensive with him" uses the future tense to project a potential context.

Understanding the basic concepts of focus is essential before focusing skills can be used effectively. Depending upon the particular affective, behavioral, cognitive, and contextual focuses addressed, a counseling session can take an infinite number of different directions. It is critical that therapists be aware of the focuses that they intend to use and actually implement in a given counseling session. If, after a session with a client, the therapist thinks "that session simply seemed to go nowhere," a focus analysis of the session may reveal that the session lacked direction because the therapist randomly shifted among foci. Or, perhaps the therapist in pursuing an affective focus in a present context was using almost all cognitive-oriented verbs and future verb tenses.

Specific focusing messages therapists can use are of three types: reflections, inquiries, and summarizations. Each is a specific kind of counselor verbal response.

Responding to Clients with Reflections

Reflection has two purposes. First, it is overly simplistic to think that therapists can completely communicate empathic understanding with only a positive listening attitude and attending to clients. While a sincere desire to listen and attending skills contribute, verbal responses are necessary to fully communicate empathic understanding to clients. Second, therapists must not only recognize the various components of client functioning but also communicate this recognition verbally to clients. Communicating this recognition to clients is the main role of the focusing skill of *reflection.* Reflection seeks to accomplish precisely what its name indicates: a mirroring of the feeling, thought, and behavior as well as the relevant context as presented in the client's message.

Each client statement or related group of statements will express, either explicitly or implicitly, information about the client's functioning and the context in which it is occurring. Thus, client communications will have a functioning component that is affective, behavioral, or cognitive (or a combination), and a contextual component. The functioning component is recognizable by the specific *verbs* employed by the client. As noted earlier in this chapter, however, clients may also express themselves in less obvious ways, particularly nonverbally.

The following illustrations distinguish the functioning and contextual components of a client's verbal message.

CLIENT: I am feeling miserable ever since I was laid off from my job at the plant.

The first part of the message ("I am feeling miserable") denotes an aspect of the client's affective functioning—misery. The latter portion of the message ("ever since I was laid off from my job at the plant") identifies the context.

The following illustrates the same client with a different functioning focus.

CLIENT: I keep thinking to myself, "You'll never find another job" since my job at the plant was eliminated.

The initial portion of this message ("I keep thinking to myself, 'You'll never find another job'") identifies one of the client's cognitions in the same context as the previous example.

Finally, the same client expresses an aspect of behavioral functioning:

CLIENT: I just sit around and do nothing since I lost my job.

The introductory portion of this message ("I just sit around and do nothing") describes a behavior being exhibited in, again, the same context. Note that in all three messages the client is maintaining a present tense focus. Even though the job loss occurred in the past, it is the client's present functioning that presents the problem. The effective therapist discriminates both the functioning and contextual parts of clients' messages because it is important that they both be responded to.

Reflections are meant to direct clients' attention to the therapist's understanding of what they have said, the purpose being to communicate empathic understanding and to help the client to discriminate and define a problem situation and specific aspects relating to it. Learning to reflect involves recalling the client's message, identifying the functioning component (or components) and context, translating the message into your own words, and then orally communicating this to the client. For example:

CLIENT: I've had it with working there! Complaints, complaints, complaints. That's all I ever hear.

The therapist goes through these steps:

1. Recall the client's message to yourself.
2. Identify the functioning component and relevant context (affective functioning; context: complaints at work, client's affective response in the present tense).
3. Translate the message into your own words. For example, "I've had it" might be translated into the feeling disgusted . . . with working there! The message "Complaints, complaints, complaints. That's all I ever hear" might be translated into "all the complaints you keep hearing at work."
4. Verbally communicate a reflection to the client: "You're disgusted with all the complaints you keep hearing at work."

Affective Reflections. Affective reflections mirror clients' affective functioning. These reflections of feeling or emotion can occur at different levels. That is, the therapist can, at the most obvious level, reflect only the surface feelings of clients. At a deeper level, therapists might reflect an implied feeling with greater intensity than was overtly expressed by the client. A basic level affective reflection occurs when therapists reflect a client's expressed affect in a manner that captures the same feeling and intensity as explicitly stated by the client.

CLIENT: I get so depressed when it rains on the weekend.
THERAPIST: You feel down in the dumps on rainy weekends.

In an anticipatory reflection, therapists respond to clients' affect that is obviously implied although not directly expressed. The most effective deeper level reflection is one that *anticipates* what the client might communicate if he or she went one step further (Hackney & Cormier, 1979). Consider the anticipatory reflection in the following illustration: note that the therapist reflects the client's implied affect, anticipating what the client would *like* to feel.

CLIENT: I feel like I have no choice but to do whatever it takes to make him happy.
THERAPIST: It sounds as if you'd feel relieved to let him take responsibility for making himself happy.

One of the major problems often faced by beginning therapists in using affective reflections is identifying an appropriate array of affect words. Cormier and Cormier (1979) identify five categories of emotion: happiness, sadness, fear, uncertainty, and anger. Identifying appropriate affective words spontaneously requires the development of a varied affective vocabulary. Commonly used affect words are listed in Table 8–1.

Another concern of beginning therapists is the wording of affective reflections. Affective reflections are not defined by beginning with "you feel" but by whether they mirror the emotional aspect of a client's communications with *appropriate affect words*. Frequently, beginning therapists will consider any response that begins with "you feel" or "you feel that" as an affective reflection (Cormier & Cormier, 1979). Just beginning a response with "you feel" does not ensure it will accurately focus on clients' feelings. For example, "You feel that she hasn't treated you fairly" reflects only context, whereas "You feel *upset* that she hasn't treated you fairly" reflects both affect and context.

Behavioral Reflections. Behavioral reflections focus on clients' actions. Their formulation and communication is the same as affective reflecting, but with a focus on behavior as opposed to affect. Behavioral reflections can similarly focus either on surface level explicit, or implicit, anticipatory client communications. For example:

CLIENT: I need to pass this course to graduate, but I just don't know where I'll find the time to study.

THERAPIST A: Passing the course and graduation depend upon your ability to find the time to study.

THERAPIST B: Scheduling your time better seems critical if you're to pass the course and graduate.

TABLE 8–1
Commonly Used Affect Words

Happiness	Sadness	Fear	Uncertainty	Anger
Happy	Discouraged	Scared	Puzzled	Upset
Pleased	Disappointed	Anxious	Confused	Frustrated
Satisfied	Hurt	Frightened	Unsure	Bothered
Glad	Despairing	Defensive	Uncertain	Annoyed
Optimistic	Depressed	Threatened	Skeptical	Irritated
Good	Disillusioned	Afraid	Doubtful	Resentful
Relaxed	Dismayed	Tense	Undecided	Mad
Content	Pessimistic	Nervous	Bewildered	Outraged
Cheerful	Miserable	Uptight	Mistrustful	Hassled
Thrilled	Unhappy	Uneasy	Insecure	Offended
Delighted	Hopeless	Worried	Bothered	Angry
Excited	Lonely	Panicked	Disoriented	Furious

SOURCE: From *Interviewing Strategies for Helpers: A Guide to Assessment, Treatment, and Evaluation*, by W. H. Cormier and L. S. Cormier. Copyright © 1979 by Wadsworth, Inc. Reprinted by permission of the publisher, Brooks/Cole Publishing Company, Monterey, California.

Therapist A reflects the client's explicit message while Therapist B helps the client anticipate what needs to be done to improve the situation. Both are appropriate therapist responses. As the therapeutic process evolves, the anticipatory reflection is often of greater utility as a focus toward specific problem definition and then consideration of goal setting are more pronounced.

Cognitive Reflections. Cognitive reflections focus on clients' thoughts, beliefs, and expectations. Like affective and behavioral reflections, cognitive reflections can be at an explicit surface level, or an implied anticipatory level. To illustrate:

CLIENT: The expectations I had going into my new job have simply not been met.
THERAPIST A: You thought things on the job would be a lot different than they turned out to be.
THERAPIST B: After being on the job for a time, you're thinking, "Is this what I really want?"

Therapist A replies to what the client has explicitly expressed, communicating to the client, "This is what I hear you saying." Therapist B reflects at an anticipatory level, implying "Given the context, logically my next thought is . . ."

Multifocus Reflections. Occasionally, especially in beginning the therapeutic process, it is appropriate to focus on more than one area of client functioning. Such multifocus reflections often communicate to clients a counselor's full acceptance of all aspects of their world. Some theoretical orientations, while focusing primarily on one specific area of client functioning, need to accumulate relevant information on more than one functioning component.

Rational-emotive theory looks at client problems in terms of its ABC model. The therapist employing this as his or her primary theoretical position focuses on a client's cognitions, the "Bs." However, in discriminating and defining Bs, As and Cs need to be explored and elaborated upon. Clients' As are frequently specific actions they have exhibited while their "Cs" are resultant emotions. Multifocus reflections addressing a behavioral A and an affective C contribute significantly to a clearer discrimination and definition of relevant Bs. For example:

CLIENT: Whenever I start procrastinating, I begin to feel depressed.
THERAPIST: [the basic ABC model having been previously explained to the client as a part of structuring] So A, your procrastination, appears to directly lead to your feelings of depression at C.

Further Investigation Through Inquiry

It may have occurred to you that many of the reflections in the previous section might have been put into the form of questions. For example:

CLIENT: I've been going round and round trying to come up with a solution to my problem.

THERAPIST A: You're confused about what path to take to solve your problem.

THERAPIST B: How specifically have you been feeling about your inability to arrive at a solution?

Beginning therapists frequently bombard clients with inquiries. This strategy often tends to create a "ping-pong" effect; the therapists asks, the client answers, and so on (Hackney & Cormier, 1979). Counselors who often ask closed inquiries to which clients respond with only one word or very brief answers find themselves having to ask progressively more and more questions in order to elicit the same information that one or two open-ended inquiries would. Egan (1982) has suggested some general guidelines on using inquiries in the counseling process. First, "when clients are asked too many questions, they can feel 'grilled.'" (Egan, 1982, p. 101). Too many questions also interfere with establishing a facilitative therapeutic climate. Benjamin (1981) addresses the issue of too many therapist inquiries:

> I feel certain that we ask too many questions, often meaningless ones. We ask questions that confuse the interviewee, that interrupt him. We ask questions the interviewee cannot possibly answer. We ask questions we don't want answers to, and, consequently, we do not hear the answers when forthcoming. (p. 71)

Using reflections as much as possible alleviates this concern. Turning potential inquiries into statements often results in a relevant reflection that communicates empathic understanding as opposed to "grilling."

Second, as the ultimate emphasis in Phase I of the therapeutic process is problem definition, the purpose of an inquiry should be to assist a client in seeing his or her problem situation more clearly. Therapists who ask too many questions are often working under the false assumption that amassing information, in and of itself, will lead to more effective problem definition.

Third, when inquiries are called for, it is generally better to employ open-ended inquiries as opposed to closed inquiries. Open-ended inquiries require more than the simple *yes* or *no* or similar one-word answer that satisfies closed inquiries. Consider the following inquiries:

OPEN-ENDED INQUIRY: What can you share with me about your relationship with Patty?

CLOSED INQUIRY: Do you and Patty get along?

The open-ended inquiry leaves room for the client to elaborate on her relationship with Patty. It will tend to almost always elicit more information from the client than the closed inquiry will.

CLIENT'S RESPONSE TO THE CLOSED INQUIRY: Sometimes, but not so well lately.

CLIENT'S RESPONSE TO THE OPEN-ENDED INQUIRY: Well, Patty and I have been roommates for four years now. We've gone through a lot during that time. Our relationship has had its ups and downs, but lately its been mostly downs. She . . .

The most effective open-ended inquiries serve as free invitations to talk and usually begin with *what* or *how*. Research has revealed that *what* inquiries best solicit facts and the gathering of information ("What happened when you attempted to be more assertive at work?"). *How* inquiries are typically associated with sequence and process or emotion ("How do you feel about your present situation?") (Ivey & Simek-Downing, 1980). Although *why* inquiries are considered open-ended, they are usually not recommended for beginning counselors as they tend to move away from critical here-and-now issues and look to the past to explain present problems. *Why* inquiries also tend to create defensiveness in clients, being inherently more difficult for them to answer. Frequently, the response to a *why* inquiry is *because* ("Why did you do that?" . . . "Because I did.").

It is important to note that an inquiry, open-ended or closed, on a topic of deep interest to a client will often result in extensive elaboration *if* it is interesting enough and important enough (Ivey, 1983). Further, there are times when closed questions are needed to elicit a brief pointed response about a specific piece of information. A closed inquiry may also work as a deterrant to further discussion. It may be used to stop clients' verbalizations if they are straying from the central issue at hand. The major point to consider is not inquiries in and of themselves, but how they relate to and promote or hinder problem discrimination and definition and other process goals within the therapeutic process.

Selecting the Dominant Foci: Summarization

Summarization is gathering together a client's verbal and nonverbal communications and presenting them to the client in outline form. Summarization involves attending to the client, recognizing the client's thoughts, feelings, behaviors and their relevant contexts, and integrating and ordering what has happened over a period of time, from a few minutes to several sessions. The therapist then selects the most cogent and important points and summarizes them for the client (Ivey & Simek-Downing, 1980).

A summarization serves as a bridging response to help clients discriminate and define their problems in a more focused and concrete way (Egan, 1982). It serves to condense and crystallize the essence of a client's communications. This essence is often seen in the themes or patterns that emerge as clients explore and elaborate on their problem situations. Typically, clients express a variety of concerns. At the outset, these concerns may appear unrelated. In seeking to determine the most critical components as concretely as possible, the relationship among various incidents, circumstances, difficulties, and experiences become apparent. For example:

SITUATION: Kathy has been describing her difficulties in her position at the agency where she works. She and the therapist explore this problem for about 20 minutes. The therapist then offers a summarization to provide more focus for her.

THERAPIST: Kathy, you mentioned that you haven't been able to approach your supervisor about a raise you surely have earned. You also noted how everyone else is dumping their work on you because they know you won't say *no*. You identified having few friends because no one seems to approach you and you don't appear to make any first efforts toward anyone else. It sounds like your nonassertive behavior is affecting all areas of your work environment.

Notice that the therapist focuses primarily on Kathy's behavioral functioning at work, and the central theme is a lack of assertive behavior. Viewing her overall situation from this concrete and concise vantage point, Kathy is ready to move on to goal setting. The primary problem has been discriminated from among the many presented and concretely defined.

Summarization, when effective, creates a more specific and intense client focus. Ineffective summarization, that is, a summarization that merely rehashes the many things the client may have communicated, can distract rather than help focus. Consider the summarization in the same case without the final essential focus.

> Kathy, you mentioned that you haven't been able to approach your supervisor about a raise you surely have earned. You also noted how everyone else is dumping their work on you because they know you won't say *no*. You identified having few friends because no one seems to approach you and you don't appear to make any first efforts toward anyone else.

Notice how without the statement, "It sounds like your nonassertive behavior is affecting all areas of your work," no specific focus is readily recognizable and thus problem discrimination and definition is not facilitated. Rather, Kathy is left feeling overwhelmed by her failures at work with no indication of how to improve her situation.

Summarizations, although they can be used at any time to assist clients in gaining focus and direction, are especially useful at certain times (Egan, 1982): at the beginning of a new session to prevent repetition of previous interchanges and provide initial focus and direction; during a session when a client is rambling and needs direction; and when a client has exhausted a certain topic and is unable to proceed with more focus and direction.

Focusing for Theoretical Implementation

Observations of counselors reveal that they selectively focus on and selectively ignore certain client messages (Ivey & Simek-Downing, 1980). The diversity of client messages presents therapists with a wide array of issues to selectively consider. Different theoretical orientations stress different information as most important as well.

When a client presents multiple issues relating to multiple areas of functioning in many contexts, the therapist can respond to all of the messages or only part of them. If only part of the client's message is responded to, that portion not responded to will likely be dropped by the client in future communications (Hackney & Cormier, 1979). Based on your primary therapeutic position, certain areas of a client's life should interest you more than others. For effective implementation of a specific theoretical orientation, it is critical this counselor focus always be kept under consideration and concretely addressed.

THERAPIST SKILLS II: THEORETICAL APPLICATIONS

Diagnosis

Traditionally, some practitioners view overt problem discrimination and definition, or diagnosis, as essential to therapeutic effectiveness. Others see it as inimical or even detrimental to the therapeutic process. The commonly espoused purpose of diagnosis in counseling and psychotherapy is to gain sufficient knowledge of a client's functioning so that goal setting and thus a treatment plan can be tailored to the client's needs (Corey, 1982). Behavior therapists epitomize this position with their emphasis on concrete specification of problem behaviors. They believe that without an objective appraisal of specific client functioning, no adequate treatment plan can be developed, nor can any evaluation be conducted on the effectiveness of intervention efforts.

Rogers (1951), by contrast, maintains that diagnosis is detrimental because it is an external way of understanding a client. It tends to pull the client away from his or her internal and subjective experience and foster an external, objective, intellectualized conception *about* the client. According to Rogers, the client is the one who knows the dynamics of his or her behavior, and for change to occur the client must experience a perceptual change, not simply receive data about him or herself.

As a proponent of existential therapy, Arbuckle (1975) similarly saw diagnosis as inappropriate in therapy, noting that "diagnosis misses entirely the reality of the inner person. It is the measure of me from the outside in, it is a measure of me by others, and it ignores my subjective being" (p. 255). Interestingly, however, both Arbuckle and Rogers do not decry an "internal" diagnosis of clients' concerns. For example, Arbuckle (1975) proposes that instead of an external, "ego-satisfying diagnostic picture" of a client, therapists should try to grasp his or her internal world. Rogers's emphasis on empathic understanding can likewise be perceived as an internal diagnosis of sorts.

Gestalt therapists also tend to avoid overt diagnosis. The Gestalt therapist's function is seen as assisting clients to more fully experience their feelings, enabling them to make their own interpretations. Clients are expected to carry out their own therapy; they make their own interpretations, create their own direct statements, and find their own meanings.

Diagnostic labels are not a part of reality therapy, viewed as at best unnecessary and at worst damaging to a client by establishing an identity that tends to perpetuate irresponsible and unsuccessful behavior. Reality therapists' "diagnosis" is more a planning for change, not a providing of rationales for past or present problems. Much of the significant work in the initial phase of therapy addresses specific ways that failure behavior can be changed into success behavior.

The cognitively-oriented approaches all are similar to behavior therapy in stressing the need to gain sufficient knowledge of clients' functioning so that goal setting and intervention can be accomplished. Whether employing the terms rational or irrational beliefs, personal rules of living, or structural or transactional analysis, these approaches' basic concepts call for overt cognitive diagnosis as a core condition for the practice of the particular approach.

Focusing Skills

Reflection is a primary therapist skill in person-centered therapy. The therapist focuses on the subjective elements of what clients say in order to communicate empathic understanding and help clients clarify their feelings as well as experience them with more intensity. The goal is to help clients move to deeper levels of self-exploration and awareness. Although reflection is a frequently used therapist rapport-building and clarification tool in all therapeutic approaches, it is emphasized the most by person-centered therapists.

Summarizations are used to a lesser degree in affectively-oriented approaches compared to the behaviorally-oriented and especially cognitively-oriented theoretical positions. None of the approaches tends to particularly emphasize, or neglect, summarization as a therapist skill.

The use of inquiries and their role in therapy presents greater divergence among theories. Inquiries are a major skill employed by rational-emotive therapists, in which therapists' questioning of clients' irrational beliefs is thought to help clients look more critically at these beliefs themselves. Likewise, the Transactional Analysis therapist uses inquiries to help clients discover early decisions and make new decisions. Gestalt therapists see *why* questions as unproductive intellectualization. They ask *what* and *how* inquiries to help clients focus on their here-and-now experience. Reality therapists too shun *why* inquiries. They believe the reasons for past irresponsible behavior are unessential. Behavior therapists use inquiries in establishing behaviors, goals, and evaluation criteria. Existential therapists use inquiries to facilitate client awareness. No particular therapist skill is stressed.

CHARLES: PHASE II

The beginning of Charles's first session with the counselor, Kay Simmons, in chapter 7 emphasized the essentials for creating a therapeutic climate. The session continues and the process proceeds into Phase II: Problem Discrimination and Definition.

THERAPIST SKILLS II

inquiry

COUNSELOR: How exactly do you perceive a need to change? What might be a specific example of how you think you must adapt to this new life situation?

CHARLES: Well, I've geared my life for a couple of years . . . I've done a lot of traveling. And I just like to travel to see new parts of the country and I geared a lot of my experience into being out in a camping situation . . . wilderness situation . . . where I could work with people who have problems or things like that . . . where I could teach them how to use recreation to help themselves. But that kind of job requires a lot of traveling . . . where I'd be gone for 30 days and then get to come home for a week . . . and then be gone again . . . and that kind of life-style is just not going to work when you have someone at home who's wanting you to be home.

COUNSELOR: Go on. Expound on what you've said a bit more.

CHARLES: It's just confusing to me because now I'm having to stay here in one city and my experience . . . everything I've done in the past that's required me to qualify for jobs . . . had a requirement of travel. So here I am . . . I can't get a job 'cause I don't have the experience I need . . . you know to be a supervisor or something. Or whatever . . . I guess I'm feeling a little inadequate.

COUNSELOR: You want to commit yourself to this one person and yet are thinking that doing so will prevent you from pursuing your present career, or even more specifically, finding a suitable job at all.

reflection/behavioral-cognitive focus

CHARLES: Right. I don't know. I'm so restless I'm not sure if I can ever be satisfied staying in one place. I don't know. This person means so much to me . . . I don't know how to work it out.

COUNSELOR: Let's look at work a bit more specifically. You seem to feel confident that you don't have the skills to find an acceptable job in this one area rather than having to do a lot of traveling. What might be some jobs that you might be interested in . . . even if you think that you don't have the skills . . . to work within this city?

reflection/affective-behavioral focus/inquiry

CHARLES: Well, as I said, I'm geared toward recreation. And a new field that's coming out is therapeutic recreation. At the time I graduated from school, they weren't really graduating people in that field. But now, they've created a field where you can graduate with a degree in therapeutic recreation. And since I don't have that specific degree, people feel like I don't have the qualifications to work with mental health, special ed., or the handicapped. Whereas, I feel I do. It's just a matter of getting a foot in the door. And I don't seem to be able to get anywhere because all of my experience was with camping situations . . . having a strong wilderness background . . . where I dealt with survival strategies . . . teaching in that kind of program, instead of adaptive recreation or whatever.

COUNSELOR: You're finding it terribly frustrating because in looking for a job in the city, you see yourself as having the skills required, but you've been unable to express this to potential employers.

reflection/affective-behavioral focus

CHARLES: Right. It's really been a pain. Especially being in a position where even those jobs I am applying for are at a low level. Having to be a bottom level person . . . I feel like I'm qualified to be up in the world, but, like I say, I'm stuck here in Jacksonville. But, I made that decision to be here, but it's driving me kinda crazy because I'm having to deal with it not working out so well and it's just confusing me I guess. I don't know what. I would hate to blame my girlfriend for all of this. And yet sometimes I feel like I'm doing just that.

COUNSELOR: So another primary concern you have is some feelings of guilt you're experiencing over the times you put the blame for job difficulties on your girlfriend . . . rather than keeping them in the proper perspective. You're thinking, "I'm terrible for feeling resentful of her desire to be near me."

reflection/affective-cognitive focus

CHARLES: Right. I would hate to mess up the relationship we've built. I don't know what to do.

COUNSELOR: How do you think you're going to mess up the relationship? I know you said you've been blaming her for your job difficulties, but what might be a specific example of when you put the blame on her that affected your relationship recently?

inquiry

CHARLES: Well, just this morning I was thinking to myself: "I'm the one that's having to take a lower position and that's really frustrating for me. And I'm the one doing the changing . . . she doesn't want to travel and get into the field I'm interested in . . . she's so set in her ways."

reflection/affective-cognitive focus

COUNSELOR: Thinking those thoughts would surely start you feeling a lot of resentment toward your girlfriend. And if you were thinking them when you were with her . . .

CHARLES: Well, Jacksonville is her home and this is where she wants to stay. This is where she wants to die! Whereas, I see so much out there. She's never considered a change of location just so I could be closer to something . . . more directed to me . . . and she could also possibly be closer to something . . . in her line of work. But she just doesn't feel like she should be doing the changing. It's me. I don't know. We try to talk about it. But we don't get very far. It usually ends up in fighting. I just want to yell out, "Be a little flexible!"

reflection/affective-behavioral-cognitive focus

COUNSELOR: So you become angry and frustrated not only when you're actually interacting with her, but also when you're thinking, "She's like a rock. I'm the one who has to do all the changing. It's just not right!"

CHARLES: Right . . . and I'm scared that down the road I'm going to rebel . . . that it's going to build up inside me . . . and I want to learn how to deal with it now so that it doesn't build up for years and years.

reflection/behavioral focus

COUNSELOR: It sounds like you see yourself not having what are called "coping skills" to deal with the different stressors that confront you.

CHARLES: Yeah. I feel like a walking time bomb. I'm just waiting for my head to blow up. I don't know . . . you never know when it's going to happen to you.

inquiry

COUNSELOR: When you say "it's" going to happen to you, what is this "it's"?

CHARLES: Well, you know . . . I start everyday just wondering . . . well, what's going to happen today? I don't feel excited about the days anymore . . . like I used to . . . and I feel like I'm just existing instead of living . . . don't know where to turn to or what to do.

reflection/affective-behavioral focus

COUNSELOR: So you find yourself at a loss at what to do. It sounds like you're experiencing some depression over the pessimism that you see as hovering over all that you do.

CHARLES: Yeah. I think the depression is coming from I've never had to sit still and think about what to do . . . here in Jacksonville. If I ever got to feeling down, I'd just cut off what I was doing . . . and I'd go do something else.

inquiry

COUNSELOR: What might be an example?

CHARLES: Head for the mountains or go camping. Leave Florida . . . get it out of my system. I spent a lot of my time leaving and going and doing what I wanted to and then coming back. But now I don't feel like I can just pack up and leave . . . I feel a lot of pressure I guess. Like I said, I feel like a time bomb most of the time . . . There's always the other side of the coin too though . . . the times I'm with my girlfriend I feel a lot of happiness. Enough to make me start to change my lifestyle. But it's having to find a happy medium.

COUNSELOR: Charles, let's see if we can summarize a bit and try to get all of what we've discussed so far into the proper perspective. You've mentioned a number of related, although different concerns: 1) You've got career concerns; determining whether to settle here in Jacksonville and if so, finding suitable employment. You see yourself as having the skills you need but have been unable to adequately present them to potential employers. 2) You've got some relationship concerns . . . feeling a real bonding with your girlfriend, but distressed about her rigidity . . . your thoughts about it and how you see it affecting your relationship, both now and especially in the future. And, 3) you're feeling depressed a lot of the time and not able to get yourself out of it. It sounds like the overriding issue with all of these concerns is what you just mentioned . . . finding a happy medium . . . being able to make satisfactory decisions that you can act on.

summarization

CHARLES: Yeah, that pretty much sums it all up.

COUNSELOR: Our time is just about up for this session. What are your thoughts about coming back again and going on further with what we began with today?

CHARLES: I'd like that.

COUNSELOR: Great. Let's set up a time. I think that we accomplished a lot in today's session.

SUGGESTED READINGS

Diagnosis

Bandler, J., & Grinder, R. (1975). *The structure of magic: I.* Palo Alto, CA: Science and Behavior Books. Bandler and Grinder offer an extensive discussion of language analysis in the therapeutic process coupled with an innovative examination of the meaning of nonverbal communication and verbal-nonverbal incongruities.

Knapp, M. L. (1978). *Nonverbal communication in human interaction* (2nd ed.). New York: Holt, Rinehart and Winston. Knapp provides some particularly informative and applicable ideas about various cues which accompany verbal speech.

Okun, B. F. (1982). *Effective helping: Interviewing and counseling techniques* (2nd ed.). Monterey, CA: Brooks/Cole. This book offers fine ideas, not only on understanding client verbal and nonverbal messages, but also the importance of counselor self-awareness as a diagnostic entity.

Patterson, L. E., & Eisenberg, S. (1983). *The counseling process* (3rd ed.). Boston: Houghton Mifflin. An excellent chapter in this book is "Diagnosis in Counseling."

Shulman, L. (1979). *The skills of helping: Individuals and groups.* Itasca, IL: Peacock. Shulman's assertions about what he terms "tuning in" and "tuning in skills" offer a superb stance for therapists to assume when seeking to form a diagnostic impression.

Focusing Skills

Benjamin, A. (1974). *The helping interview* (2nd ed.). Boston: Houghton Mifflin. Benjamin provides a graduated list of focusing responses and leads, starting with client-centered, shifting progressively to therapist-centered, then to authoritarian, and concluding with open use of therapist authority.

Cormier, W. H., & Cormier, L. S. (1979). *Interviewing strategies for helpers: A guide to assessment, treatment, and evaluation.* Monterey, CA: Brooks/Cole. This is likely one of the most complete and definitive works for the beginning therapist from a skills viewpoint. The section on "interview discrimination" is unsurpassed.

Evans, D. R., Hearn, M. T., Uhlemann, M. R., & Ivey, A. E. (1979). *Effective interviewing: A programmed approach to effective communication.* Monterey, CA: Brooks/Cole. This self-programmed text includes some superb chapters outlining various focusing skills followed by a summary chapter, "Putting it All Together."

Hackney, H. L., & Cormier, L. S. (1979). *Counseling strategies and objectives* (2nd ed.). Englewood Cliffs, NJ: Prentice-Hall. The authors' assertions about responding to client-cognitive content and client-affective content as well as discriminating between the two offer somewhat unusual ideas not often addressed so directly.

Ivey, A. E. (1983). *Intentional interviewing and counseling.* Monterey, CA: Brooks/Cole. Ivey's discussion on "Tuning in with Clients and Directing Conversational Flow" offers a sample interview to consider and practice exercises for self-assessment.

9

Phase Three: Goal Setting

Very often, the client's point of view or perspective is not enough. These perspectives are too self-limiting or self-defeating. Clients need to move beyond their own frames of reference to new perspectives on themselves and the problem situation. Old ways of thinking are not working; they are not leading to goal setting, program development, and action.

(Egan, 1982, p. 151)

Therapeutic goals are of two types: outcome goals and process goals. Outcome goals are the results clients expect to attain from counseling.

> Dennis wants a raise but is afraid to ask his boss for it. He believes that his boss, whom he describes as blunt, cold, and quick to anger, is the problem. He also has described his anxiety—a fear of authority figures—as a problem, as well as his lack of assertive behaviors. In addition, he reports relatively constant thoughts such as "It would be horrible if I asked for a raise and was told my work didn't warrant it."

Dennis's major outcome goal is to be able to ask for, and, ideally, attain, a raise in pay at work. By contrast, process goals are the objectives the therapist considers necessary if clients are to achieve their outcome goals. An affectively-oriented therapist, for example, would view Dennis's relief from anxiety and his having more confident, assured feelings as prerequisites to working toward his outcome goal. As a result of a more positive affective state, Dennis's lack of assertive behavior and his self-denigrating thoughts would likely dissipate. He would *feel* more confident and thus think "I can do it," and act in kind. The process goal of affective change is seen as instrumental in bringing about the outcome goal of asking for a raise.

The different theoretical orientations' process goals are derived from the domain of human functioning that constitutes their primary emphasis. In process goal setting, therapists' firm theoretical grounding is critical because *theory* (or theories in the case of the experienced therapist operating from a pragmatic therapeutic postion) directs the process. This is not to suggest that outcome goals are ignored, but rather that upon gaining counselor-client agreement as to specific outcome goals, process goals are necessary in order to achieve them. Therapists must help clients develop new perspectives by setting process goals. The course of goal setting in Phase III of the therapeutic process is illustrated in Figure 9–1.

RECONSIDERING CONTEXT

In Chapter 8 we discussed the importance of *context*, the degree to which environmental factors affect clients' functioning and visa versa. Its importance cannot be overstressed. Although this chapter discusses goal setting

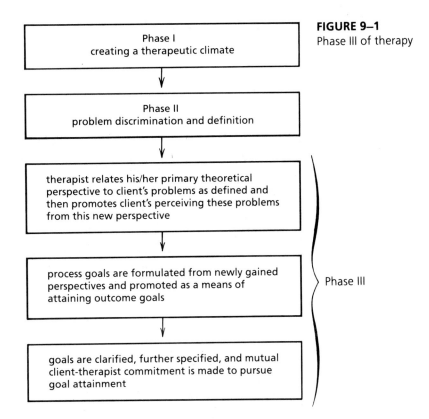

FIGURE 9–1
Phase III of therapy

for clients' *individual* functioning, the potential of environmental factors being the predominant precipitators of clients' problems must always be considered. Lewis and Lewis (1977) stress this position:

> Traditionally, it has always been assumed that the objects of change should be the attitudes, feelings, or the behaviors of the counselee. . . . We are becoming more aware every day, however, that sometimes the obstacles to a "productive and self-satisfying" life are in the environment, and not in the individual's own behaviors. Sometimes the solution to a problem is out of the counselee's hands. (p. 205)

Returning to the case of Dennis, it may be true that his boss is "blunt, cold, quick to anger" *and* completely autocratic and unyielding. Dennis may be quite correct in assuming that the boss is the primary problem. There may, in fact, be no way that Dennis will get the raise in pay he seeks at his present job. While this fact does not necessarily affect the process goals, it will likely necessitate altering the outcome goal.

Dennis' outcome goal of a pay raise being almost certainly blocked, other choices must be raised. He could still try for the raise; although he most probably won't get it, his boss might change his rigid stance. He could seek a higher paying position with another company. Or, he could learn to accept his present situation, if only temporarily, and not let himself be so adversely affected. All of these alternative outcome goals, however, still require similar process goals in order to be attained. For the affectively-oriented therapist working with Dennis, reducing Dennis's anxiety and simultaneously helping him gain confidence and feelings of comfort (with the theoretically-assumed positive behavioral and cognitive changes) is an appropriate process goal if Dennis is to either find a new, better paying job or exist more peacefully in his present job.

To paraphrase the motto of Alcoholics Anonymous, in considering context, individual counseling and psychotherapy efforts and therefore goals should seek to help clients try to change the environmental factors that can be changed, to gracefully accept those that they cannot, and be able to discriminate between the two.

PROMOTING NEW PERSPECTIVES

Many clients enter therapy with a fine realization already in hand as to what their primary problem is. They require little session time for discrimination and definition of their concerns. Their reason for coming to counseling is not a lack of awareness of the problem, but rather a lack of understanding as to what they must do to alleviate the problem. Other clients may need more session time for discriminating and defining their major concerns. All clients, however, ultimately need to develop new perspectives on their problems so they can see more clearly *where they want to be.*

These new perspectives are not sought for their own sake, but rather to facilitate goal setting. Only new perspectives with this purpose should be offered by the therapist. In providing clients new perspectives from which to view their problem situation, therapists should ask themselves, "In what way will this insight lead to change that will help the client more effectively handle this problem?" (Egan, 1982).

To illustrate this *purposeful insight* consider the case of Betsy.

Betsy, 37, has been talking to the therapist about the quality of her social life and her desire to form a more lasting long-term relationship, preferably marriage. She expresses her dissatisfaction with the string of fleeting relationships she has had over the last two years especially.

THERAPIST: Betsy, you've mentioned that your desire to get married has particularly intensified in the past two years. It seems to have done so progressively with each "fleeting" relationship that hasn't turned into a marriage proposal. It sounds like you're thinking, "This fellow has *got to* be the one" as soon as a relationship looks at all promising. Is it possible that may be pushing marriage too much on those male friends you are meeting as a result?

BETSY: (after a short silence) In thinking about it you may have something. I am 37 though and if someone doesn't come along soon, my prospects for marriage are only going to decrease.

From a cognitive orientation, the therapist focuses on Betsy's various "got to" cognitions and their effects on her feelings and behaviors. For example, her belief, "I'm 37 and if someone doesn't come along soon . . ." was examined in terms of the relevant "desperation" behaviors that result when an eligible marriage prospect does present himself. Betsy thus developed a new perspective, fresh insight into herself and her problem situation. The insight is not static; it is dynamic and directly facilitates goal setting. From within the theoretical framework chosen, Betsy and the therapist have a process goal; that is, restructuring Betsy's "got to" thinking and thereby altering her desperation behaviors and accompanying emotional distress.

Therapist skills that can be employed to promote new perspectives include information giving, interpretation, confrontation, self-disclosure, and immediacy. Each of these will now be examined in detail.

Information Giving

Information giving is the "verbal communication of data or facts about experiences, events, alternatives, or people" (Cormier & Cormier, 1979, p. 105). It includes both providing new information to and correcting prior misinformation of clients. Therapists can give information to promote new client perspectives in four primary ways. First, new information can help clients in becoming aware of possible alternatives to their present situation. As Gelatt, Varenhorst, Carey, and Miller (1973) propose, "a person's choices are increased if he can create new alternatives based on information" (p. 6). Thus, new information about possible alternatives can facilitate goal setting. For example:

Theo has been discussing with the therapist the difficulty he has had in meeting women since moving to New York City. He is especially discouraged with the bar scene which was his mainstay back in Ft. Lauderdale.

THERAPIST: Theo, you've noted how your old lines just don't appear to make it here in New York and how you find the bar scene much different. I wonder if you've considered that singles here may not frequent bars for the same purposes as they did in Florida. It may not be your approach so much as the places you're trying to use it. We might want to look at some alternative places that New York City single men and women frequent to meet new people.

New information can also create new client insights when the possible outcomes of a particular manner of functioning are shared. Giving information assists clients evaluate the different choices available to them. For example,

---

Louise, 19 and unmarried, is having her second unexpected and unwanted pregnancy. She terminated her previous pregnancy through abortion and since has been feeling deeply guilty about that course of action. She has stated that she isn't ready to accept the responsibilities of pregnancy or parenthood alone but because of her guilt is going to have the child and raise it herself no matter.

THERAPIST: Louise, you're feeling so much guilt about your previous pregnancy and abortion, seeing the abortion particularly as a mistake. At that time you say you knew what you were doing was against your value system and you would regret it. Now, in the same situation, you are going to pursue another path but one that is similarly opposed to what you see as in your best interests. Perhaps you're going to end up with the same debilitating feelings.

Information giving is also valuable in helping clients correct invalid or unreliable data and in dispelling myths that motivate maladaptive functioning.

Tina, 15, is heavily using dangerous drugs. She maintains that LSD is "super" and potential side effects are only the positive highs she gets.

THERAPIST: Tina, you've mentioned a number of times about the super highs you get on acid and how it's the thing to do. Are you aware of all the medical research that shows some potentially severe long-term problems resulting from frequent LSD use, especially during the formative years?

Finally, information is most commonly used to directly instruct clients in the content or procedures of specific theoretical orientations and intervention strategies. Behavioral- and cognitive-oriented therapists, in particular, give extensive information. For example, the therapist who primarily uses Transactional Analysis will need to teach clients the terminology necessary to analyze their concerns within a TA framework in order to facilitate process goal setting. Likewise, the behavioral-oriented therapist must teach relaxation training and hierarchy development for systematic desensitization to help the anxiously disturbed client to be able to work toward goal attainment of a more relaxed and less fearful manner of functioning.

In giving information, Lewis (1970) emphasizes that the information should be a tool for counseling, not an end in itself. As a tool, providing information is most appropriate when the need for information is directly related to a client's concerns and potential goals and when the information is expressly used to help clients achieve their goals.

Cormier and Cormier (1979) provide guidelines for therapists' use of information giving that follows a *when, what,* and *how* structure. Table 9–1 summarizes this information-giving framework.

The first guideline, *when,* is the therapist's recognition of a client's need for information. If a client does not have sufficient information about a problem or has misinformation, a need exists. The therapist then turns to the *what* guideline by identifying the kinds of information a client might use in developing a new perspective and where the information can be found. The therapist should consider presenting information sequentially; often a client will need to comprehend some things before he or she can assimilate others. Finally, the *how,* the actual delivery of the information, should be performed in such a way that it is "usable" to a client and encourages the client to "hear and apply" the information (Gazda, Walters, & Childers, 1975).

The information giving should be well-timed. Therapists should find indications of a client's receptivity before attempting to deliver it. Confusion, not knowing the next step to take, outright requests, and the like are clear signs that clients are ready for new information. Remember too that the quality and level of client readiness reflects the level to which core conditions and the therapist's social influence have been established.

Information should be presented objectively. There are usually disadvantages as well as advantages to perceiving problem situations in new ways. Objectively presenting information does not mean to overemphasize disadvantages in order to "be fair," but rather to heighten awareness of all aspects of a situation. Consider as well how much information clients can assimilate. Limiting the amount of information presented at any one time and presenting it progressively is important.

Further, discuss clients' reactions to new information and whether they will ultimately use it. Be careful, however, not to continue too long in simply discussing information as continued talking can reinforce some clients' avoidance of goal setting and action (Gelatt, et al., 1973). Make certain that data given to clients is accurate. If you are unsure of information, offer to get back to a client after consulting the appropriate

TABLE 9–1
The "When," "What," and "How" of Information-Giving

When—Recognizing Client's Need for Information	What—Identifying type of Information	How—Delivery of Information in Interview
1. Identify information presently available to client. 2. Evaluate client's present information—Is it valid? data-based? sufficient?	1. Identify kind of information useful to client. 2. Identify possible reliable sources of information. 3. Identify any sequencing of information (option A before option B).	1. Wait for client cue of readiness; don't give information prematurely. 2. Present all the relevant facts; don't protect client from negative information. 3. Limit amount of information given at one time; don't overload. 4. Ask for and discuss client's feelings and biases about information. 5. Know when to stop giving information so action isn't avoided. 6. Validate information with other sources for accuracy.

SOURCE: From *Interviewing Strategies for Helpers: A Guide to Assessment, Treatment, and Evaluation*, by W. H. Cormier and L. S. Cormier. Copyright © 1979 by Wadsworth, Inc. Reprinted by permission of the publisher, Brooks/Cole Publishing Company, Monterey, California.

resource or refer clients to other professionals for specifics. For example, medical information often affects clients' goals for therapy. Finally, providing information should not be confused with giving advice. Advice giving offers little choice to clients. Information giving challenges the client to consider a new perspective, but there is an implied choice inherent in it that is left with the client.

Interpretation

Empathic understanding is a core condition of the therapeutic process and thus is essential to a successful working relationship. Reflections are the primary verbal responses we have introduced up to this point whose major purpose is to communicate empathic understanding. Constant reflection of only expressed affect, behaviors, and thoughts, however, may limit the client's view of the problem situation. Interpretation extends a client's understanding by *going beyond* what clients have overtly said. With interpretations, therapists challenge clients to examine a new and deeper perspective of their situations. That this new and deeper perspective is described as a more intense form of empathic understanding is seen by the descriptors used to identify it: additive empathy (Carkhuff, 1969) and advanced accurate empathy (Egan, 1975).

As a therapist response that goes beyond the verbalized communications of a client and presents implications and assumptions that the client is scarcely aware of or has chosen not to explore, interpretation differs from reflection in that it deals predominantly with *implicit* client communications—what the client does not talk about directly or explicitly. Whereas reflections respond to surface level client communications, interpretation addresses aspects of a client's functioning that are somehow buried, hidden, or beyond the client's immediate reach. It is a tool to use when "the client is not clear about some issue, or if he speaks guardedly, then the helper speaks directly, clearly, and openly" (Egan, 1975, p. 147). For example,

CLIENT: My marriage hasn't been going the greatest, even though I've been working so hard to make the relationship more satisfying. My husband has been doing his best as well. I just don't know where to go from here.

THERAPIST A: It's very frustrating to see both of you work so hard and not be any more satisfied with the relationship.

THERAPIST B: It's tough to put forth all this effort and not be where you want to be in the relationship. Is it possible that no amount of effort is ever going to be enough to get to the point you want?

Therapist A uses reflection to convey empathic understanding to the client. In doing so, Therapist A responds to what the client has explicitly expressed. Therapist B, on the other hand, goes one step further. From the context, the client's nonverbal messages, and from past interchanges, the therapist recognizes a message that the client is implying, but not overtly addressing: the client and her husband have put forth their best effort and that simply hasn't been enough. Therapist B has gone beyond the expressed to the implied. Consider the client's response to each:

CLIENT TO THERAPIST A: We're frustrated and just don't know where to go.

CLIENT TO THERAPIST B: I think that you hit the nail right on the head. We really have given it our best shot and that's just not enough. I guess it's time we think about splitting.

In response to Therapist A, the client stays where she was, understood, but not moving forward. By contrast, Therapist B's interpretation stimulates the client to consider a new perspective, that points toward goal setting and change in the client's life.

As with information giving, the ultimate goal of interpretation is to give clients a new perspective so that appropriate goals become apparent. The potential for a therapist's interpretation facilitating goal setting, however, depends on many factors:

1. Timing is important. Interpretations challenge clients to critically look at themselves and their situations. A solid therapeutic climate established via core conditions and social influence will enable a client to be freer in accepting an interpretation as accurate.

2. Related to timing, clients should be ready to accept an interpretation. Generally, an interpretation is best reserved for a later rather than initial session, since data must be gathered to develop the interpretation. Also, some clients require several sessions to become accustomed to therapy. Clients will be more receptive if they are at ease with the topics being explored and the manner of exploration (Cormier & Cormier, 1979).

3. Brammer & Shostrom (1982) suggest not engaging in interpretation until a client has gained some awareness and understanding of the subject of the intended interpretation. Successive approximations can be used to help clients develop this readiness. If a client, for example, appears utterly unaware of his or her hostile rage being expressed toward a parent, this irritation and frustration might be acknowledged through reflection; then, as the client's self-understanding deepens, the hostility and anger can be interpreted (Bryer & Egan, 1979).

4. Interpretations should be offered tentatively. "I wonder if," "perhaps," "could it be," or "is it possible" reflect the reality that therapists employing this skill can never know with absolute certainty the accuracy of an implication for a client. Tentativeness allows clients to accept or deny an interpretation or alter and thus complete a partially accurate interpretation.

5. Following an interpretation, therapists should check its accuracy by observing the client carefully. Responding with a reflection to a client's reaction to an interpretation is a common practice for clarifying the client's acceptance, alteration, or rejection. Should a client reject an interpretation, the therapist can respond with a reflection, further exploration and discussion, and later restructure the interpretation with more data, provided additional data supports the original premise.

Interpretation can serve several functions: it can help clients recognize the deeper, more implicit aspects of their communications; it can call attention to deficiencies in clients' functioning that inhibit goal setting; and it can address themes, patterns, or causal relationships in a client's functioning or environment.

Identifying What Has Only Been Implied. The most basic interpretation is to tell clients what they have implied but not explicitly stated. Often this means helping clients recognize the logical conclusions that naturally flow from the premises they have offered about their problem situation.

CLIENT: I just don't think I can take living in my parents' home any longer. It's good to be there only because I can keep my living expenses down while I'm finishing college. But their constant hassles have become too much. I can't keep my mind on my coursework living there.

THERAPIST: You state that you only stay with your parents to keep living expenses low so you can finish school. Yet you also note how living there is preventing you from maintaining your studies. Perhaps the problems caused by their hassling you outweigh the advantages of staying there.

Calling Attention to Deficient Functioning. Clients frequently are inhibited in goal setting and thus problem solving because of deficiencies in their manner of functioning, be it affective, behavioral, cognitive, or a combination thereof. Calling clients' attention to these deficiencies and their effects allows for a blocked goal setting process to proceed.

Affective Deficiencies: The subject of Joan's overt communications has been her wariness about others' behaviors at social affairs.

THERAPIST: Joan, you've told me of a number of instances where you would not accept invitations to social occasions because you felt that something embarrassing was bound to happen if you attended. Is it possible that your fear of being embarrassed is not so much a matter of what others' might do as your own feelings of social ineptness?

Behavioral Deficiencies: Harry has been complaining that he has to do "every thing" around the house.

THERAPIST: Harry, you complain that you have to do the cooking, laundry, bill paying and more. You also note your displeasure with your wife's performance of these tasks and thus the need for you to do them, if they're to be done right. Is it possible your demand for perfection in your wife and your taking all responsibility for seeing things get done prevent her from even trying any more?

Cognitive Deficiencies: A majority of Corey's communications convey a poor sense of self-worth.

THERAPIST: As I listen to you, it sounds like you maintain a single thought constantly in your mind, "I can't!" I wonder how you'd be if your main thought was "I can" instead of "I can't."

Themes, Patterns, and Causal Relationships. Many clients repeatedly experience the same self-defeating problem situations without recognizing the full pattern of transactions in which the problem is embedded. Although clients often describe the visible sources of their difficulties, they do not completely specify the total network in which they occur. Recognizing the theme, pattern, or causal relationship creating this network is a prerequisite for effective goal setting. In some ways, this type of interpretation is similar to the therapist focusing skill of summarization. Interpretations, however, seek to give clients new, deeper perspectives. Consider the following illustrations:

THERAPIST A: Judy, I've heard you say that your thoughts at work revolve around how boring it is. Similarly, at social affairs and even when you are alone doing activities that most persons typically consider interesting, your main thought is "How boring." Obviously, this singular belief does little to enhance your life.

THERAPIST B: Judy, you've said a number of times in a number of different instances that your primary thought is "How boring." Is it possible that this self-defeating thinking is an excuse for not having to expend the effort and experience the initial discomfort it takes to assume responsibility for making yourself happier?

Therapist A creates a more intense, finer definition of the problem with a summarization. Therapist B takes the client one step further in promoting a new perspective that suggests potential goals.

Confrontation

One of the most useful, yet misunderstood, therapist skills is confrontation. Confrontation as a therapeutic tool has acquired a negative connotation in some circles because it is misconstrued to mean lecturing, judging, or acting in a punitive manner toward clients. Ivey and Simek-Downing (1980) address this issue, explaining:

> The dictionary defines *confront* as "1. to stand or come in front of; stand or meet facing. 2. to face in hostility or defiance, oppose" (Barnhart, 1950). . . ."A confrontation is defined as . . . *the pointing out of discrepancies between or among attitudes, thoughts, or behaviors.* In a confrontation individuals are faced directly with the fact that they may be saying other than that which they mean, or doing other than that which they say" (Ivey

and Gluckstern, 1976, p. 46). A confrontation is *not* telling a client that he or she is in error or a bad person. In counseling, the first dictionary meaning of confrontation, cited above, is central; the second meaning is potentially destructive. (p. 102)

True confrontations represent acts of caring by therapists. Johnson's (1981) characterization of the need for confrontation among friends highlights this:

If you are someone's friend, do you ignore her interpersonal mistakes, or do you confront her in a way that helps her learn not to make the same mistake in the future? (p. 229)

Effective confrontations are offered in the spirit of empathic understanding. Destructive, pseudo-confrontations communicate little or no empathy. For example:

THERAPIST A: Betsy, you keep doing the same self-defeating things over and over again. You show a complete unwillingness to cooperate. How are you ever going to change?

THERAPIST B: Betsy, you've stated a number of times your desire to change, yet you seem to keep repeating the same self-defeating behaviors we've identified. How might you explain this difference between your desires and actions?

Therapist A exhibits little empathic understanding in harshly attacking Betsy about her lack of therapeutic progress. Such harshness only produces defensiveness and alienates clients, inhibiting any potential forward therapeutic movement. Even though the therapist's observations may be correct, the style and words used to convey them are clearly inappropriate. Therapist B, by contrast, simply points out the discrepancy between Betsy's expressed desires and actual actions, confident that she can identify a goal-oriented direction to pursue.

Confrontation and interpretation are similar in some respects as therapist skills for promoting new client perspectives. Both are direct statements to a client that address specific aspects of the client's functioning or environmental context. Interpretation involves giving an explicit meaning to that which is implied in a client's communications, usually based on a therapist's primary theoretical orientation. Confrontation, however, challenges a client to provide his or her own meaning. In using an interpretation, the therapist presents a client with a hypothesis inferred from the client's communications that may explain cause and effect. In confrontation, the therapist also seeks to expressly define what the client is communicating, but asks the client to interpret and offer a cause-effect explanation. Therapists may share personal thoughts and feelings in re-action to clients' experiences or point out the potentially negative conse-quences of specific experiences, but in employing confrontation, they do not offer an explanation of meaning. That is the client's responsibility.

Operationally, in confronting a client, a therapist seeks to establish a "you said/but look" condition (Hackney & Cormier, 1979). The first part of a confrontation is the "you said" portion. The therapist reflects some aspect of a client's functioning back to him or her. The second part of the confrontation presents a contradiction or discrepancy seen by the thera-pist as being in opposition, the "but look" portion of the confrontation. The confrontation is culminated by an open-ended inquiry that requests an explanation from the client. For example:

Lois is very concerned about her deteriorating relationship with her children. She has reported on several occasions making promises to them and later not keeping them.

THERAPIST: Lois you've noted several times making promises to David and Morgan, for example, the picnic last week (reflection of the "you said"), and then not following through (the "but look"). How might this contradictory behavior be affecting the children's relationship with you? (open-ended inquiry requesting an explanation)

Thus, confrontation is used to help clients see contradictions and discrepancies that prevent them from gaining the insights necessary for therapeutic goal setting. The following situations represent occasions where confrontation would be appropriate.

Discrepancies Between Verbal and Nonverbal Communications.

THERAPIST: You say you're not worried about losing your job or finding a new one, yet your voice is slow and halting and your eyes teary. I'm not sure which message to take.

Contradictions Between the Verbal Content of Two Statements.

THERAPIST: Last session you described your wife as always warm, considerate, and loving. Now you're saying that she spent the entire week making demands on you and belittling you when you didn't comply immediately. How do you explain this change?

Incongruities Between What Is Said and What Is Actually Done

THERAPIST: Margaret, you've expressed quite sincerely your desire to finish school, especially since there's only one semester left in your degree program. Yet, you haven't gone to register for your remaining classes and they began this week. What is happening with you and school?

Discrepancies Between Statements and the Context

THERAPIST: Sam, you keep putting yourself down with statements like you just made saying you're no good because you can't find a job in your field. Yet, it's my understanding that there are hundreds of well-qualified applicants for every job opening in your area of expertise. How does job availability serve as a criterion in your self-evaluation?

Cormier and Cormier (1979) suggest some relevant ground rules to remember when preparing to use confrontation:

1. Remember that confrontation is a *description,* not a judgment or an evaluation of a client's experiencing. Using confrontation suggests doing just what the word implies and *no more.* A confrontation *describes* a client's experiencing and *presents* evidence (Hackney & Cormier, 1979).

2. In describing a contradiction or discrepancy, the confrontation should cite specifics rather than vague inferences. Concreteness is therefore critical. A vague confrontation such as "You want things to be better, yet you don't take action" offers little in the way of a new perspective to the client. What "things" and what "action" are of concern?

3. Timing is important. Core conditions and the therapist's social influence form a power base so that confrontations are taken more seriously and examined more closely.

4. Client readiness for confrontation, if not apparent, should be nurtured through successive approximation. Confronting clients with smaller issues that can be explained relatively easily and successfully gives them confidence to address greater challenges.

5. Use reflections both to introduce and follow up confrontations. An introductory reflection starts off a confrontation in the spirit of empathic understanding. A follow up reflection in response to a client's reaction helps clarify the client's explanation. As with interpretations, should a client reject a confrontation, the therapist can respond with a reflection, further exploration and discussion, and at a later time, reiterate the confrontation with more data. Carkhuff (1972) cautions against immediately successive confrontations, suggesting they are too intense.

Self-Disclosure

Therapist self-disclosure has been defined as any information therapists convey about themselves to their clients (Cozby, 1973). The kinds of therapist self-disclosure that promote new client perspectives, however, call for a more limited and purposeful definition. Egan (1982) outlines the parameters of appropriate therapist self-disclosure:

> Sharing yourself is *appropriate* if it helps clients achieve the treatment goals outlined in this helping process—that is, if it helps them talk about themselves, if it helps them develop new perspectives and frames of reference, and if it helps them set realistic goals for themselves. (p. 199)

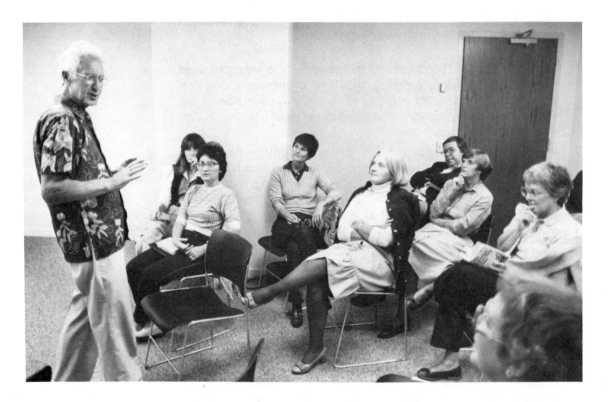

Support groups use self-disclosure to help new members learn to share their concerns with others

Thus, self-disclosures by therapists should be *goal directed*. As such, self-disclosure can take two forms. The first form, *a modeling self-disclosure*, is a way of showing clients how to tell about themselves and encouraging them to do so (Egan, 1982). Research has generally supported the positive modeling effects of self-disclosure (Doster & Nesbitt, 1979). Most clients tend to disclose less about intimate issues. Therefore, they provide less information for the therapeutic process with which new perspectives can be postulated. The therapist's ability to generate client disclosure of intimate issues can be critical for therapy to progress. The potency of modeling self-disclosures are most evident in self-help groups such as Alcoholics Anonymous where the skill is used extensively as a way of showing new members what to talk about as well as encouraging them to talk freely about themselves and their problems (Gartner & Riessman, 1977).

The second form of self-disclosure, *experience-sharing self-disclosures* helps clients develop the kinds of new perspectives that lead to goal setting. Therapists must be careful, however, to always maintain the focus on the client and his or her concerns. This focus is most effectively accomplished by ending self-disclosures with an open-ended inquiry. For example:

Greg has been discussing his recent divorce and the fact that his life has been "perfect"	in every respect since the day his marriage ended.

THERAPIST: Greg, you've mentioned no feelings of remorse or sadness over the breakup of your marriage. Although I'm presently remarried, I remember after my first wife and I divorced, I reacted on the outside as you are, showing no regret at all. Yet even though I had no doubt that we made the right choice in breaking up, inside I really was feeling a loss and just didn't want to let anyone know. I'm wondering if there might be any similarity in your reactions and those I had?

Without an open-ended inquiry, Greg is left without a new perspective to consider unless he spontaneously identifies with the therapist's disclosure. An ending inquiry concretely denotes purpose in the therapist's disclosure. Such experience-sharing disclosures suggest new perspectives in terms of clients' thoughts, feelings, and actions. Another use of experience-sharing self-disclosure is to offer a new perspective in the form of a potential solution to a problem that clients might consider. For example:

Helen has been depressed because she wishes she were more talkative at parties	and other social occasions.

THERAPIST: Helen, when I was first in college, I too found it very difficult to talk at parties. I had always known everyone in high school and was familiar with what their interests were, especially since their interests were usually mine. College represented new people with different, unknown interests. I was lost until my advisor suggested visiting the counseling center and enrolling in a social skills course they ran. There I learned new skills I had never had need of before for interacting with others. How might a course of this nature be applicable to your situation?

Egan (1982) proposes three principles to be followed to ensure that self-disclosures are used appropriately.

1. *Selectivity and Focus.* Therapist self-disclosure should not distract clients from their own problem situations. That the focus must always remain on the client is emphasized by ending disclosures with an inquiry, as discussed previously.

2. *Not Burdensome.* Therapist self-disclosure should not add another burden to an already overwhelmed client. Egan (1982) illustrates this principle with the example of a novice counselor who thought he would help make a client who was sharing some sexual concerns more comfortable by sharing some of his own experiences. The client, however, reacted with "Hey, don't tell me your problems. I'm having a hard enough time dealing with my own. I don't want to carry yours around too!" This counselor disclosed too much too soon. He allowed his willingness to self-disclose overshadow his consideration of its potential usefulness to the client.

3. *Not Too Often.* Therapist self-disclosure, when used too frequently, distracts the client and shifts attention to the therapist. Research suggests (Murphy & Strong, 1972) that therapists who disclose too often are seen as phony by clients, who suspect them of having some type of ulterior motives.

Immediacy

Of the many concerns clients present in therapy, the majority involve some form of interpersonal difficulties. Clients' interactions with a therapist often mirror their exchanges with others outside of therapy, thereby making sessions ideal situations for observing and exploring clients' interpersonal skills. Therapists who are sensitive to the dynamics of their own relationships with clients are best able to help their clients deal with interpersonal issues ranging from trust and dependency to manipulation (George & Cristiani, 1981). Immediacy is therapists' recognizing and communicating what is going on between themselves and their clients in their present therapeutic relationship.

Egan (1976) identifies two kinds of immediacy. *Here-and-now immediacy* is an open exchange with a client about "what is happening between the two of you in the here-and-now of an interpersonal trans-action" (p. 201). Here-and-now immediacy emphasizes a specific present moment transaction. For example:

Harry, a school guidance counselor, has been having trouble getting along with the teachers at his school and thus has come to therapy seeking help in remedying this situation. He is apparently trying to dominate the present session, suggesting what he thinks the therapist is thinking and feeling about him. He has just begun suggesting goals for the therapist to pursue in assisting him.

THERAPIST: Harry, I'd like to stop for a moment and look at what's happening between us in our session today. You've suggested things you think that I'm thinking about you and new goals that I should pursue to work effectively with you. These are your ideas, not mine. I have the feeling you're finding it difficult to stop being a helper and let me actually offer assistance.

HARRY: (silent pause) Maybe you're right. I guess it's hard for me to change hats.

THERAPIST: Changing hats and stepping out of your counselor's role is something you find difficult. Perhaps you're interacting with the teachers you work with in a similar manner. They might be looking for person-to-person discussion and you come on counselor-to-client?

The therapist does two things in this example. First, the here-and-now concerns of the therapy session are addressed. The therapist then extrap-olates on what has happened in therapy and offers the client a new perspective from which to view the major concern that brought him to therapy; that is, that the inappropriate way he is interacting with the therapist mirrors his interpersonal difficulties with his associates at work.

Relationship immediacy is open discussion with a client about "where you stand in your relationship to him/her and where you see the other standing in relationship to you" (Egan, p. 200). It addresses the overall counselor-client relationship as it has developed over time.

David is a high school freshman who is being sent to therapy as part of a court order resulting from his involvement in a vandalism spree. He has made it obvious he doesn't want to be in therapy. He takes every opportunity to question the value of therapy as well as the therapist's competency, often sarcastically and caustically.

THERAPIST: David, we've talked about your having to come to see me because you've been ordered by the judge to do so. From the way you put down coming here and me, I have the feeling that you see me as just another "judge" forcing you to do things you don't want to and using your comments to control what we can do. I think that if we objectively look at the power you do have here, you'll see you're not using all of it, nor are you using it for your own benefit. For instance, the faster you choose to progress, the sooner we'll be able to end your having to come.

The therapist challenges David to look at their overall relationship. The purpose in doing so is to provide him with a new perspective; with a more positive attitude he can control his time spent in an unwanted situation. As with the previous case, which illustrated here-and-now immediacy, the therapist could show the client how his response to therapy mirrors his daily life difficulties. For instance, continuing on in a later session:

THERAPIST: David, we talked last session about how you were using critical comments to control therapy and how a more positive approach is in your ultimate best interest. You agreed and now you're using your power to complete what the court has required in the shortest time possible. Perhaps what happened with us is similar to the vandalism that got you into the mess you're in. Is it possible that you and your friends were using destruction to show how powerful you were and not looking at how you could exert control in a more positive and less problematic way?

Immediacy need not only focus on blocks or strain in the therapist-client relationship. It is also a valuable tool for addressing outside-of-session difficulties by pointing to progress achieved within the therapeutic relationship. Consider the following immediacy response:

THERAPIST: We've had some rocky times over the past few sessions. You were resentful about seeking any kind of help in getting along better with your children and fought the requests I made of you with opposite requests of your own of me. We seem to have been able to settle on some fine compromises here in therapy. Is it possible that if you compromise more, as you have here, with your children, that relationship might also improve?

In reinforcing the client for therapeutic progress achieved, a counselor can foster a new perspective on the present problem.

Immediacy incorporates almost all of the therapist skills we have discussed in how it is presented to the client; for example, it can contain aspects of information-giving, interpretation, confrontation, and self-disclosure as well as attending and focusing skills. Recognizing immediacy issues can be an especially difficult task for the novice therapist. Often they tend to pay too much attention to outside-of-session client issues rather than what is occurring in the immediate therapist-client interaction, unless it directly affects the latter. Turock (1980) proposes guidelines for recognizing immediacy issues. These guidelines provide a firmer analysis of therapist-client interchanges and their influence on the therapeutic process.

1. Experiencing the Influencing Effort. Most therapists are taught to not allow clients to manipulate in therapy. It can at times be productive to temporarily allow these influencing efforts to occur in order to learn more about a client's manipulative actions and their potential impact on others. Blocking or avoiding manipulative attempts can cause therapists to lose valuable opportunities for learning about clients' interpersonal styles.

2. Abstracting. Most clients will repeat any well-practiced manipulations when they experience discomfort or vulnerability. Therapists should notice such repetitious interaction patterns, identifying clients' eliciting actions and the therapist's response to them.

3. Disengaging. One of the best ways to recognize the meaning of covert client communications is to disengage as a listener. Instead of readily giving a response expected by a client, disengaged therapists first reflect on their own experience with a client in the present moment to determine their reactions and the client's eliciting actions. Turock (1980) specifies the following self-directed questions for therapists to consider:
   - ☐ What is the client trying to tell me that can't be said directly?
   - ☐ What is the effect of the client's behavior on me?
   - ☐ What am I prompted to do, say, or feel?
   - ☐ What is the client doing or saying that leads me to choose to react this way?
   - ☐ What do I sense the client wants from me?

4. Identifying Self as Target. Some clients conceal their actual thoughts and feelings by speaking in generalities. Often these vague references directly relate to the therapist. Consider the following client comments:
   - ☐ I'm tired of other people telling me what I should do.
   - ☐ You have to watch out. Everyone has an ulterior motive for the nice things they may do.
   - ☐ I have a lot of trouble being able to trust others.

   Although the overtly expressed target of the client's statements is general (people, everyone, others), if the statements are made more concrete, the therapist might discover he or she is perceived in the same manner.

It must be remembered that immediacy is a therapist skill to facilitate goal setting and not a goal in itself. Phase III of the therapeutic process emphasizes goal setting. Immediacy used only for the sake of creating a more open, honest therapist-client relationship without the aim of gaining new perspectives and ultimately setting goals is a dead end.

Promoting a New Perspective Through Active Experiencing

Egan (1982) suggests that for some clients the best means of gaining a new perspective is through active experiencing. He offered a case illustration as an example:

> Woody, a college sophomore, came to the student counseling service with a variety of interpersonal and somatic complaints. He felt attracted to a number of women on campus but did very little

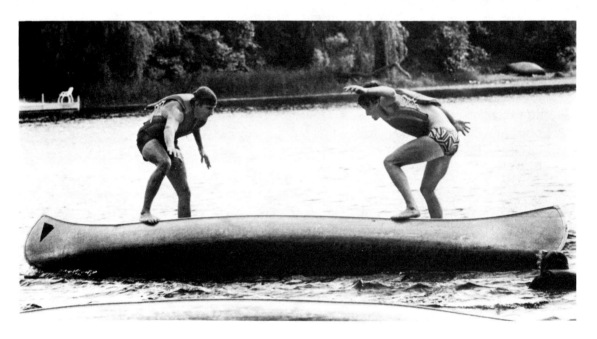

Active experiencing can help people gain new perspectives

to become involved with them. After exploring this issue briefly, he said to the counselor, "Hell, I just have to go out and do it." Two months later he returned and said that he had run into disaster. He had gone out with a few women, but none of them really interested him. Then he did meet someone he liked quite a bit. They went out a couple of times, but the third time he called, she said that she didn't want to see him any more. When asked why, she muttered something vague about his being too preoccupied with himself and ended the conversation. He felt devastated and so returned to the counseling center. He and the counselor took another look at his social life. This time, however, he had some experiences to probe. He wanted to find out what "too preoccupied with himself" meant. They could stop talking hypothetically and talk about what actually happened or did not happen. (p. 208)

Promoting a new perspective through active experiencing is often a valuable recourse to pursue with impulsive clients like Woody as well as some closed-minded clients. Giving the latter the choice of continuing as they are or seeking change is often enlightening. For example:

CLIENT: I just don't see how my changing my thinking will change how I feel.
THERAPIST: It is obviously a new way of approaching problems for you. However, you report being in a great deal of emotional pain and this is a positive alternative for alleviating that pain. You have the choice of remaining as you are or attempting new ways of functioning.

Bandura (1977) and Wessler (1982) propose that significant insight occurs as a result of new experiences and by observing one's own effica-cious actions—one experience is worth a thousand words. Respectfully letting clients continue in their maladaptive manner as well as providing them with a taste of potential intervention strategies often results in them gaining a more purposeful perspective on their problems.

COMPLETING GOAL SETTING

Clarification, specification, and commitment to mutually acceptable out-come and process goals constitute the completion of Phase III of the therapeutic process. All that has been presented up to this point has been aimed at completing goal setting. The therapeutic climate was nurtured, problem situations were discriminated and defined, and the client was challenged to develop new purposeful perspectives. These new perspec-tives show the client the direction to take for positive change to occur.

Occasionally, some therapists or clients attempt to bypass goal set-ting and move immediately toward problem intervention. Seeing a poten-tial direction to take, they impulsively move forward. More often than not, however, when both outcome and process goals are not clarified and firmly committed to, failure and unnecessary recycling result. For example:

Wendy was constantly in a state of anxiety. Her nervousness would become so intense at times that she literally "froze," unable to do anything except stay home and cry about all the responsibilities she had. In therapy, she and the therapist initially defined her problem as her excessive anxiety. In developing a new, more purposeful perspective, Wendy was aided in seeing that her anxiety directly resulted from allowing herself to take on too many responsibilities and then being unable to effectively manage them all without prioritizing. Wendy took this insight and immediately attempted to act on it. She summarily began to say no to all responsibilities she was requested to take on. Her anxiety actually worsened as her friends and associates reacted negatively to this 180 degree turnabout. Returning to therapy, Wendy completed goal setting and came to realize the necessity of establishing more appropriate process goals. One was to learn to examine her manner of accepting and refusing responsibilities placed on her in order that she need not refuse all requests. Many requests of her by others were valid and important for her to accept if she is to associate with them on a reciprocal basis, especially at work.

Wendy's incomplete goal setting resulted in inappropriate goals being set. The failure of these goals, however, illustrates promoting a new perspective through active experiencing; she learned to see the need for more planned procedures. She ultimately had to backtrack, returning to therapy to set more realistic and workable goals.

Goal setting is a highly interactive process between therapist and client. In gaining new perspectives from which to view their problems, clients will have ideally gained an understanding particularly of specific process goals to pursue. In completing goal setting, these process goals and previously defined outcome goals are clarified, specified, and firmly committed to.

Clarification

A common error made by novice therapists in goal setting is assuming that clients, because they have developed new perspectives on their problems, fully comprehend them. These therapists often fail to take enough time to ensure that clients clearly understand their desired outcome goals as well as the prerequisite process goals. Laboring under the mistaken assumption that previously discussed goals have been clearly understood, therapists are surprised in later sessions when clients indicate they have not actively attempted intervention strategies because they could not clearly relate them to their problem situations. Implicit client agreement on goals is insufficient for effective goal setting. Unless clients can repeat back precisely their outcome goals and how achieving process goals will enable them to attain their outcome goals, goal setting is incomplete. When clients restate their goals, distortions and misperceptions can be eliminated and goal setting can proceed. The first step, then, in effective goal setting is restatement and, if necessary, clarification of primary outcome and process goals.

Specification

Goals can be broad or narrow, immediate, intermediate, or long-range. The time factor implied in the concept of a broad long-range goal can provide direction to the overall therapeutic process. Beyond this, broad long-range goals offer little. Such broad goals (e.g., "I'm going to be more open," "I will stop being so shy," "I will improve what I think about myself.") are futile without specifying steps for their attainment. Rather than leading to realistic intervention strategies, these goals are merely vague descriptions of desires.

The tendency to set broad goals occurs frequently in therapy because broad goals are simply easier to identify. Getting down to details is much harder than settling for generalities for therapists and clients alike. If successful goal achievement is to be assured, however, goal-setting must be like a chain, each link a definable aspect of experience that can be carried out in a direct fashion.

Gottman and Leiblum (1974) provide a succinct goal specification plan for therapists to consider. They note:

> Goals are *discrepancy statements* which compare current functioning to some criteria of competence or to some normative standard of competence in those situations. They answer four vital questions: (1) who? (2) will do what? (3) to what extent? (4) under what conditions? (p. 48)

Dyer and Vriend (1977) suggest an additional question for therapists to add to Gottman and Leiblum's list: (5) when? They stress the importance of specifying time requirements.

Who. It is important that goals be selected that clients themselves are able to carry out. Frequently clients think that their problems will be solved only if other persons change how they function. In most cases, however, this attitude only results in failure to attain any sort of goal. For example:

Tom wanted himself and his wife to get along better with their neighbors, Sue and Fred. Insights achieved during therapy had shown Tom that he was always waiting for the neighbors to make the first overture to initiate get-togethers. Apparently, they had tired of the one-way invitations. Tom, with the therapist's help, also learned he needed to be more assertive as a process goal for achieving his outcome goal of more interaction with the neighbors. Tom expected his wife, however, who neither attended therapy nor was overly willing to increase her interaction with the neighbors, to become more assertive in being friendly to Sue, as he would with Fred. Unfortunately, she refused.

Clients can readily change their own functioning if they choose. Tom, for instance, could assertively seek a closer relationship with Fred, regardless of his wife and Sue becoming more friendly. Therapists should strongly consider confrontation as a reaction to client statements that express explicitly or implicitly the goal of having someone else change. Such statements have a high probability of impeding goal attainment (Egan, 1982).

Will Do What. Goals must be concrete and specific. The effective therapist recognizes the folly in attempting to accomplish a goal whose attainment cannot be clearly identified. If a client will not be able to say, "There, I did it and know it is done," the sought-after goal is too vague. As we noted earlier, some goals are never achieved because they are too broad and lack sufficient detail. Consider the following comparison:

BROAD: I want to find out more about colleges.

CONCRETE AND DETAILED: I will make an appointment to visit a career counselor tomorrow. I will ask the counselor about those institutions within commuting distance; their reputation, if they have the program I want, the costs, and the social advantages and disadvantages of being a commuter at each.

To What Extent. If goals are sufficiently concrete and detailed, their extent is usually not an issue. However, just as clients must know when they have accomplished a goal, they and the therapist need to know how frequently and intensely certain emotions, thoughts, and behaviors occur (depending on the therapist's theoretical orientation and the established process goals). By "marking" where a client is when a goal is set, not only can concrete goals more easily be established, but also partial as well as total progress becomes readily notable.

Dyer and Vriend (1977) suggest a number of ways to establish "to what extent":

Thus, clients can be provided with wrist counters or asked to record in a log how many times they feel angry, have suicidal thoughts, or how many times they want to speak up to a given other person and don't over a given time span. Rating scales for gauging the intensity of such behaviors can also be constructed. The client can be taught to grade each recurrence of a thought or feeling at some level of acuity. Once an accurate picture of the status quo emerges, treatment goals for change can be made more realistic with results that can be compared to baseline data. (p. 471)

Recognizing any accomplishment that results from efforts toward goal achievement is a vital part of proactive problem intervention. If clients can't see their progress, their motivation to persist in the unnatural business of functioning differently, of continuing their difficult efforts, decreases. Goals that are measurable offer this recognition.

Under What Conditions. Clients occasionally sabotage their own efforts by choosing goals beyond their reach. Some clients seek to attempt virtually impossible goals for themselves simply to please the therapist or because they have miscalculated their present capabilities; this can be exacerbated by excitement over the possibilities of being different.

A goal is not really a goal if obstacles will prevent its accomplishment; that is, obstacles that cannot be overcome with available resources. Goals are realistic if the resources necessary for their accomplishment are available to the client and not too costly. For example:

Helen recently graduated with a bachelor's degree in psychology. She found her studies very difficult and had to struggle to maintain the minimum average needed to graduate. Unable to find a job in her field, she now wants to go on to graduate school. Given her past difficulties, however, her parents are unwilling to further finance her education, and Helen lacks the funds herself.

Helen's goal of graduate school, to the objective observer, is obviously one fraught with immediate difficulties. If she is intent on pursuing this goal, however, an interim goal might be established that would bypass some of the apparent obstacles. For instance, Helen might enter graduate school part-time as a nonmatriculating student and see if she is capable and motivated enough to struggle through the difficulties. Finances would also be less of a problem on a part-time basis.

When. Establishing a reasonable time frame for accomplishing goals is critical. Many clients' major difficulty is their procrastination in actually moving to change their problem situation. Presenting themselves for therapy was likely a difficult task. Actual goal achievement often represents significant effort and initial discomfort for clients. Unrealistic or vague time frames only add to the difficulty. Goals that are to be accomplished sometime or other never seem to be achieved (Egan, 1982).

Commitment

Effective goal setting involves mutual agreement and commitment between therapist and client. Without mutuality, client commitment to working on goals can hardly be guaranteed. A goal imposed solely by the therapist, whether outcome or process, excludes clients from goal setting. The message communicated is, "I am the important person here, not you. I will do your thinking for you and when you finally change for the better, you will be grateful to me and thankful that you found me." Such ineffective therapists ultimately find themselves ordering or begging their clients "Will you give this a try?" instead of clients enthusiastically awaiting to initiate efforts themselves.

This is not to say that therapists are not responsible for fostering goal-oriented direction in therapy. As we have seen, the function of the entire therapeutic process up to this point has emphasized this purposeful therapist role. It is essential, however, that clients "own" a goal. Various questions can be asked to elicit this ownership: "How might . . . be as a way of working toward your stated outcome goal?" "Given these circumstances, would you be willing to . . .?" "Rather than react as you have in the past, could you first stop and . . .?" Clients will work harder for goals they are committed to. Having to work toward goals to which they are not personally committed lets clients blame others if they fail or if they find the effort too taxing in attempting to reach goals. This personal ownership and commitment must be made explicit. While clients may implicitly agree to work on "therapist-owned" goals, the chances for such goals being met in the world outside of therapy sessions are seriously minimized. The aware therapist respects the fact that goals must be mutually determined.

THERAPIST SKILLS III: THEORETICAL APPLICATIONS

The basic therapeutic goals of the various theoretical approaches we have presented were discussed and illustrated in Chapter 5. You are encouraged to refer back to Chapter 5 if you need to review a specific approach's basic goals. In the context of this chapter, however, it is valuable to consider the theoretical perspectives' approaches to goal setting as a procedure. Cognitive therapists, and behavior therapists especially, stress specific, measurable goals; the therapist skills addressed in this chapter are most relevant to these practitioners. The use of therapeutic contracts in many of these approaches underscores their adherence to concrete goal setting.

By contrast, the affectively-oriented approaches primarily pursue rather lofty, general process goals such as becoming full, autonomous, aware, and/or integrated. For Rogers (1961) the basic goal is to help clients become "fully functioning persons." The existentialists especially promote rather vague goals. May (1967) espouses a goal of accepting one's freedom to create a unique existence and to understand one's "being-in-the-world." Bugental (1976) describes the search for authentic existence, and Jourard (1971) writes of the "transparent self." Such general goals make using the therapist skills in this chapter a challenging endeavor for these practitioners as they are rarely employed in the format and degree of specificity we suggest.

The skills presented in this chapter, although not all-inclusive, are applicable to most theoretical approaches. Providing information is an important means of giving clients a new perspective in all the cognitively-oriented and behaviorally-oriented approaches. Cognitive therapy, rational-emotive therapy, and Transactional Analysis, in particular, each has its own terminology that is essential for pursuing relevant process goals. Thus, clients must be given this information in order to understand potential process goals and thus to carry out intervention strategies. Behavior therapy, based on principles of learning, obviously requires that therapists offer substantial didactic instruction. Information-giving is stressed less, if at all, in affectively-oriented approaches. Their position on interpretation is similar.

The Gestalt approach to interpretation presents a summative affective view. It proposes that learning is acquired through personal discovery and experiencing. The Gestalt therapist therefore seeks to create conditions in which clients can make their own interpretations. The other affectively-oriented approaches, Transactional Analysis and reality therapy, similarly allow clients to make their own interpretations. While interpretation is not a frequently employed therapist skill in behavior therapy, rational-emotive and cognitive therapy practitioners rely heavily on interpreting clients' experiences in terms of their maladaptive thinking.

Confrontation is integral to many of the approaches, regardless of which domain of human functioning they stress. Gestalt therapy is highly confrontational in that clients are continually made aware of how they are at the moment and what they are doing. The existential therapist's encounter with clients is largely a confrontational process that encourages them to become aware of their being-in-the-world and to make choices of how they want to be. Rational-emotive therapists challenge clients to critically examine their irrational beliefs and their impact on leading a satisfying life. Cognitive therapy likewise calls clients' attention to the maladaptive modes of thinking they maintain and the resultant effects. Transactional Analysis seeks to confront clients with the games that they use to avoid intimacy and challenges them to reevaluate early important decisions that still affect their lives. Reality therapy too is basically confrontational, for reality therapists continually urge clients to determine whether their behavior is realistic and responsible and to see whether their needs are being fulfilled by irresponsible behavior. Behavior therapists use confrontation primarily on an "as needed" basis. The person-centered approach alone does not emphasize confrontation as a therapist skill.

Immediacy is frequently employed by reality therapists and most affectively-oriented practitioners. Self-disclosure is a dominant therapist practice in person-centered and existential therapy. In the other approaches, these latter two therapist skills are neither emphasized nor ignored, and are employed occasionally when seen as helpful.

CHARLES: PHASE III   Charles's first session with the counselor concluded Chapter 8. This excerpt is from his second session. The therapeutic process evolves into Phase III. New perspectives are pursued, the objective being goal setting.

THERAPIST SKILLS III   COUNSELOR: Last session we considered three primary problem areas that appeared to be of the utmost concern to you: 1) career, 2) your thoughts regarding your relationship with your girlfriend, and 3) depression and your inability to adequately address it. We sort of encapsulated the three as having an overriding issue affecting them all, that being what you called "finding a happy medium;" what I reframed as being able to make satisfactory decisions that you can act on.

CHARLES: I guess dealing with my thoughts and feelings, dealing with job issues . . . seems like if I could get a grasp on things . . . making some decisions instead of floundering around . . . maybe the rest would come easier. But it's just dealing with the frustration that drives me insane, I guess . . . I'm forever having a headache anymore.

COUNSELOR: The inability to decide is causing emotional frustration and also some hard-felt physical pain.

CHARLES: Yeah.

COUNSELOR: What is it about making decisions that you find so difficult?

CHARLES: Well, I've always shied away from making any kind of important decision. I guess it scares me when I think that this is what I'm going to be doing for the next 60 years. I guess I find it hard to make that kind of commitment . . . 'cause I'm always worried if there is something else . . . something else I could have done . . . or I wonder if it was the right decision. I guess I need to learn how to accept what I decide.

COUNSELOR: It's tough to make a decision for many persons but when you're anticipating the future consequences with thoughts of "What if, what if, what if . . .", it becomes all the more difficult.

CHARLES: Yeah. I hate when I sit around and ponder about it. I guess I lack the ability to make the best of what I decide . . . 'cause I've always felt the freedom . . . of, well . . . I don't like this so I'm going on to something else.

COUNSELOR: What might be an example of a decision you made recently where you ruminated over the potential consequences causing yourself a lot of upset? Something particularly related to one of your primary concerns as we have identified them.

CHARLES: Well, coming back to Jacksonville. I was out in Colorado . . . you know . . . out in the mountains and doing everything I wanted to. But I felt this need to come back here and I decided that when I was out there, I wanted to come back. And I guess that that's why I'm experiencing so much frustration now 'cause I'm having to deal with finding a new job, finding new activities, and just being here.

COUNSELOR: You mentioned feeling a "need" to come back. What was the need?

CHARLES: My girlfriend. We met right before I left. It was kind of a weird situation . . . we were working together and it started out just being friends and then like poof . . . Cupid came out and shot us both with an arrow and we started dating. I had already made plans to go out to Colorado and spend my summer in Colorado and I was never sure I was coming back. She always knew this . . . it was always there but we never talked about it . . . and we spent a lot of time together before I left and then poof, I was gone. I decided to come back 'cause I felt that that was what I wanted. But by the time I got back, we had to start all over. We had to start rebuilding the relationship again. A lot of things were lost because I was gone for three months. I spent a lot of time fighting for it . . . you know . . . sticking in there . . . putting up with a lot so that it would work and now I'm not so sure if that's what I should be doing. If I should be changing that much 'cause I'm not sure I'll be happy. But the happiness is there when I'm with her and when I'm away from her I think about her all the time.

COUNSELOR: Charles, you seem to be saying that being sure you've made the "right" decision is all-important. Is it possible that you're demanding the impossible of yourself, always perfect decisions?

interpretation

CHARLES: Maybe so . . . I guess I need to clear my head and organize things that I want . . . otherwise there's going to be that little idea in the back of my head that maybe I should be back in Colorado.

COUNSELOR: So you feel confident that if you could control your thinking a bit better, stop the "second guessing," decision making and acceptance would be an easier task.

CHARLES: Yeah. I do second guess myself a lot.

COUNSELOR: Second guessing can be a persistent and difficult problem. Let me share a related experience I had with you. I used to second guess my decisions pretty frequently and it was causing me to feel frustrated; distressed at "What should I do?" . . . with the accompanying "what if's." I was in my counselor training program at the time and we were studying the impact of our thoughts on how we felt and acted. I learned that by blocking the "what if's" and replacing them with ideas like . . . "An imperfect decision is better than the pain of no decision" or "I've made a decision. Let me give the results a reasonable try. I can always change my mind. Nothing is permanent but death

self-disclosure

and taxes" . . . I was better able to make decisions and then accept the consequences. I even found most of my decisions were more easily made. How might what I discovered apply to you and your situation?

CHARLES: Well, a lot of people have told me I have trouble accepting things for what they are. I do do a lot of second guessing. The "what if's," as you call them, drive me mad sometimes. So being able to do what you did might help alleviate some of the frustration. Maybe I won't feel so confused.

goal setting: clarification

COUNSELOR: It sounds like this might be a good initial goal for us to pursue . . . to help you better control your thinking . . . and thereby make and accept decisions more easily and thus feel less distressed and depressed. The "what if's" probably affect your ability to present your qualifications to potential employers, too.

CHARLES: Well, if I wasn't messing up my mind with all the "what if's" I could probably concentrate on the tasks at hand better.

goal setting: clarification

COUNSELOR: These thoughts are likely to be interfering and self-defeating because you're so preoccupied with them. It would help if you could decrease them and substitute more helpful ideas. You think it would allow you to make and accept decisions and thereby affect your three primary areas of concern?

CHARLES: I think so.

goal setting: clarification

COUNSELOR: You sound a bit guarded in your acceptance of this as a goal, but still you seem willing to pursue it as a promising way to go.

CHARLES: I'm not too sure yet about what you're proposing, I guess. How will I learn to control my thinking better?

goal setting: specification ("who," "will do what")

COUNSELOR: What we'll do is talk about some strategies that you can learn to do so. You can learn how to block the "what if's" and substitute more helpful thinking.

CHARLES: Okay. Let's give it a try.

COUNSELOR: Let's look at a particular time when you're most bothered . . . affected by "what if" thoughts. What might be a specific time during your day that you're most affected?

CHARLES: Probably at night. I've always had problems falling asleep and now thinking about why . . . it's usually when I'm spending a lot of time second guessing what I've done or what I might be doing.

COUNSELOR: How much time in the evening would you say you've been spending with the "what if's?"

CHARLES: A couple of hours it's been lately.

COUNSELOR: How much would you like to decrease the amount of time you're preoccupied with "what if" thinking?

CHARLES: Well, I'm not sure. I guess it would be nice not to be preoccupied at all . . . but maybe that's not too realistic.

goal setting: specification ("to what extent," "under what conditions")

COUNSELOR: A good insight on your part . . . perfection is not a very realistic possibility. A realistic decrease, modest at first, might be a more manageable goal to pursue. You said you've been spending a couple of hours each evening. The first task you will have to accomplish is to keep a record of the amount of time you spend each evening preoccupied with "what if" thinking.

After we identify where you're at now, we can better determine a specific goal. For now, however, how does decreasing the time you spend in half sound?

CHARLES: Sounds reasonable.

COUNSELOR: So what we have established as an initial goal is to decrease the amount of time you devote in the evening to "what if" thinking about past and potential future decisions. We also said that we would start by decreasing the time you determine that you spend by half. How does this sound to you . . . an appropriate goal?

goal setting: commitment

CHARLES: Okay.

COUNSELOR: How about if we set the next three sessions and the time in between as our time frame? We can spend the next three sessions learning how to, and pursuing this goal. At the end of that time, we can evaluate our progress and make future plans.

goal setting: commitment

CHARLES: Sounds fine.

COUNSELOR: So you're committed to this course of action for the next three sessions and the time in between at least.

goal setting: commitment

CHARLES: I'm willing to work at it. I've got to do something.

SUGGESTED READINGS

Promoting New Perspectives

Berenson, B. G., & Mitchell, K. M. (1974). *Confrontation: For better or worse.* North Amherst, MA: Human Resource Development Press. Confrontation is one of the most misunderstood therapist skills for promoting new client perspectives. Berenson and Mitchell expound upon the potential strengths and hazards in employing confrontation.

Egan, G. (1976). *Interpersonal living: A skills/contract approach to human relations training in groups.* Monterey, CA: Brooks/Cole. Egan presents an extensive array of exercises for increasing therapist self-awareness and promoting new perspectives by others.

Egan, G. (1982). *The skilled helper: Model, skills, and methods for effective helping* (2nd ed.). Monterey, CA: Brooks/Cole. One of Egan's objectives in writing this book is to adequately address the therapist skills and client responses that provide the new perspectives necessary as a prelude to goal setting.

Gazda, G., Walters, R., & Childers, W. (1975). *Human relations development: A manual for health sciences.* Boston: Allyn & Bacon. The authors offer an excellent discussion relating to "responding with information."

Johnson, D. W. (1982). *Reaching out: Interpersonal effectiveness and self-actualization* (2nd ed.). Englewood Cliffs, NJ: Prentice-Hall. Johnson's book, like Egan's *Interpersonal Living* cited above, offers an extensive explanation of various exercises for promoting new client perspectives as well as enhancing therapist self-awareness.

Goal Setting

Cormier, W. H., & Cormier, L. S. (1979). *Interviewing strategies for helpers: A guide to assessment, treatment, and evaluation.* Monterey, CA: Brooks/ Cole. Cormier and Cormier offer one of the most complete skills' presentations relating to goal setting available.

Egan, G. (1982). *The skilled helper: Model, skills, and methods for effective helping* (2nd ed.). Monterey, CA: Brooks/Cole. Egan offers a fine presentation of goal setting skills and understandings through what he titles "developing and sequencing programs."

Gottman, J. M., & Leiblum, S. R. (1974). *How to do psychotherapy and how to evaluate it.* New York: Holt, Rinehart and Winston. The authors suggest some excellent ideas relating to goal setting, from "setting objectives for initial change efforts" to "negotiating therapeutic contracts."

Hackney, H. L., & Cormier, L. S. (1979). *Counseling strategies and objectives* (2nd ed.). Englewood Cliffs, NJ: Prentice-Hall. This book has a particularly fine section devoted to "Conceptualizing Problems and Setting Goals."

Krumboltz, J. D., & Thoresen, C. E. (Eds.) (1976). *Counseling methods.* New York: Holt, Rinehart and Winston. A significant number of the contributions in this edited compilation of articles address goal setting distinctly through the use of case study data.

10

Phase Four: Proactive Problem Intervention

Once specific client goals have been identified, your judgment and expertise are critical . . . you must possess a repertory of counseling strategies that can be used to help the client achieve the desired goals.

(Hackney & Cormier, 1979, p. 118)

Counseling and psychotherapy are not just discussion and planning. Clients must actively function differently if they are to live a more satisfying existence. This is the essence of the term *proactive*—actively and assertively changing the way one feels, thinks, and acts. Interventions are "modi operandi," or treatment strategies tailored to meet the specific goals of clients (Hackney & Cormier, 1979).

It might be easy to conclude from the previous chapter that clients who have effectively set goals easily move on to identifying and carrying out interventions aimed at goal achievement. Often they do, but not always without continuing therapist support and skilled help. Some clients, once they clearly understand the agreed-upon outcome and process goals, can independently move forward. They mobilize their own and other available resources to achieve these goals.

Other clients, even though they understand their problems, having identified outcome goals, and know what they must achieve in process goals, still do not have a clear idea of *how* to achieve the goals themselves. These clients critically need help in selecting, implementing and evaluating interventions aimed at goal attainment. Even clients who can help themselves can gain from therapist assistance with refinement, encouragement, and review. With both types of clients therapists' overall role and responsibilities in Phase IV of the therapeutic process model are actually quite similar. The difference lies in degree and intensity in how interventions are selected, implemented, and evaluated. Phase IV is illustrated in Figure 10–1.

SELECTING INTERVENTION STRATEGIES

Once outcome and process goals have been clearly agreed upon, appropriate interventions for achieving goals must be established. From the point of view of the therapist, selecting intervention strategies should be based on specific criteria. These important criteria include: sought-after outcome and process goals, therapist orientation, research documentation, client preference and characteristics, environmental context, and multiple interventions (Cormier & Cormier, 1979).

Outcome and Process Goals

Although it may seem obvious, interventions selected should reflect previously agreed-upon outcome and process goals. Unfortunately, this is not always the case, particularly with process goals. Some novice therapists, in less-than-fully-understood attempts to be "eclectic" in their therapeutic

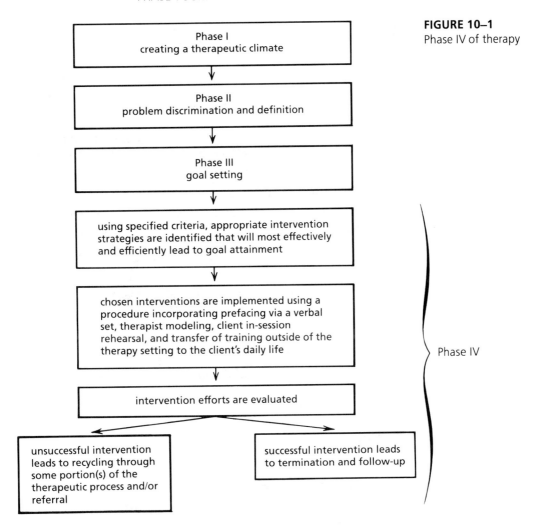

FIGURE 10–1
Phase IV of therapy

orientation, promote new client perspectives and goal-setting in one domain of client functioning and then switch to another domain without explaining this change of focus with clients. The confusion that results for the client who has committed to one goal and then must suddenly attempt an unrelated intervention strategy is disheartening. For example:

The therapist had operated primarily from an affective orientation throughout Phases I, II, and III of therapy. The client's outcome goal of feeling more comfortable at social affairs was committed to pursuing, accompanied by the process goal of reducing anxiety. No mention was ever made of cognitive components that elicit anxiety.

THERAPIST: You mentioned that you've been invited to a party this Friday evening. A fine opportunity to begin working at becoming more comfortable in such circumstances. Let's examine what you might possibly say to yourself to create the anxiety you will likely experience and how you can change that thinking.

CLIENT: (long pause) What do you mean say to myself?

While the therapist's cognitive intervention is appropriate for lessening the client's felt anxiety, and, if effective, could lead to the desired outcome goal, the client is suddenly confronted with a totally new process goal.

Therapist Orientation

Therapists emphasize the interventions based on the beliefs they have about people and how people change; that is, their primary theoretical orientation. It is critical that therapists clearly understand the interventions grounded in this dominant approach, be it affective, behavioral, or cognitive. As we have emphasized throughout this book, beginning therapists should commit themselves to one theoretical approach, even though they might disagree with some of its specifics. With experience, training, and study will come greater integration and movement to a pragmatic therapeutic approach. Developing an expertise in one approach is in the best interest of clients.

Some novice therapists who ably follow this direction through the first two-thirds of the therapeutic process occasionally fall into old "nontherapeutic" patterns when they help clients choose intervention strategies. Giving advice based on prior personal experience rather than therapeutically considered intervention concepts is inappropriate unless the two happen to coincide.

Research Documentation

Varying amounts of research and case history data exist for different therapeutic interventions. Whether a specific intervention has been documented in the professional literature should not be the only criterion in deciding whether to suggest it to a client. Strictly adhered to, such a practice restricts therapists in using their own creativity to counter client concerns. A great deal of new and ongoing research on the effects of therapist functioning and treatment strategies in producing various kinds of client change is being done (Cormier & Cormier). Sufficient data has not yet been collected to prescribe definitively which intervention is best for which person with which problem (Krumboltz & Thoresen, 1976).

Empirical support of a strategy, however, clearly enhances its utility. For example, research data can always help in determining the ways, with whom, and for what problems specific interventions have proven effective or ineffective. A good comprehension of research and case history data is also a prerequisite to helping clients with specific concerns within the different areas of human functioning. And, as Okun (1976) points out, "pretending to be an expert when you're not can backfire, and even if it doesn't, it is questionable ethics" (p. 160).

Client Preference and Characteristics

The selection of interventions, like goal-setting, is most effective when both therapist and client are actively involved. Cormier & Cormier (1979) charge therapists who select strategies or implement treatment plans independent of clients' input with misusing their social influence within the therapeutic relationship. They suggest the therapist provide a menu of intervention possibilities from which clients can select strategies rather than telling clients that only one item is "being served."

To give clients an informed choice, therapists should provide information about potential intervention options. Okun (1982) proposes an outline for providing information about interventions and thereby eliciting client preferences:

1. Explain the intervention options available
2. Provide a rationale for each option
3. Discuss the time and activities involved in each option
4. Discuss the advantages and disadvantages of each option

Clients can be particularly helped in considering the degree of discomfort or risk accompanying any intervention and weighing it against anticipated success. This important issue will be addressed in the upcoming section of this chapter on implementation.

In addition to considering client preferences, it is equally critical to review any client characteristic that might affect the efficacy of a particular intervention. For example, interventions such as behaviorally-oriented systematic desensitization requires clients to generate and sustain mental images. The therapist proposing this intervention would need to ascertain whether a client can generate clear and vivid images before committing to such a strategy.

Egan (1975) strongly urges therapists to help clients choose interventions that are consistent with their values and lifestyle. A client's values will give either a positive or negative valence to an intervention. If the essentials of the strategy run counter to the client's values, the client's motivation will surely be minimal or the use of the strategy may create even further problems.

Environmental Context

The importance of the environmental context of clients already has been discussed. Again, as in other phases of the therapeutic process, environmental context may affect whether a particular intervention is applicable or not. Egan (1982) points out that intervention strategies attempted in unbending environments are impractical. Goldfried and Davison (1976) indicate that the availability of role models and reinforcers in a client's environment may heavily affect interventions attempted. For instance, to use a strategy that requires encouragement and support from significant others when the client has no close relationship network is bound to fail.

Another important contextual consideration is the therapy setting itself. In particular, the amount of time available to spend with a client for each session and for the totality of therapy should have a tremendous impact on intervention selection. In time-limited therapy, specific, concrete strategies that are easily explained and prepared for are most appropriate. Other aspects of the setting are also relevant. For example, it is difficult to train a client in deep relaxation without a comfortable chair. It may be impossible for therapists to leave with clients in some settings to carry out any kind of "in vivo" interventions (Cormier & Cormier, 1979).

Multiple Interventions

Although interventions are best considered concretely and individually they are rarely used in isolation. A variety of interventions is normally necessary to proactively address the complexity and range of problems presented by a single client. Rarely does a client have only one very straightforward concern that can be treated successfully through a single intervention. In this regard Mahoney (1974) aptly asserts, "unidimensional presenting problems appear to be a myth propagated by research conventions. The average client is not simply snake phobic—he often expresses desires to improve personal adjustment along a wide range of foci" (p. 273).

As we discussed in the initial chapter, thoughts, feelings, and behaviors interact and affect each other. We advocate that the novice therapist focus primarily on one specific domain of client functioning and thereby affect the other two. Increasingly, evidence has indicated a strong correlation between performance changes and cognitive changes and vice versa (Bandura & Adams, 1977; Bandura, Adams, & Byer, 1977). With experience and an evolution to a pragmatic therapeutic approach, however, therapists can come to address all three domains of human functioning more directly for even more encompassing and efficient goal attainment.

Once the therapist and client have decided on a specific intervention or multiple interventions, the most effective means of its implementation must be determined. When multiple interventions are committed to, their sequence must be decided. In most cases, it is best to begin with an intervention that is directed toward the process goal most likely to relieve immediate distress and that the client is most likely to succeed at that relates directly to an identifiable outcome goal. Multiple interventions can be used simultaneously; however, it is critical that they each be kept sufficiently concrete so that clients can recognize gains toward a goal.

     After the sequence of interventions is agreed to, their implementation should proceed. Complete and thorough implementation comprises prefacing via a verbal set, then modeling, rehearsal, and transfer of training (Cormier & Cormier, 1979).

IMPLEMENTING INTERVENTION STRATEGIES

Verbal Set

Cormier and Cormier (1979) stress the importance of a verbal set for prefacing the implementation of intervention strategies. They define this procedure as encompassing three aspects: a rationale for the intervention, an overview of the intervention, and a confirmation of the client's willingness to use the strategy. These three components are ideally addressed during intervention selection; therefore, implementation normally entails merely a brief review and recommitment. For example:

THERAPIST: Mary, when we discussed the intervention options available to us for relieving the anxiety you have at job interviews, you'll remember I explained the purpose of and how we could use role playing to help you become more confident and comfortable. Now that we've agreed to begin with that, I'd like to review our previous discussion. I'll play the role of you and show you how to approach a prospective employer, and then you can pretend that I am an employer and approach me in the manner I will have just shown you [overview]. If you can pretend that I'm an employer and approach me confidently and comfortably with new skills, then later you will be able to do so in a real situation much easier [rationale]. How does this sound to you? [client's willingness].

Modeling

Modeling is a procedure by which a person can learn through observing the actions of another person (Cormier & Cormier, 1979). Models can be either live or symbolic. Live models are people: a friend, relative, or therapist. Therapists especially serve as live models "by demonstrating a desired behavior and arranging optimum conditions for the client to do the same" (Nye, 1973, p. 381). Most behaviorally- and cognitively-oriented therapists explicitly explain interventions as they model them for clients. An example would be live modeling by the behaviorally-oriented therapist working with Mary from the previous case illustration:

THERAPIST: Mary, let's give the role play a first trial. I'd like you to play the part of a prospective employer. You've gone to a number of interviews. Just pick one interviewer in particular that you remember and act as she did. I'll role play you. Only instead of sitting meekly by and staring away at the floor and barely speaking, I'll sit up straight, maintain eye contact, and in a clear and firm voice respond directly and ask questions when a lull occurs. Now you begin the interview.

MARY (as a prospective employer): Well, Ms. Willis, what do you see as your major qualifications for this position?

THERAPIST (as Mary): (sitting squarely, maintaining eye contact, and speaking firmly) I have investigated the position opening as well as your company and find my background well suited. . .

After the demonstration, the therapist can suggest that Mary summarize the main points of the modeled demonstration. Also, general principles that she should remember when she acts upon these new learnings can be reviewed. These guidelines can help Mary code the therapist's modeled behavior in a way that will help her recall it. If she has difficulty summarizing or reviewing, additional modeling may be required before she can actually act on the new learnings herself. Further, Mary should be encouraged to select for her own use only those parts of the modeled demonstration that she finds acceptable, unless to do so would change the scope of the intervention (Cormier & Cormier, 1979). For example:

THERAPIST: Let's talk about what we just did. Do you think that you accurately acted the part of the employer?

MARY: Yes, I do. I remember one interview I went to at. . . I acted just like I remember her doing.

THERAPIST: What did you see me doing as I played you that you didn't do at that particular interview?

MARY: Well, you looked right at me and you sat up straight in the chair leaning toward me. You sounded sure of yourself too when you talked about investigating the company.

THERAPIST: Are you ready to act as I did, this time being yourself with me role playing the employer?

MARY: Okay.

Affectively-oriented therapists also use modeling as a significant therapist skill for helping clients implement intervention strategies. Often, their modeling is not overtly stated but rather implied in their role as therapist. Carl Rogers, although not categorizing his actions as modeling per se, nonetheless describes a modeling procedure quite distinctly in the following illustration:

> So then what is the process of counseling and therapy. . . . To the therapist, it is a new venture in relating. He feels, "Here is another person, my client. . . . I realize that at times his own fears may make him perceive me as uncaring, as rejecting, as an intruder, as one who does not understand. I want fully to accept these feelings in him, and yet I hope also that my own real feelings will show through so clearly that in time he cannot fail to perceive them. Most of all I want him to encounter in me a real person. I do not need to be uneasy as to whether my own feelings are 'therapeutic.' What I am and what I feel are good enough to be a basis for therapy, if I can transparently be what I am and what I feel in relationship to him. Then perhaps he can be what he is, openly and without fear." (Rogers, 1961, p. 27)

Typically, whether explicitly or implicitly identified, therapist modeling results in the client practicing the newly learned ways of functioning in the therapy session. The rationale is quite simple for using therapist modeling in this preparatory manner: if the client wants to function differently but doesn't know how, without some type of modeled demonstration it is almost impossible to do so. Should live modeling by the therapist not be appropriate, nor observation of some relevant significant other, clients can use symbolic models. Written materials such as pamphlets and books, films, audio and video tapes, slide tapes, or photographs are all potential substitutes or adjuncts to live modeling demonstrations. Symbolic modeling can also occur by having clients imagine functioning in a particular manner (Cormier & Cormier, 1979).

Rehearsal

Most interventions involve some form of rehearsal in which the client practices the new desired form of functioning in therapy before attempting to do so in everyday living. Rehearsals can be overt or covert. A client can rehearse covertly by imagining and then critiquing the desired changes. Or, in overt rehearsal, the client can verbalize and act out the sought-after changes. Both overt and covert rehearsal have research support; the choice depends upon the theoretical approach of the therapist, timing, the client, and desired changes.

Before and during rehearsals, it is often helpful for therapists to prompt or coach clients, giving the client instructions or cues to help them make the desired changes. Verbal suggestions and verbal and nonverbal minimal encouragers can help clients make the necessary discriminations between old and new ways of functioning as well as encourage them to persist in completing the practice attempt. Gestalt experiences are well known for the therapist's use of prompts and coaching to facilitate client change. Consider the following excerpt from Fritz Perls's work with a client, Jean, during a workshop demonstration:

PERLS: So, let's switch back to Jean. Jean, would you talk again, tell again the dream, live it through as if this were your existence, as if you live it now, see if you can understand more about your life. . . .

JEAN: I don't—it doesn't really seem clear until I find myself—the place has become kind of a top of the chute. I don't remember whether at first I was afraid or not, possibly—oh, I should say this now?

PERLS: You are now the chute. Are you afraid to go down?

JEAN: (laughs) I guess I am a little afraid to go down. But then it seems like . . .

PERLS: So the existential message is, "You've got to go down."

JEAN: I guess I'm afraid to find out what's there.

PERLS: This points to false ambitions, that you're too high up.

JEAN: That's true.

PERLS: So the existential message says, "Go down." Again our mentality says, "High up is better than down." You must always be somewhere higher.

JEAN: Anyway, I seem a little afraid to go down.

PERLS: Talk to the chute.

JEAN: Why are you muddy? You're slippery and slidy and I might fall on you and slip.

PERLS: Now play the chute. "I'm slippery and . . ."

JEAN: I'm slippery and muddy, the better to slide and faster to get down on. (laughs)

PERLS: Ahah, well, what's the joke?

JEAN: (continues laughing) I'm just laughing.

PERLS: Can you accept yourself as slippery?

JEAN: Hm. I guess so. Yes . . . (Perls, 1969, p. 145)

Following a rehearsal, the therapist should provide *feedback* to help clients recognize successful performance and correct any difficulties they encountered. Feedback should be designed to improve performance by helping clients recognize the desirable and undesirable aspects of their rehearsal. Continuing with the previous excerpt of Fritz Perls and Jean, they went on to consider Jean's relationship with her mother. Perls concluded the rehearsal by stating:

> I'm very glad that we have this last experience—we can learn such
> a lot from this. . . . Very few people can really visualize, conceive
> themselves as adults. . . . A person doesn't want to take the
> responsibility of the adult person, and thereby rationalizes, hangs
> on to the childhood memories, to the image that they are a child,

and so on. Because to grow up means to be *alone,* and to be alone is the prerequisite for maturity and contact. Loneliness, isolation, is still longing for support. Jean has made a big step toward growing, tonight. (Perls, 1969, p. 148)

Cormier and Cormier (1979) identify a number of conditions that help feedback after rehearsal attempts be of the greatest benefit:

1. The client should be given the first opportunity to assess his or her performance. If a client is responsible for a large portion of the feedback, this sensitizes him or her to the optimal ways to function and improves performance outside of the session (Rose, 1973).
2. The client should be encouraged for some or all of his or her performance during the rehearsal. It is important not to wait for perfect performance before offering encouragement. Any progress should be noted.
3. The feedback should provide suggestions for how the client might improve his or her performance. Cormier and Cormier (1979) suggest the use of the "sandwiching" technique for therapist feedback. The first part (a slice of bread) is an encouraging remark, followed by a suggestion or a constructive criticism (the filling), followed by another encouraging remark (the other slice of bread).

Transfer of Training

Helping clients transfer their changes in functioning from within the therapy session to real life completes the implementation process. With many clients this generalization occurs without direct therapist help. Affectively-oriented therapists in particular tend to trust their clients to transfer in-session gains naturally. In this regard, Carl Rogers described how the typical client experiences therapy, stating:

"You know, I feel as if I'm floating along on the current of life, very adventurously, being me. I get defeated sometimes, I get hurt sometimes, but I'm learning that those experiences are not fatal. I don't know exactly *who* I am, but I can feel my reactions at any given moment, and they seem to work out pretty well as a basis for my behavior from moment to moment. Maybe this is what it *means* to be *me*. But of course I can only do this because I feel safe in the relationship with my therapist. Or could I be myself outside of this relationship? I wonder. I wonder. Perhaps I could." (Rogers, 1961. p. 28)

Therapists ordinarily help their clients transfer training in therapy with *homework* experiences. Homework experiences are tailored to enable clients to use their new functioning skills in low-risk situations in which the probability of recognizable success is high. Gradually, the client can then experience more unpredictable and threatening situations. The particular homework given depends on the therapist's theoretical orientation, the client, and their goals. Cognitive and behaviorally-oriented approaches use homework extensively to transfer training.

Walen, DiGuiseppe, and Wessler (1980) propose that therapists ask themselves, "What can my client *do* this week to put into practice what we have discussed during this session?" (p. 216). In considering homework, they suggest that such outside-of-session experiences share several important characteristics:

1. *Consistency.* Homework should be consistent with the work done in the session and not be irrelevant or arbitrarily assigned. Assignments that lead naturally from the main theme of the session are best.

2. *Specificity.* Homework should be given in sufficient detail and with clear instructions. For example, if a client is asked to come up with possible solutions to a problem, a vague request like "Think of as many as you can" is less preferable to the concrete "Think of at least five potential solutions."

3. *Systematic Follow-Through.* It is critical that homework be systematically agreed upon and discussed at the beginning of the next therapy session. Otherwise, therapy sessions often become an end in themselves rather than focusing, as they should, on helping the client attain goals in daily life.

EVALUATING INTERVENTION STRATEGIES

The importance of monitoring and evaluating the effects of intervention strategies cannot be overstated. Evaluation not only indicates the extent to which therapeutic goals are achieved, but it also provides continuing encouragement to client and therapist alike as progress is clearly seen.

Throughout this book are many references to clinical research studies as well as case histories that have demonstrated successful goal attainment resulting from a particular intervention strategy being applied to certain clinical problems. The experimental terminology and designs used in these research studies have been described in a variety of sources and will be addressed in a later chapter in this book. It is not the purpose of this present section to discuss evaluation as it relates to detailed experimental research design. Rather, the objective here is to provide a practical method with which therapists can evaluate the effectiveness of strategies for achieving agreed-to therapeutic goals.

It should be noted that experimental research evaluation and therapy evaluation often use similar methodology and assessment schemes.

Their purposes, however, frequently vary. Empirical research may be considered a quest for causality or "truth." In contrast, therapy evaluation is more of a hypothesis-testing procedure (Shaprio, 1966). The data collected for therapy evaluation are used to make decisions about the effectiveness of intervention strategies and the extent to which outcome and process goals are achieved (Cormier & Cormier, 1979).

Therapy evaluation is used to see whether an intervention strategy is helping a client as it was designed to and whether the client is using the strategy accurately and systematically. Evaluating the effectiveness of intervention strategies helps the client and therapist determine the type, direction, and amount of change in functioning demonstrated by the client. Although this form of evaluation can yield valuable information, it is naturally not so rigorous as an evaluation conducted under carefully controlled experimental conditions as it is not meant to be. Mahoney (1977) addressed this issue in stating:

> The most efficient therapist is sensitively tuned to the personal data of the client. He is not collecting data for the sake of scientific appearances or because that is what is considered proper. . . . The effective therapist uses data to guide his or her efforts at having an impact, and . . . . he adjusts therapeutic strategies in tune with that feedback. (p. 241)

The Egan Model

Egan (1982) proposes three principal areas of inquiry to guide therapy evaluation efforts: quality of participation, quality of intervention strategies, and quality of problem resolution.

1. *Client Participation.* Is the client participating in the intervention efforts? To what extent?

    Losing weight is one of Gloria's outcome goals. Progressively reducing her caloric intake to 1000 calories per day constitutes her process goal. She and the therapist devised a schedule for gradually reducing consumption to the 1000 calorie limit. Gloria has maintained the schedule, reducing her daily intake 50 calories per day in pursuit of the process goal. Clearly, she is fully participating in the intervention efforts.

2. *Intervention Effectiveness.* Are the agreed-to outcome and process goals being accomplished through the client's participation in intervention efforts? To what extent? (The emphasis here is not necessarily on total goal attainment, but *progress toward* goal achievement.)

    Gloria's outcome goal is to reduce from 170 pounds to a maximum 130 pounds body weight. Her process goal is to gradually reduce her daily caloric intake until reaching a 1000 calorie limit and then maintaining that until the desired 130 pound body weight is achieved. Not only has she maintained her scheduled decrease in daily caloric intake for the past 2 weeks, but also she simultaneously has lost 6 pounds. Gloria's progress and the effectiveness of the current intervention strategy is readily recognizable.

3. *Problem Resolution.* Is the problem that was originally defined being satisfactorily handled through achievement of the goals that had been established? To what degree? (This is the ultimate inquiry, for it deals with the reason for beginning therapy in the first place.)

    Gloria went to therapy because she saw herself as a loser, a failure in life. The original discrimination and definition of her problem indicated that Gloria possessed little self-control; her overeating, excess weight, and poor physical appearance made her see herself as a failure. The weight loss program was geared not just to improving her eating habits and physical appearance, but to her overriding outcome goal of increased self-control and thus a sense of mastery and success. Gloria has found that changing her behavior in the area of eating has had a generalization effect: she feels more self-confident and her thoughts are now "I can" instead of "I give up." She now sees herself as a person with potential.

Gathering Evaluation Data

Evaluation via the Egan Model may seem relatively simple given only three very basic areas of inquiry to pursue. Evaluation can be easily conceptualized; however, it often is not viewed that way because of the difficulty many therapists have in systematically gathering evaluation data. This gathering process includes selecting an appropriate type, method, and time schedule for measuring evaluation data. Cormier and Cormier (1979) summarize the major indices for gathering evaluation data. These include the type of data, method of measurement, and time schedule: they are illustrated graphically in Figure 10–2.

Types of Evaluation Data. Information that falls into Egan's three areas of inquiry must be gathered in such a way that the client's functioning at Point A (minimally, prior to intervention) can be compared against that same functioning at Point B (minimally, after intervention). This information can be assessed using one or more of the following measures:

☐ *Verbal Self-Report.* Client verbal self-reports are likely the easiest and most convenient type of evaluation data to gather. Although client verbal reports are not typically regarded as the most reliable measure of evaluation data, "from a purely clinical perspective, measurement

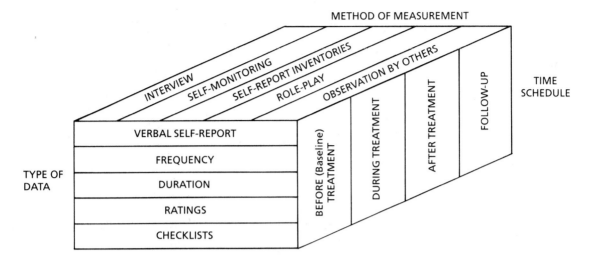

FIGURE 10–2

Major indices for gathering evaluation data

that is independent of the patient's report is superfluous" (Tasto, 1977, pp. 153–154). Tasto further asserts in this regard:

In the realm of clinical practice *the operational criteria for the existence of problems are self-reported verbalizations.* If a patient says there is a problem, then there is a problem. And conversely, when the patient claims there is no problem, then there is no problem. Therapeutic intervention is considered to be progressing to the extent that the patient (and others who may also be involved) report that things are better and conversely, therapeutic intervention may be considered to be of no value or even harmful as a result of the patient's (and sometimes others') report. (p. 154)

Client verbal self-reports, however, are often too vague to offer enough information to make accurate comparisons. For example, a client may report after intervention strategies have been implemented, "I'm feeling less depressed now." The client may be unable to identify *how much* his or her depression has actually decreased. For this reason, client verbal self-reports are frequently supplemented with other types of measurement that produce more concrete and quantifiable data (Cormier & Cormier, 1979).

☐ *Frequency Counts.* Frequency counts reflect the number of times (how many, how often) that specific types of functioning occur. The number of anxiety attacks, self-denigrating thoughts, or inappropriate behaviors experienced within a given time are examples of forms of client functioning that can be assessed with frequency counts.

☐ *Duration Counts.* Duration counts reflect the length of time a particular response or collection of responses occurs. For example, the amount of time spent speaking with another person, how long depressive thoughts are compulsively repeated, and the length of time an anxiety attack lasts are forms of client functioning that can be appropriately measured using duration counts.

Frequency counts and duration counts are commonly obtained in two ways: continuous recording and time-sampling. In continuous recording, the client records *each time* the specified response occurs. Often, this is impossible, particularly when the response occurs frequently or when its onset and ending are difficult to ascertain. Time sampling is therefore usually the procedure of choice. In time sampling, a client keeps track of the frequency or duration of the selected response only during specific time intervals. For example, a client might record the number of self-denigrating thoughts he or she had from 10 to 11 A.M., 3 to 4 P.M., and 8 to 9 P.M. each day for a specified period. Time sampling is not as precise as continuous recording in that many responses will possibly be missed; however, the former is clearly the more practical.

☐ *Rating Scales.* The intensity or degree of specific responses can be assessed with a rating scale. For example, the intensity of anxious feelings might be measured by using a rating scale with gradations from 1 (calm) to 5 (panic-stricken). Cronbach (1970) suggests in regard to rating scales that what is to be rated should be well-defined. For example, if a client is to rate self-denigrating thoughts, examples of what constitutes these types of thoughts should be concretely identified and agreed-to (e.g., "I hate myself," "I'm no good," etc.). Cronbach also emphasized the importance of descriptions for each point on a rating scale. Episodes of depression, for example, might be graded from 1 to 5 and described as 1 (no depression), 2 (some depression), 3 (moderate depression), 4 (severe depression), and 5 (incapacitating depression). Finally, rating scales should have at least four gradations and no more than seven. Cronbach proposes that less than four points limits a client's capacity to discriminate and more than seven cannot be rated reliably because too many discriminations are called for.

☐ *Checklists.* Checklists are somewhat similar to rating scales. The type of judgment required, however, differs. Rating scales assess degree or intensity. Checklists simply seek to determine the presence or absense of a certain response. For instance, consider the client seeking to display more assertive behaviors in interactions with others. The verbal and nonverbal behaviors associated with assertive action would be listed on a checklist. If the client demonstrates a specific assertive behavior in an observed setting, it is recorded on the checklist.

Methods of Measurement. Each type of data just described is characteristically gathered using a specific method. Client verbal self-reports, for example, are commonly assessed regularly during therapy sessions as an intrinsic part of the therapeutic process. Consider the four-phase therapeutic model:

Phase I: In creating a therapeutic climate, core conditions, social influence, structuring, and therapist attending all lie on a continuum— the more these therapist skills are in evidence, the better will be the atmosphere in which the therapeutic process evolves.

Phase II: In discriminating and defining the problem situation, the manner in which a client is functioning before interventions are implemented is clearly identified. Thus, a standard is established against which change can be compared.

Phase III: In setting goals that are concretely clarified, specified, and committed to, another standard is set. If outcome and process goals are readily recognizable, then their attainment or nonattainment will be as easily noted.

Phase IV: In intervention strategies that are well-considered and planned, client participation will be obvious. Vague and ill-considered strategies create problems in determining the extent of client participation.

Frequency counts and duration counts are gathered through *client self-monitoring,* a process in which clients observe and record aspects of their own functioning. Monitoring usually involves observing specific responses and recording them with pencil and paper, mechanical counters, timers, or electronic measuring devices (Ciminero, Nelson, & Lipinski, 1977). Rating scales and checklists form the basis for *self-report inventories,* written questionnaires that clients complete. Self-report inventories can be developed by a therapist and client that specifically address the client's particular circumstances; professionally published versions are also available. Published inventories include such measures as the Beck Depression Inventory (Beck, 1972) and the Assertion Inventory (Gambrill & Richy, 1975).

Cormier and Cormier (1979) also suggest within-session *role play* procedures and *observation by others* as methods of gathering evaluation data. Role play consists of scenarios designed by the therapist to evaluate a client's functioning in a theoretical situation. For instance, role play scenes might be created to gather data on a client's functioning in stressful or painful situations, or in a specific problem situation such as a social exchange or parent–child or other relationship (Nay, 1977). Role plays can be conducted before, during, and after intervention.

While finding reliable and willing observers in a client's environment may be difficult, their observations of a client's functioning can provide valuable evaluation data. This is especially true where clients have changed their "negative" forms of functioning, but may still be mislabeled by persons in their environment. As Kazdin (1977) suggests:

> The evaluation of behavior by others is important independently of the behaviors that the clients perform after treatment. The problem with many deviant populations is not merely their behavior but how they are perceived by others and perceive themselves. . . . Thus, it is possible that changing behavior of clients will not necessarily alter the evaluations of individuals with whom the target clients have interacted. (pp. 446–447)

A client's problem may be more with the environment than the way in which the client is functioning. Often others' observations and feedback are critical in effectively recognizing and reacting to this fact.

Time Schedules. Evaluation is a critical part of the entire therapeutic process and thus should not simply be left until after intervention strategies have been applied. In its most effective form, evaluation and thus data gathering for evaluation purposes is ongoing. At the minimum, evaluation information should be gathered at the *beginning of treatment* (prior to any intervention being applied), *during treatment* (while an intervention is being implemented), and *after treatment* (at the conclusion of the intervention strategy). We stress the value of *follow-up* as well.

Many practitioners see follow-up as a critical component of the therapeutic process that is frequently ignored. As Bandura (1976) convincingly states, the value of therapeutic intervention must be judged not only in terms of successful "initial elimination" of a client's problem but also in terms of the client's "vulnerability to defensive" or maladaptive "re-learning" after therapy is terminated (p. 261). Follow-ups can be long- or short-term. Follow-up methods will be presented later in this chapter.

RECYCLING AND REFERRAL

If, after evaluating the effectiveness of intervention strategies, it is determined that the client is not participating fully, that a particular intervention shows little efficacy in achieving a goal, or that the original problem is not being satisfactorily resolved, the steps taken in all phases of the therapeutic process should be reexamined, a process known as recycling. The problem may not have been properly defined, or the most important problem may not have been identified, or process and outcome goals may not have been concretely specified. Interventions may have been impulsively selected or poorly implemented. And, possibly, everything worked out as planned, but the resolution of one problem produced another (Patterson & Eisenberg, 1982).

Egan (1982) addresses this last issue in stating:

> I have frequently suggested that problem solving is not a magic linear process that works automatically, but then there are few such magical processes in life. Just as researchers recycle their experimental processes (with an occasional dramatic breakthrough) until they achieve their experimental goals, so people recycle problem-solving procedures (with an occasional dramatic breakthrough) until they are satisfied with the way they are meeting their needs and handling their problem situations. (p. 285)

Throughout this book and most all resources relating to counseling and psychotherapy, oversimplified examples, usually with quite successful reported results, are the norm. This presentation is chosen to help the reader understand the optimal possible outcomes. It is a teaching tool. In clients' (and therapists') daily lives, however, most therapeutic efforts result in moderate successes; spectacular successes are the exception rather than the rule. For example, a client who is severely anxious in all social situations will be able to lessen significantly the level of felt anxiety in most social encounters. To expect that the client will feel no anxiety, however, is unrealistic if not simply foolish.

When expectations are not met as a result of therapeutic efforts, the therapist must decide whether recycling is appropriate, based on a realistic expectation that more effort will result in proportionate progress. Therapists must decide whether they can continue to be of significant assistance to a client. That client must decide whether what might be realistically achieved is worth the extra expense in terms of time, energy, and money.

Recycling, then, is not a sign of failure. Rather, it is a part of the human condition (Egan, 1982). Perfection is rarely attainable. This is not to say that initial therapeutic efforts cannot nor should not be optimally efficient and effective; rather, that it is impossible to consider all that has happened, is happening, and will happen. Recycling is, however, an opportunity to review, revise, and reinvest when client and therapist see it as worthwhile.

Even with recycling, therapy is not always a singularly successful endeavor by itself. The therapist and client may have incompatible personalities (Goldstein, 1971), the client's problems are discovered to be beyond the therapist's level of competence to deal with, or the client's concerns require a specialized treatment approach (e.g. chemical dependency). Under such conditions, complete or concurrent referral to the appropriate resources is the correct course of action. Referral requires an honest acknowledgment from the therapist that some other person or resource can provide more efficient or effective help to a client.

The therapist can smooth the transition to a referral by offering a client more than one meaningful possibility for additional assistance. This procedure often prevents the client from feeling shunted from one professional to another with little input into or control of the situation (Hansen, Stevic, & Warner, 1982). The therapist should be familiar with the referral sources suggested and promote the best possible fit between the client and resource selected. The therapist can also help the client and the referral source by providing information, with the client's permission and within the limits of confidentiality, so that the referral source can begin immediately to mobilize appropriate resources to help the client.

Successful therapy is often related to using various resource personnel. Every therapist will eventually find himself or herself calling on outside assistance for a client.

TERMINATION AND FOLLOW-UP

If evaluation has indicated that intervention strategies have been successful in achieving desired outcome and process goals and the presenting problem has been sufficiently resolved, termination of therapy is natural. Such a positive termination will likely involve some sadness because of the loss of a meaningful relationship. Both therapist and client may experience some separation anxiety about the impending end of their relationship. Eisenberg and Delaney (1977) describe the circumstances normally present:

> For counseling to be of maximum impact, the relationship must be uncommonly close and intense. When counseling goals have been attained, it is time for the intense relationship to be terminated. As anyone who has experienced the separation of a loved one can attest, terminating an intense relationship is not easy for anyone involved. (p. 206)

Thus, clients especially must be proactively prepared for therapy to end. Termination is considered an intervention strategy in itself for readjusting to a new life situation in which clients are less reliant on their interactions with the therapist.

There are many similarities between ending a single therapy session and ending the therapeutic relationship. In both situations, it is important that clients be made aware of the impending termination so they can anticipate and prepare for what they may experience during termination and afterward. It is also important to acknowledge that terminations are not always permanent. Follow-up sessions can be conducted and therapy can always be reentered if circumstances call for it. It is important, however, that clients realize their own independent strengths and capabilities and that therapy not be a permanent condition (Hackney & Cormier, 1979).

Preparation

Clients should be made aware throughout therapy that there will come a time when the therapist's assistance is no longer appropriate. This time is not necessarily when the client's life is idyllic; it is when clients have more to gain from being independent of the therapist than they would gain from continuing therapy. We agree with Hackney and Cormier (1979) who take the therapeutic position that "human beings are happier and more self-fulfilled when they are able to trust their own resources" (pp. 58–59). While happy and self-fulfilled persons often rely on others, they do so out of self-perceived choice rather than self-perceived necessity.

Some therapists contract with clients during the initial phase of therapy to end their relationship after a stated period of time. In some cases, this is out of necessity. For example, a couple may be seeking premarital therapy to conclude just before their wedding. Or, a college student will be leaving for summer vacation when a school term ends. In other cases, time-limited therapy is contracted to as a motivational procedure for facilitating client effort ("We've got just 8 sessions to accomplish your goals. Your full effort will be needed."). In such cases, it is appropriate to acknowledge throughout the therapeutic process that these time constraints exist (Hackney & Cormier, 1979).

When the therapeutic relationship is more open-ended and determined by the client's progress, termination should still begin well before complete goal attainment. Most therapists begin lengthening the time between sessions as the latter portions of the proactive problem intervention phase are entered. Weekly sessions can be reduced to bi-weekly, then monthly. Extending the time between sessions has the advantage of reducing potential separation anxiety while providing continuing support and encouragement as well as enabling a more accurate evaluation of the client's ability to independently maintain changes made during therapy.

Termination as an Intervention Strategy

A critical issue that frequently emerges during termination is that of client dependency. This issue is often a complex one (Eisenberg & Delaney, 1977). Therapists generally believe in the desirability of clients' self-reliance; they should not be dependent on others to attain goals that are important to them. By coming to therapy for help, however, a client implies dependency on the therapist for aid in dealing with whatever concerns he or she wishes to present. In defining problems and setting goals, the client is clearly dependent on the therapist for assistance. By continuing therapy, the client further implies that he or she has a better chance of attaining stated goals with the therapist's help than without it, again a distinctly implied statement of dependency (Eisenberg & Delaney, 1977).

After the stated therapeutic goals are attained, the therapist must still work with the client to regain a stronger sense of self-reliance. The therapeutic relationship, no matter how intense, is always temporary. At therapy's natural conclusion, clients must be able to function on their own without being dependent on the therapist for further assistance. The outcome goal is to terminate the therapeutic relationship. The process goal aimed at achieving this outcome goal is to help clients gain a greater sense of self-reliance at the expense of any implied dependency on the therapist.

Patterson & Eisenberg (1983) propose an intervention outline for ending an intense therapeutic relationship in a positive manner. They address eight specific guidelines for therapists to consider in structuring termination to achieve the process and outcome goals just noted.

1. *Be clearly aware of the client's needs and wants.* If dependency is present, termination may significantly affect the client. It may be necessary to explore and elaborate on what it will mean. New perspectives can be fostered about feelings of dependency and perceived needs for support.

2. *Be clearly aware of your own needs and wants.* Therapists too need to end the relationship for themselves as well as the client. A need to be wanted, admired, or to control may cause a therapist to resist termination. Awareness of these needs can elicit greater control over them.

3. *Be aware of your previous experiences with separation and your inner reactions to these experiences.* If the therapeutic experience has been intense, therapists can expect reactions to termination similar to those elicited by previous separations. Expecting and being aware of these reactions enables the therapist to competently cope with them.

4. *Invite the client to share how he or she is responding to terminating therapy.* Closure, or ending the therapeutic experience, is important for the client. Sharing inner experiences, thoughts and feelings, is an essential part of this closure. Immediacy is a most helpful therapist skill to employ here.

5. *Share honestly with the client your responses to this therapeutic experience.* If therapy has been intense, there will have been moments of excitement, anxiety, stress, and confusion for the therapist. Reviewing these various reactions to experiences that occurred during therapy will help both the therapist and the client with closure. Both

parties will have gained from the relationship. The therapist's information-giving and self-disclosure in this regard can have an affirming effect on a client.

6. *Review the major events of the therapy experience and bring the review into the present.* Reviewing with the client major themes, changes that have occurred, and critical moments through the use of focused summarizations brings the experience full circle. It helps the client elaborate on and enhance the positive changes in his or her functioning that have taken place. Seeing self over time also significantly fosters closure.

7. *Supportively acknowledge the positive changes the client has accomplished.* Implementing intervention strategies to bring about changes in how one functions is never easy, natural, or automatic. Discomfort and difficulty are prerequisites. Maintaining these changes requires continued effort. Recognizing and affirming the changes the client has made as well as the stress involved in achieving them encourages the client to maintain changes after therapy has concluded.

8. *Invite the client to keep you up to date on what is happening in his or her life.* While the formal therapy experience ends, respect and caring need not. A genuine (as opposed to doing one's "therapeutic duty") invitation for follow-up is a valuable expression of respect that challenges the client to continue to enhance his or her functioning in the future.

Follow-up

Follow-up is an important part of the termination experience. Yet this is a procedure that many therapists do not use (Okun, 1982). Follow-up means checking to see how a client is progressing with his or her problem situation and the outcome goals that were pursued during therapy. Follow-up can be both short-term (1, 3, or 6 months) and long-term (9 months, 1 year or longer) and can be conducted in several ways. The kind of follow-up depends upon a client's availability to participate, the therapeutic issues that were involved and current time demands on the therapist. Possible follow-up procedures include the following (Cormier & Cormier, 1979):

☐ Invite the client to come in for a follow-up session to assess how the client is coping with his or her "former" problem. In the session, the client could demonstrate changes in functioning in simulated role plays with the therapist.

☐ Mail a self-report inventory to the client requesting information about his or her current status in relation to the original presenting problem.

Cormier and Cormier (1979) caution to remember to include a stamped, self-addressed envelope.

☐ Send a letter to the client asking about the current status of the problem and the client's continuing progress.

☐ Telephone the client for a report.

It is important for the therapist to distinguish between genuine follow-up and any attempt to extend a client's possible dependency. The purpose of follow-up is to evaluate the continuing progress of the client and thereby the effectiveness of therapy efforts as well as the therapist's skills. Occasionally, follow-up will result in a client temporarily returning to therapy if the client is experiencing notable difficulties from prior problems or from a new problem; this too is an important function of follow-up.

THERAPIST SKILLS IV: THEORETICAL APPLICATIONS

This chapter investigated proactive problem intervention; that is, actively and assertively seeking to produce change in the ways clients feel, think, and act. Depending on a therapist's theoretical perspective, this chapter may have many or few applications. We believe that these therapist skills have significant value for all therapists. The deciding variable is how "intervention" is defined. For the purpose of this discussion, we define intervention as a purposeful procedure tailored to meet the specific goals of the client.

Given this definition, the specific theoretical orientations presented in this book may be placed on a continuum ranging from implicit, client-controlled intervention to explicit, therapist-controlled intervention. This continuum and relevant placement of the various theoretical approaches is illustrated in Figure 10–3.

Person-centered therapy, at the far left of the continuum, has almost no emphasis on explicit intervention. Intervention is assumed to be initiated by the client as a result of actualizing his or her potential through exploration that occurs within a facilitative therapeutic climate. Thus, successful interventions can be inferred to result from the therapist's providing appropriate conditions that encourage a client's natural tendency toward personal growth. Like person-centered therapy, existential therapy places little importance on explicit intervention. Rather, its emphasis is on flexibility and versatility; what the therapist does depends entirely on the nature of a client's present experience. The therapist does, however, take a greater role in explicitly facilitating clients' self-awareness and commitment. Existentialists can be quite confrontive.

Gestalt therapists and reality therapists are close together on our intervention continuum. Gestalt therapists deliberately try to force clients

Person-Centered Therapy	Existential Therapy	Gestalt Therapy Reality Therapy	Transactional Analysis Cognitive Therapy	Rational-Emotive Therapy	Behavior Therapy

IMPLICIT,   EXPLICIT,
   CLIENT-CONTROLLED   THERAPIST-CONTROLLED
      INTERVENTION STRATEGIES   INTERVENTION STRATEGIES

to confront and acknowledge feelings they have been arduously trying to avoid. Interventions are aimed at helping clients fully live the present. A variety of exercises are employed to foster clients' increased awareness and subsequent reintegration. To a similar degree, reality therapists attempt to put responsibility on clients. More explicit teaching, however, is employed by reality therapists.

Transactional Analysis and cognitive therapy occupy the same basic position on the continuum. The interventions and accompanying terminology specific to each are explicitly advocated as necessary client change components. Rational-emotive therapy differs from its cognitively-oriented counterparts only in that rational-emotive therapists assume a greater role in initiating and monitoring interventions.

Behavior therapy more than any other approach emphasizes very explicit intervention strategies and advocates greater therapist responsibility for initiating these strategies. Behavior therapy is also set apart in that it stresses the evaluation component of proactive problem intervention to a far greater degree than all of the other approaches combined, with the possible exception of Beck's cognitive therapy.

We stress again that the therapist skills in this chapter are applicable regardless of theoretical approach. In the chapter we presented a number of examples from the left end of the continuum approaches, stressing implicit strategies. While they are not explicit in addressing intervention strategies and advocating less therapist responsibility, nonetheless, these approaches can help practitioners significantly through their constant consideration if not overt implementation. The evaluation component most notably is of concern in this latter regard.

FIGURE 10–3
Continuum of intervention strategies

An excerpt from Charles' second session with the counselor concluded Chapter 9. A commitment was agreed on that called for decreasing the amount of time spent in dysfunctional (for Charles) "what if" thinking. The therapeutic process now proceeds into Phase IV, Proactive Problem Intervention, in the session excerpt that follows.

COUNSELOR: Charles, in terms of decreasing the amount of time you spend in the "what if" thinking we have discussed as being a problem for you, there are several strategies we could employ. One that I am most familiar with and have found to be effective with other clients with similar concerns is called

CHARLES: PHASE IV

THERAPIST SKILLS IV intervention selection (explanation of options)

thought-stopping. I'd like to give you some information about thought-stopping so we might judge together whether it would be appropriate with your circumstances.

CHARLES: I'd be willing to try whatever you suggest.

COUNSELOR: Well, I think that it's important that you have information about procedures we can use so that you can decide if something sounds like it might be effective or possibly you could recognize a problem with it.

CHARLES: Okay.

intervention selection (rationale, time & activities, advantages & disadvantages)

COUNSELOR: As I mentioned earlier, an effective strategy might be thought-stopping. It's a way to stop yourself from constantly ruminating "what if this, what if that." It will take one session to learn the procedure and then time and practice on your part outside the session as well as maintaining the record you have begun on the amount of time you spend each evening in "what if" thinking. Reviewing and refining of your efforts could constitute the focus for at least the following two sessions. That would keep us within the three-session timeline we agreed to after which we'll evaluate where we're at and then what we might further pursue. The one potential risk in using thought-stopping may be that it alone won't be sufficient to change your thinking. However, I would see it as more efficient to not expend a lot of extra time and effort in beginning a number of strategies at this point when we might not have to employ anything else but this one. If it's sufficient, you should be able to get the time you spend in "what if" thinking decreased by the one half relatively easily which is our immediate goal.

CHARLES: Let's give it a try.

COUNSELOR: So you're confident at this point that thought-stopping might work for you. Do you have any questions at all?

CHARLES: Not really at this time.

intervention implementation (verbal set)

COUNSELOR: Why don't we proceed then. We talked about how your "what if" thinking about decisions you have made or might make creates problems in a number of areas in your life. Up to now, you might say that your thoughts have been controlling you. Thought-stopping is a way for you to control your thoughts.

CHARLES: So I'm going to tell myself to stop thinking certain thoughts.

intervention implementation (verbal set)

COUNSELOR: Right. A good way to look at it. We'll focus on using the word *stop* to interrupt your "what if" thinking. However, it's not only a matter of telling yourself to stop, but practicing to the point where, upon your command, you can break your habit of continually ruminating "what if, what if" and also begin to substitute more productive, positive thinking. How does that sound to you?

CHARLES: Okay.

COUNSELOR: First I am going to model for you how you can interrupt your "what if" thinking. Ready?

CHARLES: Yes.

intervention implementation (modeling)

COUNSELOR: Relax as much as you can and imagine yourself being home alone in the evening. Think of a situation you've been "what iffing" about a lot . . .

perhaps your relationship with your girlfriend . . . "Should I be doing all the changing . . . what if I don't?"

CHARLES: (pauses, contemplating) Well, what if I go back to Colorado? Will I lose her? Will she follow me? Probably not. Oh, darn. What if I stay here, though?

COUNSELOR: (yelling) *STOP!*

CHARLES: Hey! I sure wasn't expecting that.

COUNSELOR: I realize it's startling, but the surprise element when first learning the procedure seems to make it more effective. How did the "stop" effect your thinking?

CHARLES: I just realized. I stopped the "what if" thinking and switched to something else immediately.

COUNSELOR: Great. Let's try it again, a bit differently though. This time again imagine yourself alone at home in the evening thinking those "what if's" about you and your girlfriend, but keep them to yourself. As soon as you really get into the "what if's," signal to me by raising your index finger on your right hand. Okay?

intervention implementation (modeling)

CHARLES: (pausing, contemplating; then raises his index finger)

COUNSELOR: (yelling) *STOP!*

CHARLES: It worked again.

COUNSELOR: Perfect. You seem to be able to interrupt your thinking very well with this procedure. Let's practice a couple more times.

[Additional practice follows during which Charles is shown and practices going through the same procedure, but yelling the "STOP!" himself, rather than the counselor doing the interrupting]

COUNSELOR: Of course, it won't always be possible to yell *stop* out loud. Your neighbors may come banging on your front door wondering what's happening. So what we'll do is go through the same procedure, only this time when you get into the "what if" thoughts, yell "STOP!" to yourself so that no one else but you knows you're doing it.

intervention implementation (rehearsal)

CHARLES: (pauses, contemplates) I did it. I think I've got thought-stopping well in hand.

COUNSELOR: Great. So far you've passed with flying colors. Now let's look at how after you stop your negative "what if" thinking, you can immediately substitute more productive, positive thoughts with which to occupy your mind. This will fill the void left by blocking your negative thoughts. How does this sound?

[Charles and the counselor then proceed with the second part of the thought-stopping procedure via a therapist modeling/client rehearsal/feedback paradigm]

COUNSELOR: You've really done a great job with learning this. As you can imagine, it may take some time and repeated practice to get this solidly in place in your frame of thinking. Could we agree on how often you might be willing to practice this week?

intervention implementation (transfer of training)

CHARLES: What do you suggest?

COUNSELOR: Since our agreed-to focus for now is the time you spend in "what if" thinking in the evening, how about if you utilize thought-stopping between nine and ten P.M. each evening this week and we'll proceed from there after we get together again next week.

CHARLES: I'll agree to that.

COUNSELOR: Fine. Don't forget to maintain your record of the amount of time you spend each evening in "what if" thinking. It will be important to have this information when we evaluate in three weeks.

SUGGESTED READINGS

Selecting, Implementation, and Evaluation of Intervention Strategies

Eisenberg, S., & Delaney, D. J. (1977). *The counseling process* (2nd ed.). Chicago: Rand McNally. Eisenberg and Delaney's discussion of specific strategies is particularly valuable as they punctuate it most specifically in offering six "principles" by which clients change.

Hackney, H. L., & Cormier, L. S. (1979). *Counseling strategies and objectives* (2nd ed.). Englewood Cliffs, NJ: Prentice-Hall. This book addresses selection, implementation, and evaluation as well as offering a counseling strategies checklist for assessing one's performance in proactively intervening with client problems.

Okun, B. F. (1982). *Effective helping: Interviewing and counseling techniques* (2nd ed.). Monterey, CA: Brooks/Cole. Okun devotes a significant portion of this book to introducing and applying intervention strategies.

Recycling and Referral

Gottman, J. M., & Leiblum, S. R. (1974). *How to do psychotherapy and how to evaluate it.* New York: Holt, Rinehart and Winston. Gottman and Leiblum propose that reevaluation of client goals be pursued "with the understanding and consent of the client" who is "free to exert 'counter-control'—that is, to challenge, refute, or refuse to comply with the therapist's suggestions."

Ivey, A. E., & Simek-Downing, L. (1980). *Counseling and psychotherapy: Skills, theories, and practice.* Englewood Cliffs, NJ: Prentice-Hall. Ivey and Simek-Downing's discussion of the therapeutic process as a "decision-making model" incorporates numerous suggestions and examples of recycling and referral.

Van Hoose, W., & Kottler, J. (1977). *Ethical and legal issues in counseling and psychotherapy.* San Francisco: Jossey-Bass. An important topic addressed in this book is that of the ethical responsibilities associated with referral.

Termination and Follow-up

Eisenberg, S., & Delaney, D. J. (1977). *The counseling process* (2nd ed.). Chicago: Rand McNally. Termination and follow-up are well covered in this book. Of special value is a case study illustrating a termination session with a client.

Patterson, L. E., & Eisenberg, S. (1983). *The counseling process* (3rd ed.). Boston: Houghton Mifflin. Patterson and Eisenberg address issues of readiness and resistance in termination as well as "ending in a positive way."

Shulman, L. (1979). *The skills of helping: Individuals and groups.* Itasca, IL: Peacock. The author provides some interesting insights into the dynamics and skills of what he terms "endings and transitions."

Part Four

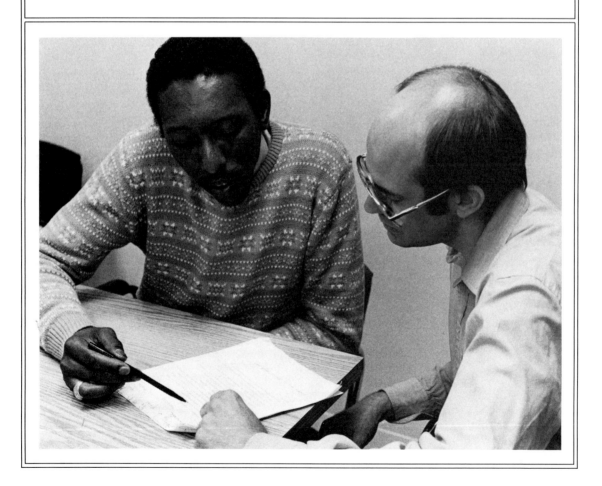

Clinical Accountability

The practice of counseling and psychotherapy is widely recognized as a significant part of the larger mental health field. Along with this recognition comes the responsibility of therapists to be accountable for the services offered. This section examines two primary considerations in this regard: (1) the expectation that obstacles to therapeutic progress are an inherent part of practice and must be adequately addressed if positive client change, which forms the foundation of the profession, is to be realized; (2) that as professionals, therapists must maintain recognized standards of competence and respected credentials, practice in accordance with stated ethical standards, and constantly seek to improve their services by assuming roles as therapist/researchers and research consumers.

In Chapter 11, we look at some of the problems that can arise during therapy that block positive client progress. In doing so we consider procedures and alternative directions to use in overcoming any obstacles encountered. Chapter 12 explores major professional issues: (1) therapists'

development, maintenance, and enhancement of professional competence: academic training, clinical supervision, mentoring and networking, licensure and certification, the necessity of continuing education, and professional affiliations; (2) ethical considerations pertaining to client welfare, informed consent, and confidentiality; (3) research, often perceived as the key element in promoting clinical accountability. These two chapters offer realistic and relevant information to the practitioner. The portion of Chapter 12 dealing with research, in particular, offers frameworks for practitioners to make more pragmatic use of research as opposed to suggesting academic studies to pursue.

In many ways Part Four is the most important in this book. The public seeks effective and efficient services. Similarly, both insurance companies and state and federal governments are concerned about paying for therapy that individuals have received but for which there was no benefit or no documentation of benefit. It is vital that therapists clearly convey a strong sense of clinical accountability.

11

Overcoming Obstacles and Considering Alternative Therapeutic Directions

Counseling and psychotherapy are interpersonal processes
that have identifiable barriers.

(Brammer & Shostrom, 1982, p. 211)

Much of what has been presented in the preceding chapters has been based on the assumption that clients who enter counseling and psychotherapy are relatively willing to cooperate in the therapeutic process. This is usually the case; initiating and maintaining a working relationship with clients usually presents no major problems and therapeutic progress is evident. However, not all persons participate in therapy willingly.

Some clients, if given the choice, would not talk about themselves, behave differently, or be in therapy at all. A significant number of clients in certain therapeutic settings come reluctantly, only because they are urged or occasionally forced to do so. And, in some cases, clients come to therapy willingly, but with misguided expectations. For example, many clients enter therapy believing that the therapist will magically bring about desirable changes in the client's life with little or no effort on the client's part.

Those persons who enter therapy under pressure or with misguided intentions are likely to exhibit attitudes and behaviors that tend to limit progressive therapeutic movement. They come to sessions with an orientation toward self-protection, being defensive and quick to place blame for any problems somewhere outside of themselves. Many resent the person or authority who pressured them to come to therapy and transfer that resentment to the therapist. Often clients perceive no need for help and therefore do not view the therapist as a helping person.

Problems that such clients present in initiating or maintaining therapeutic progress are expressed in a variety of ways. Some persons show defiance: "I don't want to be here and I don't have to cooperate." Others exhibit their defiance in passive-aggressive ways: continually leading the discussion away from themselves to some irrelevant topic, being unwilling to communicate anything beyond brief and inadequate answers to direct questions, or sitting silently with a disgusted demeanor. Still others, so as to be free of any responsibility, try to manipulate the therapist into providing all the effort.

Clearly, therapists encounter some genuinely difficult clients and it is tempting to always attribute lack of therapeutic progress to the particular mode of functioning presented by a troublesome client. Yet therapists can also contribute to lack of therapeutic progress. As the expert provider of therapeutic services, the therapist has the major responsibility for structuring the therapeutic process. Lack of progress may often be due to the therapist's manner of functioning in seeking to develop and facilitate this process and the specific interaction that occurs in sessions.

Since therapists ask clients to examine how they are living their lives in order to understand themselves, their problem situations, and the direction for positive change, it is incumbent upon therapists to develop and maintain a similar level of awareness in their own lives. Without such self-awareness, a therapist may shift the focus of therapy from working to meet the client's needs to meeting the needs of the therapist, thus obstructing the client progress that is supposedly the purpose of their interaction. Consequently, therapists' own needs, personal conflicts, areas of vulnerability, and defenses can also create significant obstacles to therapeutic progress.

Finally, certain client problems are simply less appropriate or inappropriate for individual counseling and psychotherapy, and alternative therapeutic directions are then called for. Focusing therapeutic efforts on changing specific environmental circumstances or significant persons in clients' lives rather than directly toward clients themselves can benefit clients more directly in many cases. Certain other problems need to be addressed prior to individual counseling and psychotherapy. Psychosis, for example, is either demonstrably physical in origin or has a significant physical, biochemical basis. Individual therapy can be of benefit to the client with this condition, but only after overt symptomatology has been stabilized through medical treatment.

LACK OF PROGRESS: CLIENT VARIABLES

Certain problems posed by clients occur with some regularity in most practitioners' caseloads. These problems significantly interfere with therapeutic efforts and must be dealt with successfully if therapy is to be of any benefit. They include the battle for structure, resistance, transference, and premature termination.

The Battle for Structure

Therapy actually begins before a client is ever seen. It begins with the initial contact made with the therapist, usually by telephone. The family theorist and therapist Carl Whitaker (Keith & Whitaker, 1980) claims that his work with families always begins with a "battle for structure"; that is, a contest over who controls the context of therapy. He proposes that a family must agree to the therapist's mode of operating. The therapist is the expert from whom the family is seeking assistance, and thus it is appropriate that the therapist has leverage over those factors necessary for effective therapy to occur. The importance of this battle for structure is the same for individual therapy.

There are a number of issues on which clients will stage a battle for structure with a therapist. The most common is who decides the content of therapy and how it is to proceed. Clients will often test a therapist to see whether he or she can withstand the manipulations they are likely using to create the present concerns that carry them to therapy. This testing can be compared with the manner in which preadolescents often test their parents. They seek reassurance that, if self-control is lost, their parents can be firm enough to take over. Within an umbrella of trust thereby established, these youths, or presumably, clients beginning therapy, can begin to take initiative toward more constructive action.

It is important to remember that many clients enter therapy with ambivalent feelings. They are experiencing difficulties in their lives and desire change, yet they are also afraid that change may mean the loss of what they presently possess in terms of acceptance, affirmation, and identity. They come half convinced of the potential value of therapy, but also half scared. If they sense that the therapist is confident and firmly committed, they are more likely to put forth the energy needed for positive therapeutic progress to occur. The ability of a therapist to display a significant degree of social influence early in therapy is a critical component in the battle for structure.

For all of the reasons clients might be reluctant to enter therapy, it is critical that the battle for structure be immediately won by the therapist. A clearly understood initial agreement should be made with the client that delineates details of time, fees, and purpose. When the client is obviously reluctant, the therapist should be resolute in stating that if therapy and positive change are considered important, arrangements can be worked out. Of course, tact and realistic flexibility must characterize the therapist's response to potential reluctance. Nevertheless, the importance of agreeing to a set of criteria before therapeutic efforts are initiated cannot be minimized.

Although the battle for structure may appear to end, the same dynamics can recur in other forms later in therapy. Some clients, at this point, will simply abandon the present therapist and shop for one who is willing to be more supportive in meeting their demands, no matter that they lead only to continuing personal dissatisfaction and dysfunction.

Feminist Therapy

A parallel to the battle for structure can be described in terms of a growing movement known as *Feminist Therapy*. Many women who enter therapy define themselves as traditional, possessing certain attitudes that may no longer be adaptive and thus cause difficulties in their lives. These women believe that they are supposed to be only submissive, passive, dependent, and nurturing. They narrowly perceive roles of homemaker and mother as singularly appropriate for themselves (Dworkin, 1984; Steinman, 1974).

Translated into modern times, these traditional roles pigeonhole women in supportive as opposed to power positions, causing many to experience a discrepancy between their ideal self-image and the image they perceive as necessary to fulfill traditional role functions (Dworkin, 1984).

Feminist therapy asserts that women and men have similar roles and traits. The feminist therapist seeks to free women clients from these roles that restrict their opportunities. The feminist therapist believes in the potential of women and sees that potential as frequently being thwarted by oppressive sex-roles. This is not to suggest that women give up traditionally feminine behaviors and adopt masculine behaviors, but rather that mental health for adults equally combines feminine and masculine characteristics (Thomas, 1977).

As the feminist therapist and traditionally defined female client enter into therapy, the process will likely be different from what the woman expects. Instead of letting the client submit to the authority of the therapist, the feminist therapist refuses to accept the absolute power such women usually try to project onto them. Instead, a cooperative, equalized relationship is emphasized and established. feminist therapy focuses on the client learning about and claiming her own power. The therapeutic process becomes a study of the psychological effect of social conditioning, sex roles, and women's secondary status (Klein, 1976; Radov, Masnick, & Hauser, 1977). It has been recommended that a major part of this study arises from the therapist's own disclosure of experiences of sexism and feminism. For this reason, it may well be that the feminist-oriented therapist will have to be a woman herself (Johnson, 1976; Kronsky, 1971; Thomas, 1977).

Resistance

Resistance within the context of therapy refers to a lack of agreement between the goals of the client and those of the therapist. As such, it is often manifested in a client's opposition to the therapeutic process. The therapist needs to reduce this opposition as much as possible. Resistance usually occurs in response to one or both of two primary issues:

1. Opposition to the basic concepts of the overall therapeutic approach being employed.
2. Opposition to one or more of the intervention strategies being attempted.

Whenever resistance is detected, it is important to interrupt the therapeutic process and try to negotiate a new basic structure or set of goals that both the client and therapist can accept. Therapy can then proceed. There will be times, however, when negotiation leads to an agreement that consensus on the direction for therapeutic efforts is not possible. In such cases, referral to another therapist or termination is indicated (Dinkmeyer, Pew, and Dinkmeyer, 1979).

Resistance may be present to some degree in beginning most client-therapist relationships. Because it is so prevalent, therapists should be aware of its potential—especially in initial therapy sessions. Any indication of arising resistance should be dealt with immediately. The therapist skill of immediacy is especially appropriate in this regard. By taking preventive measures, however, the therapist can significantly reduce the likelihood of resistance occurring.

Lieberman, Wheeler, deVisser, Kuehnel, and Kuehnel (1980) propose a number of activities therapists can implement to prevent or overcome resistance to therapeutic efforts. These include providing an orientation to and rationale for therapeutic procedures, facilitating favorable expectations, offering an opportunity for catharsis, employing a "customer approach," and making therapy special.

1. *Orientation and Rationale.* A potentially resistant client should be carefully oriented to the overall therapeutic process as well as specific intervention strategies as they are planned. It is important that the rationale be understood and accepted by the client. Therapy can progress only if it deals with specific issues that clients recognize as important and want to work to change. No movement can occur until the goals of therapy, and the means of achieving those goals, are explained and mutually agreed upon.

2. *Favorable Expectations.* The key variable in facilitating favorable expectations for therapy is the therapist's attitude, expressed in both verbal and nonverbal ways. The means of expression minimally include words, tone of voice, gestures, and facial expressions. The therapist can convey a sense of optimism by looking forward to working with a client and by proposing that therapy will be challenging, worthwhile, and fun. Anecdotes and positive statements anonymously quoted from former clients can also help create an optimistic atmosphere.

3. *Catharsis.* Catharsis involves giving clients an opportunity to ventilate their accumulated feelings of hurt or anger and to express any complaints or accusations they feel are relevant before structuring therapy or setting firm goals. Some clients will be more receptive to identifying and agreeing to work toward positive changes if they have ample opportunity to express negative ideas and emotions. Catharsis can also be of significant value in early sessions for it offers the therapist

a source of information in helping clients discriminate and define their primary problems that then become the target of later goal setting and intervention efforts. As a result, the goals of therapist and client become more closely aligned.

4. *Customer Approach.* The customer approach involves a therapist's active and vigorous solicitation of a client's desires, hopes, fears, and wishes for therapy. The therapist works to have the client clearly identify his or her major concerns and formulate specific objectives for therapy. Common therapist inquiries when employing a customer approach include: "What would you like to get from therapy?" "What would you like to see changed?" "How might we work together to improve your life circumstances?" Discrepancies between the therapeutic objectives of the client and those of the therapist and possible resistances are thus kept to a minimum.

5. *Making Therapy Special.* A final way of preventing or overcoming a client's resistance to therapy is to establish this experience as different from other attempts at positive change that may have failed in the past. Many clients who have sufficient problems to compel them to therapy have tried a variety of approaches for dealing with their difficulties; these include speaking to friends and family, reading self-help books, or even prior therapeutic endeavors. If previous attempts a client has made to resolve problems included methods similar to those of the present therapist, it might be pointed out that the present therapist's approach is more comprehensive and intensive. In addition, the therapist can have the client explain or show how he or she attempted certain procedures that were unsuccessful. Almost all reasonable methods and suggestions for improvement have some validity. The usual reason for their lack of effectiveness in improving some aspect of the client's life circumstances lies not in procedures as much as in the client's implementing them incorrectly, inconsistently, or for too short a time. By stressing the value of the therapist as an expert and objective observer who can offer feedback and follow-up, the current therapeutic experience can come to be seen as a special one.

Transference

Most clients' perceptions of situations and other persons are relatively objective and realistic; others have distorted views of their surroundings and those around them. The more troubled clients are, the greater their tendency to perceive the therapist in a distorted manner. Transference refers to an unconscious process whereby clients project onto their therapists past feelings or attitudes they hold toward significant persons in their lives. The concept of transference stems from psychoanalysis, which stresses clients' unrecognized or unresolved feelings about past relationships, but the phenomenon is not restricted to psychoanalytic therapy (Corey, Corey, & Callanan, 1984).

Brammer and Shostrom (1982) describe the basis for transference in stating:

> People do not come empty-handed from their past. They bring various means of manipulating their environments. But they tend to lack self-support—an essential quality for survival; their manipulations minimize their self-support; and these manipulations are endless. For example, people break promises, play stupid, forget, lie, and continually ask questions . . . . clients are not persons who *had* problems, they are persons with continuing here-and-now problems. (p. 216)

In transference, clients distort their perception of the therapist, viewing him or her from a past subjective referent rather than in a present, objective manner. The thoughts and feelings and behaviors may be positive or negative; loving, hostile, dependent, ambivalent, and others. The essential point is what they connected with the past is now directed toward the therapist (Corey et al., 1984). Since a climate of mutual trust and acceptance is important for successful therapy to occur, transference, especially of the negative or hostile type, is a significant obstacle to therapy. Similarly, transferences reflecting past dependency or unmet needs for affection can also block positive client change from occurring.

In responding to suspected client transference, it is important that the therapist not provide the client with the response he or she expects. For example, the client who presents himself or herself as extremely dependent, constantly seeking advice from the therapist for even minor decisions, may be looking to the therapist to provide the "right" answers as significant persons have been relied on since childhood. The therapist must not respond by taking responsibility for making the client's decisions. Instead, the therapist should recognize the client's transference as dysfunctional and help the client to understand it as such with its detrimental effects on his or her current life circumstances and on the therapeutic efforts. As Brammer and Shostrom (1982) note, "The general principle here is that counselors should not fit themselves to the client's projections, so as to satisfy the client's neurotic needs. If the counselor fulfills the client's expectations, there is the possibility they will be perpetuated by virtue of having been reinforced" (p. 219).

Brammer and Shostrom (1982) suggest that although transferences may create obstacles to therapeutic progress, they can also serve significant positive functions in therapy if the therapist responds to them appropriately. Transference can help facilitate the development of a working relationship between the therapist and client by allowing the client to express distorted feelings without experiencing dysfunctional responses. Appropriate therapist reactions to client transference can also promote clients' confidence in the therapist who responds in an accepting but firm manner rather than being manipulated. Finally, transferences therapeutically dealt with enable clients to see the origin and significance of chronic manipulative interpersonal patterns they employ and the effect they have on their present life (Hansen, Stevic, & Warner, 1982).

When transference presents obstacles to therapeutic progress, Brammer and Shostrom (1982) identify the therapist's main task as encouraging client expression and exploration while simultaneously keeping distanced enough to prevent the emerging transference from developing into a deep transference. They propose several therapist procedures to do so:

1. *Simple Acceptance.* The client is allowed to live out any projected thoughts and feelings and within the therapeutic interchange comes to recognize that these ideas reside in self, not in the therapist.

2. *Clarifying Questions.* Questions can be used to help clients interpret the basis and current impact of transferences. For example, "You seem to be unloading on me today. What do you suppose is behind this?"

3. *Reflection.* Reflections provide the client with a better understanding of their own internal frame of reference. For example, "You're anxious about discussing this because you think it may make *me* feel uncomfortable."

4. *Interpretation.* Interpretation can be especially useful in developing a new perspective on clients' earlier interpersonal experiences and their present manner of functioning. For example, "You appear worried that you may have been telling too much to me and that you shouldn't have. Is it possible that this insecurity has been something you've been experiencing in relationships for some time?" It is important that the new perspective should emphasize present problems and not merely dwell on earlier experiences; on the "what" and not the "why."

5. *Reversing the Projection.* By regarding the transference as a projection, the therapist can request that the client reverse the projection, encouraging repetition of the projection until it is correctly experienced by the client as emanating from himself or herself. For example:

CLIENT: You don't like me.

THERAPIST: How might you reverse that statement?

CLIENT: You mean, I don't like you.

THERAPIST: Yes, how about saying that again louder?
CLIENT: I don't like you.
THERAPIST: Even louder and with more determination.
CLIENT: I don't like you!
THERAPIST: True or not true?
CLIENT: I guess it's true.

While transference is an obstacle to therapeutic progress, it is not a catch-all intended to explain all the thoughts and feelings clients express toward their therapists. Corey et al. (1984) address this issue quite aptly:

> If a client expresses anger toward you, it may be justified. If you haven't been truly present for the client, responding instead in a mechanical fashion, your client may be expressing legitimate anger and disappointment. Similarly, if a client expresses affection toward you, these feelings may be genuine; simply dismissing them as infantile fantasies can be a way of putting distance between yourself and your client. (p. 44)

In order to differentiate between the obstacle of transference and objective, present-oriented experiencing, therapists must actively work at being open, vulnerable, and honest with themselves. Although they should be aware of the possibility of transference existing, they must also always consider the danger of discounting the genuine reactions clients may have toward them.

Premature Termination

At times, clients may seek to terminate therapy before goals have been attained. Premature termination can occur at any time during the therapeutic process. Frequently clients showing little motivation or commitment to work on improving their present circumstances may communicate an inclination to terminate therapy from the very beginning. Some may communicate their rejection of therapy and the therapist as a helper at a later phase of the process. One mechanism is for a client simply not to return for later sessions. Another is for clients to tell the therapist directly that they feel therapy is not of much benefit to them so they see no point in continuing. Occasionally such a statement by clients may be appropriate—therapy indeed is not being of any significant benefit. But, especially when change is difficult for clients to experience, such a statement may suggest that they are fearful about the impact therapy may have on them, or that they are just not putting forth the necessary effort to change. Obviously, when these conditions hold, benefits do not accrue.

Initially, a therapist confronted with a client choosing to prematurely terminate therapy should identify his or her own thoughts and feelings about the client rejecting therapeutic assistance. Apprehension and anger toward the client are often therapist responses. Beginning therapists especially are apt to react with anxiety, because rejection by a client is often seen as reflecting therapist ineffectiveness. The therapist's goal is to help clients achieve therapeutic objectives; being told therapy is not being of assistance may represent a serious block to goal attainment for therapists, leading to frustration, anger, and anxiety. Ironically, these maladaptive modes of response are sure to interfere with the therapist's effectiveness. Thus, when such stress occurs in the therapist-client relationship, it is important to face it openly rather than to avoid dealing with it. Responding openly to stress in the relationship is far more likely to result in favorable consequence than will the avoidance of existing stress (Eisenberg & Delaney, 1977).

Assuming the therapist is aware of the impact that a client's rejection has on him or her and copes with it effectively, the next step is to determine why the client wants to terminate therapy. The major means for accomplishing this is through the use of the therapist skill of immediacy. For example:

THERAPIST: You've stated that you don't see our work together as having been of much benefit to you so far. I am disappointed to hear this, but I am glad that you're telling me. I do feel it's important that we explore how you arrived at this conclusion.

Depending on the client's response and further discussion, the therapist can then decide whether the client's criticisms are valid or whether they are statements of resistance. If they are the latter, the therapist should try to intervene using the strategies previously discussed in the section on client resistance. If the therapist decides that the criticisms are valid, the therapist must reevaluate his or her therapeutic approach in working with the client. Where the structure of therapy has been inappropriate or inefficient, the therapist must be willing to adapt. Communicating this to the client may avert premature termination. Otherwise, referral to another therapist whose orientation is more likely to suit the client's desires is indicated.

Other Obstacles Clients Create

For beginning therapists, certain obstacles clients create blocking therapeutic progress cause more concern than others; new therapists' lack of experience in dealing with these particularly unyielding interpersonal patterns makes them frustrated and anxious, desirous of success but unable to achieve it. Even for experienced therapists, however, particular client behaviors are cause for serious concern.

Argumentativeness. Therapists occasionally encounter clients who are excessively antagonistic during therapy. Their voices always seem on edge. The therapist feels fatigued by the therapeutic interaction—there appears to be almost more arguing than cooperating. This client seeks to make an issue of any point with which he or she even slightly disagrees. The therapist's initial response upon recognizing this argumentativeness should be to stop fighting in any way with the client. In a sense, the therapist and client are tugging at opposite ends of a rope. The therapist need only let go of one end to terminate the tug-of-war. The therapist should go through one or more sessions without trying to suggest, advise, or convince the argumentative client of anything. Suggesting ideas or possible changes only intensifies the potential for quarrelsome reactions. Instead, the therapist can work to attain the client's cooperation, simultaneously progressing toward therapeutic goals; this is accomplished by focusing on the strength and power of the client, seeking cooperation through inquiry. For example, "What do *you* think you might do to cope more effectively in that situation?" "What might *we* come up with to help you deal with that difficulty?"

Yes-But. Clients who counter therapists' ideas and recommendations with "yes-but" responses are demonstrating a more subtle form of argumentativeness. They present themselves as seeking assistance but then proceed to show the therapist how ineffective the therapist's advice is, how suggested strategies will not work, and so on. The yes-but is actually an implicit no. By playing helpless, these clients attempt to render therapists helpless. It is important that therapists examine yes-but responses and determine whether this form of resistance is attributable to their own style; are they off-task, or have they focused discussion on an irrelevant issue? If not, perhaps the most likely explanantion for a client's "yes-but" is that he or she simply does not want to change. For instance, a client may be afraid of changing and try to use a smoke screen, such as yes-but responses, to hide this fear from the therapist. Such a client uses communication in order not to communicate (Beier, 1966).

With a client who uses yes-but responses chronically, the therapist must first consider what the payoff is for the client. It is important to identify the positive or negative consequences that maintain the dysfunctional beliefs this behavior is based on. In doing so, the therapist skill of confrontation is most timely. Confrontation can be followed by the use of immediacy to help the client see how resistant behavior is occurring in the therapist-client relationship. This technique can lead to the client lessening yes-but defensiveness. The therapist can go on to enumerate the strengths and capabilities the client possesses but has not used effectively; although the client still has to make a decision to change, listing his or her personal resources after confrontation and exploration of a yes-but behavioral pattern in itself challenges the client to act in a more adaptive manner (Egan, 1975).

It's Not Working. Some clients who are very capable of changing burden themselves with the belief that immediately upon beginning therapy they should experience positive changes. This impatience and short-term hedonism often is translated into patterns of poor self-discipline and low frustration tolerance. For example:

CLIENT: I know what we discussed in the session makes sense, but when the real situation occurred, what we had planned that I would do didn't work for me at all.

When such an opinion is expressed, chances are that the client spent little time actually practicing the therapeutically planned response. By this neglect the client puts total responsibility for his or her changing on the therapist. The expectation is that the therapist will come up with magical and immediate solutions to all problems presented.

It is possible that the agreed-to plan was inappropriate. However, it is essential that the therapist never automatically assume responsibility. The client should be asked to explain in detail exactly what happened. The therapist should listen for any obvious flaws in the client's handling of the situation. Assuming there were flaws in the client's carrying out of the original plan, the procedures agreed to can be discussed again and rehearsed during the session until the therapist is assured of the client's competency in implementing them. The client should then be asked to practice the procedures and, should a similar problem situation arise, to *make* them work. Simply, the therapist helps the client understand that it may take several attempts for any plan to work effectively, and that the responsibiity to make it successful is ultimately the client's.

THE THERAPIST AS AN OBSTACLE TO CLIENT CHANGE

Although clients can create obstacles that impede therapeutic progress, therapists too can contribute to lack of success. Throughout this book, we have described what the therapist should ideally be doing to facilitate positive client change. Therapists, being as human as their clients, however, have their own idiosyncratic natures, their own set of particular needs, and their own problems, any of which may work to the detriment of the therapeutic process. Some common therapist obstacles to client change include therapists' personal problems, countertransference, inappropriate expectations, and problems with procedure.

The Therapist's Problems

It would be ideal if therapists were void of all personal problems and adjustment difficulties or that these conflicts could be put aside so that they would not interfere with therapeutic efforts. Unfortunately this ideal (while not an impossibility, nor even a rarity) is often only occasionally realized by many therapists. Therapists frequently bring to the therapy setting all of their personal difficulties, and despite efforts to the contrary, these personal problems exert a powerful force during therapy. Experienced therapists can control these factors so that they do not disrupt therapeutic efforts, but to do so they must first be intimately aware of the types of problems they have and the types of interference these problems can create (Belkin, 1980).

Therapists experience the same difficulties as everyone. There are health problems, family problems, financial difficulties, insecurities about self-esteem and social competence, and the like. While circumstances beyond therapists' control may dictate the extent to which these difficulties interfere with their daily living and professional practice, it is incumbent upon therapists to take responsibility for governing their own lives in as intelligent, effective, and productive a manner as possible. This is not to say that therapists must resolve all of their personal difficulties before they begin to counsel others; such a requirement would likely eliminate the practice of counseling and psychotherapy. The critical issue is not *whether* a therapist is struggling with personal problems, but rather *how* those problems are being addressed (Corey et al., 1984).

Therapists must therefore, if they are to serve their clients well, seek to constantly promote harmony in their own lives. Their work with clients will in many ways reflect the manner in which they approach their own life circumstances, particularly in regard to stability, purpose, constancy, and direction (Belkin, 1980). As Carkhuff and Berenson (1967) state, "Counseling is as effective as the therapist is living effectively" (p. 197).

Countertransference

Countertransference occurs when therapists' own needs become entangled in the therapeutic relationship, interfering with the therapist's objectivity (Corey et al., 1984). Therapeutic progress is blocked when therapists use clients to fulfill their own unmet needs. For example, needing to feel powerful or even to be nurturant, some therapists believe they have the ultimate answers concerning how clients should live. They constantly give advice, trying to direct clients' destinies. This relationship can be especially harmful because many clients enter therapy primarily because of nonassertiveness and a lack of trust in themselves. Therapists who assume a parental role with such clients cause them to become even more dysfunctionally dependent and only perpetuate their presenting problems. Therapists who need to feel powerful or important frequently think that they are indispensable to their clients or, worse, make themselves so (Corey et al., 1984).

In a similar manner, therapists with unmet needs for approval strongly seek clients' acceptance, admiration, and awe. Some therapists may be primarily motivated by a need to receive confirmation of their value as persons and professionals. The therapist role allows them to control therapy sessions in such a way that these needs are continually reinforced. Successful therapeutic efforts result in clients having less and less need for their therapists. Therapists who use sessions to enhance their own sense of worth diminish the autonomy of their clients and actually encourage increased dependence and thus lack of therapeutic progress.

A common manifestation of this form of countertransference is the development of romantic or sexual feelings toward clients. When this occurs, therapists can exploit the vulnerable position of clients, whether consciously or unconsciously. Especially if a client is experiencing a transference of a similar nature to the therapist's countertransference, seductive behavior on the part of the client can readily be reacted to in a seductive manner by the therapist and vice versa. In a less intense way clients occasionally let their therapist know that they would like to develop more of a relationship than is possible in the limiting environment of the office. They may, for example, express a desire to get to know the therapist as a "regular person."

It is natural for therapists to be attracted to some clients more than others, and the fact that they have sexual feelings toward some clients does not mean that they cannot effectively counsel them. More important than the mere existence of such feelings is the manner in which therapists deal with them. Feelings of attraction can be recognized and even acknowledged frankly without becoming the focus of therapy. Likewise, even experienced therapists sometimes struggle with the question of whether to blend a social relationship with a therapeutic one. When this question arises, therapists should assess whose needs would be met through such a friendship and whether an effective therapeutic relationship can coexist with a social relationship. In regard to the question of simultaneous therapeutic-social relationships, Corey et al. (1984) proposes that therapists consider the following questions:

☐ Will I be as readily inclined to challenge clients in therapy if I also engage in social relationships with them?

☐ Will my desire to preserve a friendship interfere with my therapeutic activities and possibly defeat the purpose of therapy?

Projections by the therapist are another form of countertransference. Therapists see themselves in their clients (Corey et al., 1984). This is not to suggest that feeling close to a client and identifying with his or her struggle in an empathic and genuine manner equates with countertransference. One problem many beginning therapists have, however, is that they identify with clients' problems to the point that they lose their objectivity. They become lost in their clients' worlds, unable to separate their thoughts and feelings from those of their clients. Or they may perceive in their clients traits that they dislike in themselves.

Brammer and Shostrom (1982) illustrate the difference between genuine therapist expression and countertransference in the form of a projection:

Genuine Expression:
THERAPIST: You are very pretty.
CLIENT: Thank you.
THERAPIST: You're welcome.

Projection:
THERAPIST: You are very pretty.
CLIENT: Thank you.
THERAPIST: I suppose you react that way to all men who say that?

To deal with their projections, therapists must have insight into their own immaturities, prejudices, objects of disgust, anxieties, and punitive tendencies. No therapist is free of these reactions. Unless they are aware of their basic attitudes, however, therapists may respond to client statements with their own biases. These negative attitudes tend to have a destructive effect on therapeutic efforts by arousing negative transference or, in fact, warranted negative reactions by clients. Positive countertransferences by therapists can be even more deleterious, since they are less apt to recognize them and clients are more confused and upset when they are withdrawn.

Therapists of course do have personal needs. It is critical from a therapeutic standpoint, however, that these needs do not become more important or impede clients' growth. Individuals who become therapists do need to experience the satisfaction that comes from promoting positive client change. Excitement, enjoyment, and a significant sense of reward come as clients move from being victims to assuming control over their lives. Some therapists believe, however, that this satisfaction is experienced only when clients overtly tell of their achieved successes. They fail to remember that more effective client living, not verbal confirmation, is evidence enough.

To keep their needs from becoming obstacles, therapists should be clearly aware of the dangers inherent in working primarily to be appreciated by clients rather than helping clients appreciate themselves and the therapeutic progress they attain. If therapists can recognize the potential danger in the former and the benefits to be accrued from the latter, they will likely not seek to use clients to meet their own needs.

Inappropriate Expectations

Some therapists burden themselves with the belief that they must be perfect. They think that they must always have the appropriate response for any situation that arises and never make errors in judgment. Yet the fact is that all therapists will occasionally err.

Beginning therapists often become readily discouraged when they don't see positive change almost immediately in their clients. After expecting to perfectly handle any problems clients bring to sessions, therapists soon realize that most clients simply do not make instant progress. Indeed, it is far more common for clients to report an increase in anxiety and confusion in the early phases of therapy as they become more vulnerable by giving up their old defenses and try out new ways of functioning. Therapists often place obstacles in their clients' therapeutic path by reacting to this lack of instant change with undue demands on clients as a result of their own unrealistic expectations. Covering too wide a variety of client concerns in too short a time or overloading clients with inappropriate outside-of-session homework assignments are common reactions (Wessler & Wessler, 1980).

By contrast, other therapists fail to do their clients justice in thinking them so fragile that they will fall apart if the therapist makes the slightest mistake. They concentrate so strongly on avoiding mistakes themselves that they diminish their clients' role in taking responsibility for their own therapeutic successes or setbacks. Furthermore, by putting all their energies into portraying the role of the polished professional, they have little left for actually working with clients. This misdirection can particularly impede positive client change. It is difficult to imagine the core therapeutic conditions of empathic understanding, genuineness, and respect even minimally present in such circumstances. As a result, therapeutic progress will similarly be minimal.

All therapists must learn their own limits and those of their clients. They will not succeed with every client. Even experienced therapists sometimes doubt their effectiveness with certain clients who seem unwilling or unable to change. For beginning therapists, an inability to positively change clients is even more threatening. Many beginning therapists tell themselves that they should like all the persons who come to them for assistance and that they should be able to work with anyone (Corey et al., 1984). At some point the therapist will consider whether it is better to begin, or continue to work with a client not relating well or to admit to oneself and the client that a referral to another therapist is in the client's best interest. Or simply, the therapist must acknowledge that positive client change will take more effort and time than originally expected.

Personal Therapy for the Therapist

It seems obvious that if therapists are to promote positive client change, they must promote positive change in their own lives by exploring themselves and by striving to become more aware of how their personal problems and unmet needs obstruct opportunities for enhancing their current life circumstances. The willingness to practice what you preach and thus to be a positive model for clients is what distinguishes the effective from the ineffective therapist. Through being a client themselves, therapists can better come to know what it is like to look at oneself as one really is.

Personal therapy can especially help beginning therapists honestly look at their motivations for entering the profession. It allows therapists to explore how their needs influence their actions, how they use power in their lives, what their basic beliefs are, and whether they have a need to persuade others to live by them. Personal therapy offers objective feedback that can help identify any dysfunctional needs. It is also a means by which therapists can explore painful memories and past experiences that have shaped the way they now live and the influence these memories and experiences still exert.

All therapists have blind spots that may interfere with their effectiveness in helping clients. All have areas in their lives that are not as fully developed as they might be and that can prevent potentials from being realized, both personally and professionally. Personal therapy is one way of coming to grips with these and other issues that can obstruct therapeutic progress. While especially valuable for the beginning therapist, personal therapy can provide experienced practitioners with periodic and ongoing introspection. At times, even the most mature professional therapists can profit from a program of personal therapy that challenges them to reexamine their feelings, beliefs, and behaviors, particularly as they pertain to their effectiveness in working with clients.

Problems with Procedure

Some clients may not progress in therapy because therapists fail to be sensitive to clients' responses to various therapeutic procedures. Probably the most common error that therapists make in this regard is not asking the client what progress is being made. Walen, DiGiuseppe, & Wessler (1980) summarize several issues that therapists should consider in this regard:

1. *Failure to listen.* Misdiagnosis is likely if therapists fail to listen carefully. Clients may say that they are angry, for example; it is important

that it be clearly understood what meaning this has for them because if they or the therapist mislabel their condition, therapy can take off in the wrong direction.

2. *Failure to develop goals.* It is important that therapist and client clearly agree on what a client's goals are, rather than assume them. It is also critical to determine the client's expectations of therapy. Clearly understood client goals can be clarified, confirmed, or corrected, or, if agreement cannot be reached, the client can be referred elsewhere.

3. *Errors in information gathering.* New therapists in particular may err in one of two directions: spending too many sessions gathering data before moving on to proactive problem intervention, or failing to get sufficient information and too quickly implementing intervention strategies. In either case, they run the risk of alienating or losing the client or at least of doing inefficient therapy.

4. *Errors in assertiveness.* Again, errors can be made in either direction: allowing clients to vaguely ramble or extracting concreteness at a cost of being rudely abrupt.

5. *Errors in questioning.* The following is a list of potential mistakes to be avoided: 1) asking irrelevant or overgeneralized inquiries (e.g., "How've you been?") instead of directly relevant inquiries, 2) overusing rhetorical inquiries (e.g., "Where does your getting upset get you?"), 3) using too many "why" inquiries that generally lead only to "because" excuses; it being better to concentrate on "how" and "what" questions, 4) overusing closed yes/no inquiries rather than open ones that require fuller participation or richer answers, 5) asking multiple inquiries, bombarding clients with three or more questions without allowing them to answer any one of them, 6) answering clients' questions for them instead of allowing them time to grapple with the inquiries on their own or helping them to break inquiries down into simpler components, and 7) failing to note whether the client has, in fact, answered the inquiry asked or zigzagged off into a rambling story. If an inquiry is unanswered, the therapist should bring the client back to task by repeating it.

6. *Errors in information-giving.* Avoid lengthy lectures, particularly if the client is not consulted to see if he or she is following. Most of the information presented in a long didactic lecture is forgotten before the lecture is even completed. Clients' recall is increased by short, crisp, concrete presentations.

7. *Failure to check understanding.* It is important that therapists get frequent feedback from clients to assure that they are understanding the focus of present therapy efforts. It is useful to periodically ask clients to summarize by inquiring, "What's your understanding of what we've just been discussing?"

8. *Errors in being too wise.* Therapists should avoid being the wise potentate. It may be more profitable to request that clients seek to convince the therapist of the virtue of a specific perspective, goal, or intervention strategy.

OVERCOMING OBSTACLES: ALTERNATIVE THERAPEUTIC DIRECTIONS

The sensitive therapist recognizes that some client problems will not yield to individually-oriented counseling and psychotherapy. Individual therapy is primarily intended for reducing psychological disturbance. Thus, when problems of a social/environmental or biological origin are the core of a client's difficulties, alternative therapeutic directions must be considered. While such problems likely have a psychological component, often the biological or environmental impact is of such significance that meaningful positive change in clients' lives can only come about through addressing these nonpsychological realms.

Biologically Based Treatment

Therapists in psychiatric settings are sure to fully consider the possible biological bases for their clients' problems. Psychopharmacology, the use of medication in the treatment of mental illness (biopsychological dysfunction) has been shown to be of unequivocal value. In fact, psychotropic

Medical information can help therapists understand biologically based problems

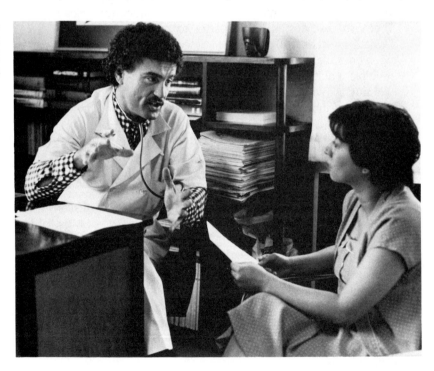

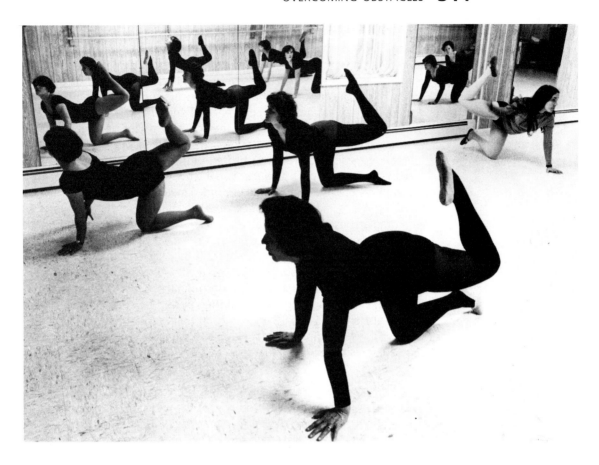

medication for biological deficits is the only treatment that has been consistently proven effective with schizophrenia and manic-depressive disorders (Fay, 1976). A particular therapeutic setting tends to attract people with specific types of biologically-based problems and thus suggests the type of knowledge a therapist must possess.

Yoga can help individuals control their biological states

Therapists in a drug abuse treatment program should possess some pharmacological knowledge of different drugs and chemical substances and how they affect client functioning. An alcoholism counselor should know about the impact of alcohol and alcoholism on related illness, altered states of functioning, addiction and consequential withdrawal, potential brain damage, and related physical disorders. Therapists in rehabilitation settings need to understand biologically-based problems such as paralysis, paresis, sensory disorders such as blindness and deafness, and mental deficiencies, among others. In hospitals and clinics, biologically-based patient concerns such as asthma, allergies, low blood sugar, obesity, and the like all have accompanying psychological components that therapists are called upon to treat concurrently or after the biological problem has been addressed.

Even in school settings a knowledge of the biological causes of problems is important, such as how prescribed medications affect children's learning and social behavior. Counselors must understand the expected illnesses of growing children and the changing metabolic and neurological structures that explain their developing forms of functioning. Moreover, counselors may be approached by teachers and parents for therapeutic assistance to help children better cope with numerous psychophysical conditions such as hyperactivity and petit mal epilepsy. Through secondary school and beyond, biologically based phenomena such as puberty and increasing sexual desires have a significant impact on emerging adolescents, young adults, and the counselors from whom they may seek therapeutic assistance.

How therapists deal with biologically based client conditions is influenced by the setting in which they find themselves and the nature of the client's problem. Harper (1981) proposes that therapists must function responsibly in conducting individual therapy by detecting biologically related client problems and then suggesting and monitoring treatment for their resolution and prevention. He posits five approaches as alternatives or as adjuncts to individual therapy.

1. Use *referral* in cases where the client's presenting needs or problem transcends the capability and role of the therapist or is not covered by the services provided in the therapist's work setting. Sources for referral may be various specialists, medical/health services, and special treatment services.

2. Serve as a leader or *trainer* in treatment groups that help clients better control internal biological states. Examples of these self-regulatory treatment-training activities include meditation, yoga, biofeedback, and exercise therapy.

3. Establish *growth groups* for psychophysical development and enhancement, for example, focusing on common problems or combining activities and interviews. A common problem group might be structured around common biologically related concerns such as controlling body weight, achieving sexual adequacy, or managing internalized reactions to stress. Harper (1978) combined jogging with group discussion in an activity-interview group to enhance the psychophysical development of college students.

4. Act as a *consultant* to significant others in clients' lives on biologically-based problems of clients. As a consultant, the therapist can function as a change agent, trainer, resource person, and direct provider of services (Kurpius & Robinson, 1978). In this framework, the therapist

can play a pivotal role in treating and preventing disruption in clients' lives as a result of treatable biologically based conditions.

5. Provide biologically related *information* on specific conditions, drugs, sexuality, nutrition, exercise, and the like. Information can be disseminated first-hand or by referral to appropriate sources.

Social-Ecological Approaches

Economic, educational, cultural, and political factors all significantly affect human functioning. Clients do not live in isolation. Their environment is an important aspect of their current reality and greatly affects their development and well-being. Lewis and Lewis (1977) call attention to therapists' need to assess environment in noting:

> Their work brings them face to face with the victims of poverty; of racism, sexism, and stigmatization; of political, economic, and social systems that allow individuals to feel powerless and helpless; of governing structures that cut off communication and deny the need for responsiveness; of social norms that stifle individuality; of communities that let their members live in isolation from one another. In the face of these realities, human service workers have no choice but to blame those victims or seek ways to change the environment. (p. 370)

Direction for implementing environmental change comes from the work of social ecologists. Social ecologist Rudolph Moos (1973, 1974) reports numerous examples of how human functioning is best understood by considering the characteristics of persons and their environments jointly. In contrast to the primarily personality-based focus that theories of counseling and psychotherapy have, social ecology suggests that individuals' functioning varies from setting to setting. The particular environment clients are in places specific demands upon them, and they respond differently to different environments. A tenet of social ecology is that more effective human functioning comes about only through environments designed to foster the development of positive interpersonal relationships, individual personal growth, and social system orderliness and change (Moos, 1974).

The social-ecological focus is on changing environments to change people. This change is facilitated by gathering, analyzing, and acting upon environmental impact data in order to make the environment more conducive to those persons who function in it (Conyne, 1977). The approach is very similar to that used in identifying and modifying individuals' psychological functioning. Like clients, environments have unique personalities. Some clients are supportive; likewise, some environments are supportive. On the other hand, some clients desire to dominate and control others rather than coexist with them in an egalitarian manner. Similarly, some environments are extremely controlling and rigid and would need greater flexibility.

Huber (1983) posits that the use of a social-ecological perspective in the therapeutic process involves five basic procedures: 1) identifying the problem as being primarily in the environmental setting, 2) gaining environmental support, 3) assessing the dynamics of the setting, 4) instituting social change strategies, and 5) evaluating the outcome.

Problem Identification. Problem identification considers both clients' presenting problems in terms of how they are reacting and a measure of the environmental variables affecting them. In regard to the latter, therapists should ask two questions. First, in how many and what kind of settings does a specific problem occur? The more a client's problem is limited to a particular setting, the less likely it is that the difficulties directly result from some deficiency in the client's functioning. The following situation illustrates this point:

Jim, age 14, was sent to the principal's office three times from the same class with various reports of misbehavior. The principal supported the teacher and disciplined Jim. Following the third incident, Jim was seen by the counselor in his school. Jim maintained that there was a group of students in that class who constantly harassed him. The counselor checked with Jim's other teachers. In no other class was Jim seen as a problem of any kind. In fact, one teacher described him as a real leader in class.

A second question for therapists to ask is: How many and which individuals in a setting express experiencing a problem? The greater the number of persons who say they are experiencing a problem in a certain setting only, the more likely it is that the characteristics of the setting itself are the prime determinants of the problem.

A therapist working in a juvenile court setting was struck by the large number of adolescents being arrested by a certain police officer. These youths, in meeting with the therapist, complained about the harsh demands and strictness of this particular officer. When approached about this by the therapist, the officer's initial response was to ask those youths about "their" unwarranted actions. It began to seem increasingly likely to the therapist that in this situation the problem lay more with the officer's methods than with these young persons.

As can be seen in both examples, the clients' problem was first explained as arising from them as individuals. On closer examination, however, variables in the environment in which the problems were occurring came to be seen as the primary instigators. These illustrations support the importance of considering social and ecological context; that is, clients' presenting problems may be a response to the characteristics of the environment in which they occur. If this is determined to be the case, a therapist's next step is to explain to significant persons in that environment how the environment affects the client.

Environmental Support. As noted in the discussion of problem identification, initial evaluations of clients' concerns by significant others in their environment are likely to focus on clients themselves. It is critical that the therapist gain the support of both clients and significant others about the impact environmental factors may have on the problem situation and the importance of also viewing the environment as client. This environmental support, however, is not always easily attained.

Significant others making judgments about individuals they are involved with in their environment often have difficulty in being objective. Such an evaluation demands that the evaluator maintain an autonomy of perception and judgment that few persons meaningfully involved with an individual in the same setting are able to sustain. In short, it is clearly much easier to view problems as "in the person" rather than as an indication of possible problems in the social setting or in the fit between individuals' needs and the social context (Tricket & Todd, 1973). Consider, for example, the marriage partner whose spouse is experiencing emotional difficulties. It is much easier to focus on that spouse as having a problem than on the notion that there is some weakness in the marriage itself, thus involving that significant other.

Questioning these role-related beliefs often leads to conflicts in role relationships. Therapists trying to implement social change strategies from an ecological perspective must analyze correctly the communications sent by these persons. They must also accurately communicate back to them. Thus, the ability to establish and maintain an effective working relationship with significant others in a client's environment is essential in initiating social change.

Given that an effective working relationship is established, environmental support is further enhanced by the therapist conveying two basic assumptions to the client and significant others: 1) the cause of the problem may be as much in the social context as in the client, and 2) sufficient data can be gathered assessing the contributions of both the individual and the setting to the problem. Once a meaningful level of environmental support is achieved, the next step in the process is to conduct an environmental assessment.

Environmental Assessment. A major reason for considering a social-ecological perspective is that the therapist is aware of the effect of environmental factors on the client's concerns. During environmental assessment, the therapist systematically assesses and confirms prior observations as well as gains a greater understanding of all factors that might affect the problem. In particular, persons' perceptions of current circumstances as opposed to what they see as ideal circumstances are evaluated.

Data collection alone, however, does not create an optimal environment. The therapist's next step is integrating the data from problem identification and environmental assessment into a program where the probability of the desired environmental modification being accomplished is as high as possible.

Environment shapes people's functioning and view of the world

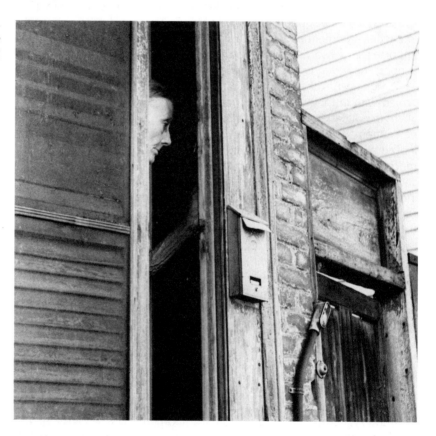

Social Change. Once the integration of relevant information has been completed, the following methodology by Moos (1974) provides an outline for facilitating social change.

1. The therapist gives feedback to all involved, paying particular attention to similarities and differences in the perceptions of the various individuals within the setting. For example, in a family, parents versus children and husband versus wife would be examined; in a school, students versus teachers or teachers versus administrators. In addition, emphasis is placed on the differences and similarities between what might be viewed as the reality of the present versus a potential "ideal" and resultant implications for change.

2. Practical planning of specific methods by which this change might occur is then initiated. This planning is coordinated by the therapist.

3. The change process is assessed by the persons involved to determine the degree to which the current environment is coming to approximate their previously proposed ideal environment. Feedback is continuously provided to participants, offering an ongoing, systematic approach to achieving an optimal environment.

Evaluation. There are no clear, well-defined criteria for the ideal environmental setting that will meet everyone's requirements. Individuals in different social settings have different criteria and different goals. During environmental assessment, however, involved persons' perceptions of the current circumstances and what might be the ideal circumstances are collected. The analysis of the environmental data taken in the initial assessment and sequentially throughout this social-ecological change process, showing a convergence of the "current" and "ideal," explains how well those persons in the particular environment have been helped in achieving their ideal environment.

CLINICAL SUPERVISION

To work with clients when obstacles block the path of therapeutic progress is not easy. The process of helping clients improve can be emotionally and physically draining. This is especially true for the therapist inexperienced at recognizing, let alone appropriately dealing with, therapeutic obstacles. It is similarly often frustrating for the novice therapist to apparently be proceeding with therapy in the "right" way from his or her primary theoretical orientation when, in fact, addressing biologically-based or environmental variables would be the more helpful. When such circumstances arise clinical supervision is most helpful, and in many cases necessary.

Clinical supervision is crucial in helping therapists understand all of the dynamics potentially affecting therapy and the means of making positive movement a reality. The clinical supervisor is a resource person and educator capable of teaching therapists what they need for both immediate and ongoing clinical development.

As a resource person, the supervisor may suggest specific strategies to deal with special problems. Or he or she may focus on basic therapeutic skills such as conveying core conditions, communicating a greater sense of social influence, or properly assessing clients' concerns that need to be reviewed or stressed even more by the therapist. The supervisor may propose alternative therapeutic directions with which to clarify clients' current circumstances, particularly in planning intervention strategies.

In the educator role, the supervisor is removed from the therapeutic relationship between therapists and their clients and can thus help therapists gain a more objective view. From this position the supervisor can also better offer therapists feedback on the tone of therapy, apart from its content, and observe subtle changes in therapists' style or technique. All these variables can significantly affect therapists' ability to effectively respond to obstacles that arise during the course of therapy. Clinical supervision, then, is a key factor in effectively delivering therapeutic services. The supervision process will be again and more fully addressed in Chapter 12 in considering professional and ethical issues in counseling and psychotherapy.

SUMMARY

This chapter looked at a variety of obstacles that can block or retard therapeutic progress. These difficulties include client-initiated obstacles, obstacles that emanate from the way the therapist is approaching therapy efforts, and biologically-based and social-ecological concerns.

The value of clinical supervision was stressed for helping therapists deal with obstacles that may arise in therapy sessions. Supervision can significantly aid therapists in maximizing their therapeutic understandings and skills.

Therapists must always seek to work toward a holistic understanding of clients. In using a primary theoretical approach with a particular client, problem discrimination and definition can be conducted according to the basic tenets of the theory model. As with any model, however, the deductions had best be tested against reality for goodness of fit. It is critical that therapists listen with all of their senses because cues clients present, for example, nonverbal ones, although elusive, provide critical information affecting the course of therapy. Bit by bit, a mosaic representing this particular client, his or her problem, and how the therapist is interacting in response is formed. The mosaic will only be suggestive at first and may take some time to complete. But only by completing it can the client achieve more meaningful and lasting positive change.

SUGGESTED READINGS

Lack of Progress: Client Variables

Greenspan, M. (1983). *A new approach to women and therapy.* New York: McGraw-Hill. Greenspan contrasts the tenets of traditional therapeutic approaches with those of feminist therapy and offers a framework from which to conduct the latter.

Strong, S. R., & Claiborn, C. D. (1982). *Change through interaction.* New York: Wiley. Counseling and psychotherapy operate within the framework of social influence. Its importance is most evident when clients present obstacles that block goal attainment. This book identifies critical opportunities available to therapists to exert influence through interaction with clients, thereby creating an environment where positive change can occur.

Wolman, B. B. (Ed.). (1983). *The therapist's handbook: Treatment methods of mental disorders* (2nd ed.). New York: Van Nostrand Reinhold. The editor and his contributors provide a broad spectrum of treatment techniques for dealing with various client problems.

The Therapist as an Obstacle to Client Change

Corey, G. (1978). *I never knew I had a choice.* Monterey, CA: Brooks/Cole. This book provides a superb basis for personal reflection and enhanced professional growth. Corey has summed its central theme in noting: "As we recognize that we are not merely passive victims of our circumstances, we can consciously become the architects of our lives. Even though others may have drawn the blueprints, we can recognize the plan, take a stand, and change the design."

Pines, A., & Aronson, E. (1981). *Burnout: From tedium to personal growth.* New York: Free Press. The authors offer a particularly pointed presentation on the nature and causes of professional burnout and recommend ideas on effectively countering this continuing challenge.

Rogers, C. (1980). *A way of being.* Boston: Houghton Mifflin. Rogers writes about new challenges to the helping professions and trends in the field of counseling and psychotherapy. In doing so, he invites therapists to examine and enhance their own lives if they are to effectively help others.

Alternative Therapeutic Directions

Kelly, D. (1980). *Anxiety and emotions: Physiological basis and treatment.* Springfield, IL: Thomas. Kelly considers the biological mechanisms that affect human emotion and discusses the implications for planning and initiating intervention strategies.

Lazarus, A. A. (1981). *The practice of multimodal therapy.* New York: McGraw-Hill. Lazarus presents a therapeutic approach that addresses not only individual clients' psychological functioning, but gives equal consideration to biological variables as well as the environment within which clients experience their problem situations.

Sanborn, C. J. (Ed.). (1983). *Case management in mental health services.* New York: Hayworth Press. In a time of ever increasing caseloads, reductions in staffing, and proliferation of agencies, case management as a means of providing effective service delivery has become critical if therapists are to adequately assist clients. This book provides a solid base for conceptualizing the many functions of successful case management.

12

Professional Issues

In the long run, however, if counseling is to be maintained, developed, and accepted by the general public, institutions, governmental credentialing agencies, funding sources, and members of allied professions, it must possess credibility as a profession.

(Boy & Pine, 1982, p. 114)

No presentation of the theory and practice of counseling and psychotherapy is complete without discussion of contemporary professional issues. Counseling and psychotherapy entail more than theoretical concepts and skills applications. Public acceptance of the profession demands that its practitioners acquire and maintain meaningful and relevant credentials. Such acceptance further depends to a large measure on the profession's practitioners adhering to a high level of ethical standards. Finally, the continued maintenance of the profession itself calls for sustained research and evaluation efforts to improve the services it offers to the public.

In this chapter, issues relating to professional training and competence, ethics, and the importance of relevant research efforts are examined.

PROFESSIONAL COMPETENCE

Counseling and psychotherapy as a profession is truly a melting pot of talent (Belkin, 1980). It includes practitioners who have gone through a wide variety of training programs in one or another of the allied mental health fields (counseling, psychology, social work, psychiatric nursing, etc.). Their training, orientation, and professional recognition may be similar to or very different from others within the profession.

Academic Training

Primarily related to the issue of professional competence is the academic training received by practitioners. Typically, therapists are trained in university graduate programs by a qualified professional staff, frequently with a wider diversity of background and specialization than is ordinarily found in a single academic department. The faculty training students to practice counseling and psychotherapy may include counselors, nurses, psychologists, and social workers. This diversity is credible inasmuch as counseling and psychotherapy are interdisciplinary in scope and practice (Belkin, 1980).

Training programs vary in emphasis, in depth, and in what they require of students. Some place primary emphasis on personal development and the ability to relate to others. Some programs posit the purpose of training to be the development of research skills, the ability to generate and test hypotheses, emphasizing the quantitative aspects of training. The ideal program of training is likely a balance between the two.

Belkin (1980) suggests that the scope of training in counseling and psychotherapy can be set down in four general categories: (1) self-awareness and the willingness to be introspective, to grow and, when necessary, to change; (2) mastery of theoretical concepts relating directly to the therapeutic process; (3) technical proficiency in the therapeutic setting, a relevant repertoire of therapist skills and intervention strategies; (4) the ability to administer programs and to interact effectively, both orally and in writing with professional colleagues, clients, and significant others in clients' lives.

The types of understanding and skills required for mastery in these four areas represent an amalgam of knowledge—theoretical and practical—that transcends any single discipline or specialization. Trainees must become proficient in the theoretical foundations of counseling and psychotherapy, as well as in the real-life applications offered through experiential practica and internships. Furthermore, however, trainees should be exposed to the liberal arts, psychology, sociology, anthropology, learning and teaching principles in education, the myriad cultural influences that affect society, and to the interrelationships of all these disciplines and ideas. From an intimacy with critical concepts throughout these disciplines, trainees should be able to synthesize and extrapolate findings and relevant issues that pertain to their effectiveness with the therapeutic setting.

Clinical Supervision

After students are trained in the appropriate academic areas, they need to gain a strong experiential background and put theory and skills into practice under close supervision. The primary goal of clinical supervision is therapists' enhanced development—the ability to assess, offer new perspectives, set goals, intervene, and evaluate more efficiently and effectively in order to best help clients improve. Trainees are working with actual clients experiencing real concerns. Client welfare is always the overriding issue.

Clinical supervision typically involves an individual (one-to-one) or small group (three to five members). A group setting allows for the addition of peer interaction as well as other benefits inherent in group learning. Supervision sessions are best scheduled regularly. Trouble-shooting supervisory sessions held on the run are sometimes necessary when crises arise; however, they don't offer a consistent and coordinated critique. Refinement and growth as well as effective crisis consultation are best achieved through ongoing supervision conferences. For example, should a crisis arise with a client a trainee has already discussed with his or her supervisor, the supervisor has an understanding and background from which to respond immediately. In addition, when supervisory sessions are a regular ongoing process, the clients' concerns can be better anticipated and prepared for.

As in structuring therapy, certain aspects of supervision need to be established in beginning the process. The more specific and explicit the ground rules, the less the likelihood that misunderstandings might interfere with attaining the goals of both supervisor and supervisee. Considerations include where supervision will take place; the time, frequency, and duration of supervisory sessions; and any procedures to be followed in the event of cancellations or missed appointments. There should be agreement on the minimum number of clients the supervisee is expected to work with.

It is particularly important for the beginning therapist serving in a practicum or internship to establish responsibility for obtaining clients. In some training settings supervisors assign clients to supervisees; in others the supervisee selects potential cases and then obtains the supervisor's approval. It is usually best, however, for the novice therapist to always clear any choice of clients with the supervisor before initiating contact unless relieved of such responsibility by the supervisor during initial structuring of the supervision process. Discussing all potential first client contacts will ensure that the supervisee does not become involved in cases that are inappropriate for his or her present level of expertise.

Depending on the individual supervisor, there is much variation in what materials and information are used in supervision and how they are obtained. Some supervisors require only a verbal report of therapy sessions based on written process notes. Although oral reports and process notes are most valuable in teaching supervisees to conceptualize their client contacts, such summaries (by definition) leave out a large portion of the basic therapist-client interchange and are invariably subject to distortion by the selection process itself (Schaefer, 1981). The less experienced the supervisee, the more advantageous it is for the supervisor to have direct access to the actual therapeutic interaction. Video and audio tapes are the norm in this regard, although some supervisors employ direct or indirect observation of therapy through a one-way mirror; cotherapy in which the supervisor and supervisee work together with a client; and on-the-spot supervision in which a supervisor stays in direct communication with the supervisee during a therapy session by earphone or telephone from behind a one-way mirror.

While supervisees' actual work with clients is the basis for supervisory sessions, many supervisors also recommend readings relevant to specific cases in order to broaden supervisees' general therapeutic knowledge and skills base. Supervisors may also elaborate on certain theoretical points and explain specific skills and intervention strategies. It should be remembered, however, that while didactic teaching has a valid place in the supervision process, it does not by itself constitute adequate clinical supervision. Supervisees can demonstrate an impressive range and depth of knowledge and be inept in actual practice (Schaefer, 1981).

Clinical supervision, however, is not just for the trainee. As noted in Chapter 11, clinical supervision is similarly valuable and at times even necessary for the experienced practitioner. For purposes of supervision, therapists can be categorized in three distinct types, based on their levels of experience and expertise: beginning therapists, experienced therapists, and mature therapists.

Beginning therapists often have narrow and rigid notions of the best approach to therapy, especially when obstacles block client progress. This inflexibility is usually due to inexperience. For example, a novice therapist may feel that confronting a client's resistance is the best tack. However valid or invalid this assumption may be with a particular client, a supervisor's familiarity with alternatives can help the beginning therapist see the diversity of available courses to pursue. In addition, therapeutic assets such as humor, vivid imagery, or an active combination of warmth with assertiveness can be modeled by the supervisor.

Experienced therapists have fairly well-formulated, flexible sets of strategies to deal with difficulties that may arise during therapy. These therapists have likely encountered a number of distressing circumstances, overcome most of the anxiety that arises about intervening, and gained a sense of confidence and responsibility. Supervising the experienced therapist involves identifying and enhancing specific areas of clinical concern. The supervisor tasks differ with an experienced therapist from what they are with the beginning therapist; they involve sharpening, accentuating, and integrating the competencies the therapist already possesses.

Mature therapists are highly functioning clinicians; many probably fill supervisory roles themselves. Therefore, the process of clinical supervision with a mature therapist involves an open-ended relationship, with the supervisor and therapist functioning as equals. The supervisor serves as an ally, resource person, and peer who shares ideas and information on his or her own manner of responding in specific circumstances. This relationship is creative and stimulating for both parties, with particular potential for growth and enhancement of competence.

Kadushin (1973) points out a number of positive sources of satisfaction that can be derived from all levels of clinical supervision:

- [ ] A resource person is available to discuss client behavior.
- [ ] Critical feedback is provided.
- [ ] Clinical responsibilities can be shared.
- [ ] Discussion of the theory and practice of therapy is stimulated.

☐   Emotional support is available.
☐   Professional development is enhanced.
☐   A forum for person growth is provided.

Mentoring and Networking

Getting ahead, moving up, and climbing the ladder are common metaphors for career advancement. Few professions require or expect their members to progress alone. A growing body of research substantiates the crucial value of finding a mentor and developing a network of associates if professional and career goals are to be attained (Rawlins & Rawlins, 1983).

Mentors teach, advise, open doors for, encourage, promote, cut red tape for, show the politics and subtleties of their job to, and believe in protegés, thus helping them to succeed. Mentors can explain the unwritten traditions and laws within organizations. They show their protegés, both the overt and covert decision-making processes that are in the profession and the ways to achieve rewards and payoffs (Schmidt & Wolfe, 1980).

Mentors may be the same age as or younger than their protegés; typically, however, they are 8 to 15 years older (Rawlins & Rawlins, 1983). More important than age are mentors' skills, knowledge, or power that protegés lack and need. Usually, mentor-protegé relationships last 2 or 3 years. These liaisons do not have to be particularly close; some are clearly formal arrangements (Phillips-Jones, 1982). As protegés develop greater competence and mature professionally, mentoring relationships gradually realign themselves as peer relationships.

Beginning therapists in search of mentoring should look to experienced colleagues with qualities such as recognized expertise, involvement in professional activities and organizations, a history of mentoring with other novice professionals, willingness to give time, and compatible value systems (Schmidt & Wolfe, 1980). The mentoring relationship is not one-sided. Mentors also benefit from the process by having help with their work, thus accomplishing more; gaining satisfaction from developing new talent; achieving goals vicariously; getting future paybacks as a result of investing in protegés; and paying back past debts incurred from their own mentors (Rawlins & Rawlins, 1983).

Networking is a systematic process of developing helpful contacts, linking with other professionals for assistance, support, and sharing of resources in the form of information, professional opportunities and feedback. Networking reduces isolation and builds participation and self-confidence (Rawlins & Rawlins, 1983). To construct a successful network, the beginning therapist should seek out opportunities to help others, keeping in mind that the greater strength of networking is in mutual support, not

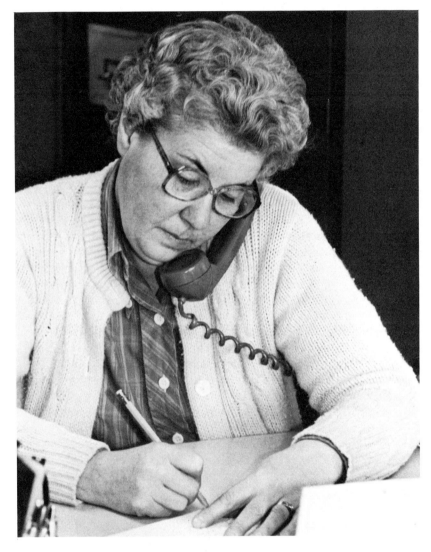

Networking enables professionals to help each other

paybacks (Gillis, 1980). It is also important to remember that the goal of networking is professional development; gossip, criticisms, confidences, or controversial issues unrelated to work are not appropriate discussion topics.

Lunches, after-work drinks, and telephone calls to report back or to share information are the essence of networking. Welch (1980) suggests that three special-contact lunches per week are the prescribed norm for the active networker; networking takes time, so being excessively task oriented and not wanting to waste time are drawbacks. The larger the network, the better the chance for enhancing professional development. Remember former bosses, colleagues, professors, and department chairs and keep them updated on current activities. Courteous feedback to helpful persons maintain their interest and involvement. Network members should be contacted at times other than when making a request. When seeking help, ask for one thing at a time and ask separate individuals for select, small portions of assistance.

Finding a mentor can be the most important initial strategy a beginning therapist can consider for climbing the career ladder. For maintaining and enhancing professional development, an extensive network is a necessity.

Licensing and Certification

Licenses and certificates inform the public that a practitioner has received specific training and supervision in the profession he or she seeks to practice. Although a license or certificate does not guarantee professional competence, practitioners must be prepared to address this issue regardless of their anticipated practice setting.

While licensing and certification differ in purpose, they have basic commonalities. Both require applicants to meet specific requirements in education and training; both rely on tests of competence to determine whether applicants have met the standards and deserve to be granted a credential (Shimberg, 1981). Licensure is "the statutory process by which an agency of government, usually of a state, grants permission to a person meeting predetermined qualifications to engage in a given occupation and/or use a particular title and to perform specified functions" (Fretz & Mills, 1980, p. 7). Certification is "the nonstatutory process by which an agency or association grants recognition to an individual for having met certain predetermined professional qualifications" (Fretz & Mills, 1980, p. 7). Simply stated, licensing gives practitioners the legal right to practice via governmental legislation, while certification is a standardized recognition of competence awarded by a professional organization.

The licensing and certification of counselors, psychologists, social workers and other mental health professionals is an area of intense professional interest, primarily because professionalism tends to be associated with some type of license or certification (Corey, Corey, & Callanan, 1984). Indeed, practitioners who misrepresent themselves are subject to legal penalties in most states. Certification by one's relevant professional organization can greatly affect a practitioner's credibility among colleagues and the community at large; professional certification equating with professional competence, lack thereof suggesting less ability to provide acceptable services. Thus, the major advantage of licensing and certification is that entry into practice can be either formally or informally restricted, and, in the case of licensure, those denied entry who persisit in the activities defined by statute can be prosecuted (Davis, 1981).

Continuing Education

Every therapist needs to develop a program of continuing education. Earning advanced degrees and achieving certification or licensure only minimally assures that an individual possesses necessary skills and knowledge; continuing education is essential to staying current with the ever-evolving and expanding field of counseling and psychotherapy. Most professional organizations require periodic proof of continuing education to maintain professional certification. Similarly, state licensing boards require continuing education as a regular part of licensure renewal. Formal coursework, professional workshops, professional conferences, and similar activities all are avenues for continuing education for the practicing professional.

Professional Associations

Professional associations provide counseling and psychotherapy practitioners with a variety of services. First, they bring together colleagues with similar interests and investments. They are dedicated to maintaining and improving the science and practice of the profession. As a response to this mandate all have established codes of ethics that provide guidelines

Peer review in professional associations can help in establishing appropriate professional conduct

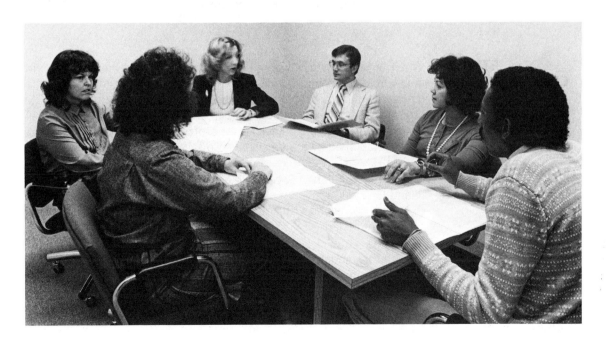

for practitioners. Further, all publish professional journals and sponsor conferences where relevant research and practice is reported, keeping them abreast of critical issues within the profession. Journals and conferences are necessary and significant resources for practitioners to update and enhance their knowledge and skills base.

Professional associations provide national and regional leadership, creating greater credibility and public acceptance of their members. They can provide a political strength as a body of professionals trying to affect legislative processes that cannot be individually attained. The potential to enhance the professionalism of service delivery to clients is thus significantly strengthened by membership in professional associations.

All practitioners of counseling and psychotherapy should be active in professional associations. Three of the major ones are:

American Association for Counseling and Development
5999 Stevenson Avenue
Alexandria, Virginia 22304

American Psychological Association
1200 Seventeenth Street, N.W.
Washington, D.C. 20036

National Association of Social Workers
7981 Eastern Avenue
Silver Springs, Maryland 20910

ETHICAL CONSIDERATIONS IN COUNSELING AND PSYCHOTHERAPY

When an aspiring professional group undertakes activities that involve public trust and confidence, translating prevailing values into ethical standards that guide how its members practice is a necessary first step. As the group develops toward professionalism, these ethical standards are generally codified, providing guidelines for professional behavior. Those ethical codes established by the American Association for Counseling and Development (AACD), the American Psychological Association (APA), and the National Association of Social Workers (NASW) are listed in Appendices A, B, and C.

Van Hoose and Kottler (1978) posit three reasons why professional codes of ethics exist:

☐ Ethical standards are designed to protect a profession from government interference. Professional codes assert the autonomy of the profession through stated self-regulation as opposed to being regulated by legislative bodies.

☐ Ethical codes establish common norms and thereby protect a profession from self-destructive internal bickering.

☐ Ethical standards are designed to protect the therapist from the public. If therapists act within their code of ethics, they are afforded greater protection if sued for malpractice.

Although there are distinct advantages in having an accepted code of ethics to guide one's practice, they impose several limitations as well. Two of the most frequently mentioned limitations are conflicts within the standards, and that there are legal and ethical issues not covered by the standards. Therefore, professional codes of ethics must be supplemented by other information (Talbutt, 1981).

Daubner and Daubner (1970) define a code of ethics as "principles or norms that ought to govern human conduct" (p. 433). It is incumbent upon the practitioner to exercise professional judgment in applying them to specific situations. Stude and McKelvy (1979) summarize this matter aptly: "They [ethical codes] are statements of principle, which must be interpreted and applied by the individual or group to a particular context. They present a rationale for ethical behavior. Their exact interpretation, however, will depend on the situation to which they are being applied" (p. 453).

The three major ethical issues most frequently of concern to beginning therapists are client welfare, informed consent, and confidentiality.

Client Welfare

All ethical codes affirm that a therapist's *primary* responsibility is to the client. This means that the needs of the client, not the therapist, assume primary importance in the therapeutic relationship. It also implies that the therapeutic relationship should be maintained only as long as the client is benefiting from it. Guidelines of the AACD, APA, and NASW in this regard are excerpted in Table 12–1.

It is important that therapists be able to concretely evaluate clients' progress. They must recognize the boundaries of their own competence as well as clients' realistic needs and, when appropriate, either refer to another professional or terminate therapy. In both situations, however, a problem of ethics arises should the client resist referral or termination. While the therapist has a primary responsibility to the client, neither the client nor the therapist live in a vacuum; they are affected by other relationships. The therapist also has a responsibility to his or her own agency, to any referring agency, to society, and to the profession (Corey, 1982).

TABLE 12–1
Ethical Considerations Relating to Client Welfare

American Association for Counseling and Development (1981)

The member's *primary* obligation is to respect the integrity and promote the welfare of the client(s), whether the client(s) is (are) assisted individually or in a group relationship.

American Psychological Association (1981)

Psychologists respect the dignity and worth of the individual and strive for the preservation and protection of fundamental human rights. They are committed to increasing knowledge of human behavior and of people's understanding of themselves and others and to the utilization of such knowledge for the promotion of human welfare. While pursuing these objectives, they make every effort to protect the welfare of those who seek their services.

National Association of Social Workers (1979)

The social worker's primary responsibility is to clients.

The general principle of the primacy of the client's welfare may appear clear, but is often easily clouded by the therapist's other responsibilities. Consider the following case example:

Larry, 16, has been working with a counselor at Youth House, a drop-in recreational center in his community. Short-term crisis counseling is a part of the agency's services. Larry has seen the counselor each day for the past week and feels that the sessions are extremely helpful to him. The counselor agrees that Larry is making progress but is also aware of some other realities: the counselor's time is limited because she has both administrative and therapeutic demands placed on her; the agency has a policy that long-term counseling should not be provided and referrals should be made instead; and that while Larry's therapy enabled him to cope with the immediate crisis, more intensive and long-term therapy is clearly indicated. Because of these realities, she suggests a referral to Larry and gives him reasons for the referral.

Larry might respond in two ways. He might agree to accept the counselor's referral to another therapist or agency. In this case, the counselor's responsibility for the client's welfare would continue until he could begin seeing the other therapist. Even after that, some form of consultation with the other therapist might be in order. On the other hand, Larry might refuse to accept the referral, emphasizing his desire to continue the present relationship. The counselor must weigh the potential harm to all concerned and the likely consequences that would ensue should the

TABLE 12–2
Ethical Considerations Relating to Client Referrals

American Association for Counseling and Development (1981)
☐ If a member determines an inability to be of professional assistance to the client, the member must either avoid initiating the counseling relationship or immediately terminate that relationship. In either event, the member must suggest appropriate alternatives. (The member must be knowledgeable about referral resources so that a satisfactory referral can be initiated.) In the event the client declines the suggested referral, the member is not obligated to continue the relationship.

American Psychological Association (1981)
☐ Psychologists terminate a clinical or consulting relationship when it is reasonably clear that the consumer is not benefiting from it. They offer to help the consumer locate alternative sources of assistance.

National Association of Social Workers (1979)
☐ The social worker should terminate service to clients, and professional relationships with them, when such service and relationships are no longer required or no longer serve the clients' needs or interests.
☐ The social worker should withdraw services precipitously only under unusual circumstances, giving careful consideration to all factors in the situation and taking care to minimize possible adverse effects.
☐ The social worker who anticipates the termination or interruption of service to clients should notify clients promptly and seek the transfer, referral, or continuation of services in relation to the clients' needs and preferences.

relationship continue. Relevant excerpts from the ethical codes of the AACD, APA, and NASW are in Table 12–2.

Informed Consent

Issues of clients' rights are an important part of the ethical codes referred to in this chapter. Clients frequently present themselves for therapy vulnerable and desperate for help. They may perceive the therapist and the therapeutic process through rose colored glasses, exaggerating the potential benefits and minimizing the efforts required. For most clients, the therapeutic situation is a new one, so they are unclear about what is expected of them, what they should expect from the therapist, what they should expect from therapy, and what their rights as clients are (Corey et al., 1984).

The ethical codes of the AACD, APA, and NASW all require that clients be given adequate information in order to make informed choices

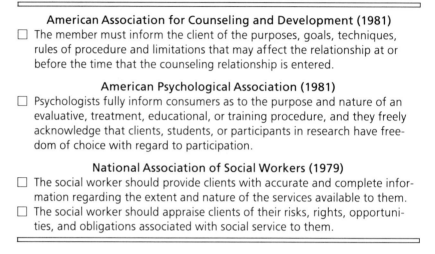

TABLE 12–3
Ethical Considerations Relating to Informed Consent

American Association for Counseling and Development (1981)
☐ The member must inform the client of the purposes, goals, techniques, rules of procedure and limitations that may affect the relationship at or before the time that the counseling relationship is entered.

American Psychological Association (1981)
☐ Psychologists fully inform consumers as to the purpose and nature of an evaluative, treatment, educational, or training procedure, and they freely acknowledge that clients, students, or participants in research have freedom of choice with regard to participation.

National Association of Social Workers (1979)
☐ The social worker should provide clients with accurate and complete information regarding the extent and nature of the services available to them.
☐ The social worker should appraise clients of their risks, rights, opportunities, and obligations associated with social service to them.

about entering and continuing the client-therapist relationship. This responsibility is referred to as the ethical issue of *informed consent.* Relevant excerpts from the aforementioned three organizations' codes of ethics are in Table 12–3.

Hare-Mustin, Marecek, Kaplan, and Liss-Levenson (1979), in asserting that ethical principles require that clients be given sufficient information to make informed choices about entering and continuing in therapy, identify three areas of prerequisite background for such choices: (1) the procedures, goals, and possible side effects of therapy; (2) the qualifications, policies, and practices of the therapist; and (3) the available sources of help other than therapy.

Clients considering therapy should be told that they may experience changes that could produce disruptions and turmoil in their lives. The potential for positive change and the probable personal and financial cost should be frankly discussed during initial sessions. While it may be difficult to give clients a detailed description of what may occur in therapy, some general procedures and goals should be explained, especially if any unusual or experimental methods may be used. Therapists should describe to clients their training and education, any specialized skills they have, and the types of clients and problems that they are best trained to deal with. In addition, relevant information on limits to confidentiality, particularly potential consultation with supervisors or colleagues, and video or audio tape recording and its purposes are important to clients.

A number of writers have discussed the preparation of a "Professional Disclosure Statement" (Gill, 1982; Gross, 1977; Swanson, 1979;

Winborn, 1977). This statement may be used as one means of meeting informed consent provisions of the ethical standards. Winborn's (1977) professional disclosure statement in figure 12–1 is a model to consider in this regard.

FIGURE 12–1
Winborn's Professional Disclosure Statement

Some Things You Should Know About Your Counselor and the Counseling Process

Since counseling is conducted in a number of different ways, depending on the counselor, this description has been prepared to inform you about my qualifications, how I view the counseling process, and what you can expect from me as your counselor.

My Qualifications. I received a doctorate from Indiana University with a major in counseling and a minor in psychology. During my 16 years as a counselor I have served as an assistant director of counseling centers at two major universities and as a professor in a university department that trains counselors. I am a licensed consulting psychologist in Michigan.

Most of my experience in counseling has been with teenagers and adults. I also have had experience in counseling elementary school pupils, but this has been a small amount of my practice. Although most of my experience has been in counseling members of the white race, I have had some experience in counseling Blacks and Americans with Spanish surnames. I am not, however, bilingual. Having been reared in Oklahoma, I have some knowledge of the American Indian culture in addition to that of Black and Latin cultures.

I have counseled individuals who have various kinds of vocational, educational, and personal, social problems. My training and experience provides me with the skills to work with people who have concerns that range from what type of job they should seek or how to overcome problems associated with school achievement, to marital problems, fears, and anxious feelings. I have also worked with individuals who have been referred to me by the Probate Court, Vocational Rehabil-

itation Service, Veterans Administration, and Social Security Disability Determination Program.

In summary, my qualifications enable me to counsel people who are able to function at home, school, or work even though they may have serious problems. I am not qualified to work with individuals who need hospitalization or similar care, or who need the care of a psychiatrist. In certain situations, however, I can work with individuals under the supervision of a psychiatrist.

What is counseling? Counseling is a learning process whereby you may learn to make personal decisions or learn skills, such as how to become comfortable in social situations. You may have some behavior you want to eliminate such as the fear of flying in an airplane. You may want to learn how to communicate with your husband or wife, or how to cope with situations that cause you to be depressed or anxious.

There are several steps in the counseling process. First, we will probably spend some time talking about your problem. I need to get to know you and how you view yourself. You will probably come to understand yourself better as we talk. Obviously, we need to discuss your concerns openly and honestly. This means that we will need to develop a special kind of relationship between us so that you will feel free to tell me about yourself. My responsibility at this point in the counseling process is to listen to you, to help you communicate with me, and to provide an environment of trust so that you can freely tell me how you feel and what is on your mind.

All of our interviews will, of course, be confidential. A professional code of ethics prevents me from discussing our interviews with anyone or from releasing any records without your permission. The only exception to this is if you indicate that you are going to harm yourself or someone else. In such cases I am ethically bound to report such a situation to someone in authority or someone responsible for you.

After we have information about your concerns, we will decide upon goals and objectives to work toward to relieve these concerns. Then, we will develop a plan to achieve these goals and objectives. Such a plan may require that you perform certain activities such as obtaining information, taking tests, practicing skills you want to learn, thinking certain thoughts, and keeping records of your behavior.

We will evaluate your progress in terms of whether the plan is helping you to attain your goals and objectives, and then compare your progress with your behavior when you first came in to see me.

The last step in counseling involves some brief follow-up sessions. Quite often this is done by telephone or in short interviews. At this time we will determine if you are maintaining your progress. In other words, after you have attained your counseling goals and objectives, we will have an occasional contact to make sure that everything is going according to our plans.

Time and Money. You may want to know how many counseling sessions will be needed and how long each session will last. Normally, we spend a maximum of one hour during each interview. Needed exceptions can be made but interview time of more than one hour is often nonproductive. Depending on the nature of your problem, counseling sessions may be needed once or twice a week.

It is difficult to predict how many sessions will be needed, as this varies with each person and the type of problem. I will be glad to discuss with you the number of sessions that might be needed after I understand why you are coming to see me.

(At this point, for clients I see in private practice, I explain my fee structure and how payments can be made. Counselors who work for institutions where counseling services are free, but charges for tests and so forth are made can explain any such charges at this point.)

Please Ask Questions. You many have questions about me and my qualifications, or about the counseling process that are not discussed in the above paragraphs. *It is your right* to have a complete explanation for any of your questions at any time during the counseling process. Please exercise this right if you have any doubts or concerns about our counseling relationship and the counseling process.

SOURCE: From "Honest Labeling and Other Procedures for the Protection of Consumers of Counseling" by B. B. Winborn, *Personnel and Guidance Journal,* 1977, *56,* 206-209. Copyright 1977 by American Personnel and Guidance Association. Reprinted by permission.

FIGURE 12–1
Winborn's Professional
Disclosure Statement
(continued)

To make a fully informed choice, clients need to know about alternative sources of help other than therapy. Therapists must therefore be knowledgeable about available resources so that they can present these alternatives to clients. Hare-Mustin et al. (1979) suggest these alternatives to therapy:

☐ *Individual self-help:* the use of self-help reading materials, recreational and religious activities, changes in social relationships, work, or place of residence.

☐ *Training for personal effectiveness:* parent effectiveness training, assertiveness training, marriage encounter, Transcendental Meditation, yoga.

☐ *Peer self-help groups:* Weight Watchers, Alcoholics Anonymous, Parents Without Partners, and similar support groups for individuals to better deal with particular problems in their lives.

☐ *Crisis intervention systems:* Suicide hotlines, rape crisis centers, shelters for abused spouses, pregnancy and abortion counseling centers.

☐ *Psychological/psychiatric helping systems:* hospitalization, partial hospitalization, day treatment programs, physical interventions based on psychotropic medications.

☐ *Other institutional helping systems:* social welfare agencies, legal assistance, vocational rehabilitation.

An open discussion of therapy and potential alternatives may, of course, lead some clients to choose assistance other than that offered by the therapist. For beginning therapists, giving clients' such open choices can create anxiety in that their livelihood depends upon their client caseload. However, the practice of openly discussing therapy and its alternatives will likely strengthen the commitment of clients who do choose to continue with the therapist.

Confidentiality

Perhaps the greatest single ethical issue in counseling and psychotherapy is confidentiality. Confidentiality in therapy had its genesis in the physician-patient relationship. In the 16th century, physicians began to practice confidentiality when they realized that contagious diseases were spread extensively by persons who feared that detection of their affliction would remand them to social isolation (Slovenko, 1973). More recently, professional reasons for guaranteeing confidentiality are being augmented by legal mandates under the term *privileged communication.* The terms confidentiality and privileged communication, however, should not be used interchangeably because they have different meanings.

Shah (1969) defines confidentiality in stating: "Confidentiality relates to matters of professional ethics. Confidentiality protects the client from unauthorized disclosures of any sort by the professional without informed consent of the client" (p. 57). Confidentiality is a standard established and maintained by the ethical codes of professional organizations. Denkowski and Denkowski (1982) identify two primary reasons that militate the need for client confidentiality: (1) confidentiality protects clients from the social stigma that is frequently associated with therapy, and (2) confidentiality is based on promoting vital client rights, which is integral to therapists' professed concern for the welfare of clients. Relevant excerpts from the AACD, APA, and NASW codes of ethics are in Table 12–4.

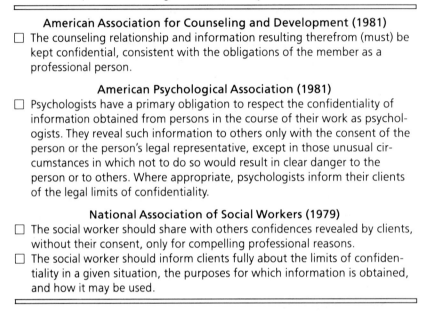

TABLE 12–4
Ethical Considerations Relating to Confidentiality

American Association for Counseling and Development (1981)
☐ The counseling relationship and information resulting therefrom (must) be kept confidential, consistent with the obligations of the member as a professional person.

American Psychological Association (1981)
☐ Psychologists have a primary obligation to respect the confidentiality of information obtained from persons in the course of their work as psychologists. They reveal such information to others only with the consent of the person or the person's legal representative, except in those unusual circumstances in which not to do so would result in clear danger to the person or to others. Where appropriate, psychologists inform their clients of the legal limits of confidentiality.

National Association of Social Workers (1979)
☐ The social worker should share with others confidences revealed by clients, without their consent, only for compelling professional reasons.
☐ The social worker should inform clients fully about the limits of confidentiality in a given situation, the purposes for which information is obtained, and how it may be used.

Rules of confidentiality have legal status through licensing laws for physicians, psychologists, social workers, and counselors, through patient rights legislation, and through court decisions that have considered the unauthorized disclosure of information as an invasion of privacy. Thus, privileged communication is "a legal right which exists by statute and which protects the client from having his confidences revealed publicly from the witness stand during legal proceedings without his permission" (Shah, 1969, p. 57). Privileged communication is a narrower concept than confidentiality and deals with the admissibility of evidence into court. Privileged communications laws typically are not relevant to disclosures unrelated to legal proceedings (Knapp & Vandecreek, 1982).

When privileged communication laws apply, clients can prevent their therapists from testifying about them in court without their consent. If the client waives this privilege, the therapist has no grounds for withholding information. Thus, the privilege belongs to the client and is meant for the client's protection, not for the protection of therapists (Corey et al., 1983). Since the therapist-client privilege is a legal concept, there are certain circumstances under which information *must* be provided by the therapist. These situations are summarized in Table 12–5.

Related to the issues of confidentiality and privileged communication are the regulations established by some governmental and private agencies that define therapists' primary obligations as being to the insti-

TABLE 12–5
Exceptions to Privilege

☐ When the therapist is acting in a court-appointed capacity—for example, to conduct a psychological examination (DeKraai & Sales, 1982).

☐ When the therapist makes an assessment of a foreseeable risk of suicide (Shultz, 1982).

☐ When the client initiates a lawsuit against the therapist, such as for malpractice (Denkowski & Denkowski, 1982).

☐ In any civil action when the client introduces mental condition as a claim or defense (Denkowski & Denkowski, 1982).

☐ When the client is under the age of 16 and the therapist believes that the child is the victim of a crime—for example, incest, child molestation, rape, or child abuse (Everstine, Everstine, Heymann, True, Frey, Johnson, & Seiden, 1980).

☐ When the therapist determines that the client is in need of hospitalization for a mental or psychological disorder (DeKraai & Sales, 1982; Shultz, 1982).

☐ When criminal action is involved (Everstine et al., 1980).

☐ When clients reveal their intention to commit a crime or when they can be accurately assessed as "dangerous to society" or dangerous to themselves (DeKraai & Sales, 1982; Shultz, 1982).

SOURCE: From *Issues and Ethics in the Helping Professions*, 2nd Ed., by G. Corey, M. S. Corey, and P. Callanan. Copyright © 1984, 1979 by Wadsworth, Inc. Reprinted by permission of the publisher, Brooks/Cole Publishing Company, Monterey, California.

tution as opposed to the client (Shah, 1970). In such situations, therapists may be faced with conflicts between their obligations to their employer and obligations to their client. For this reason, it is critical that possible conflicts should be clarified before therapists enter into therapeutic relationships with clients. In short, clients should be informed about the limits of confidentiality.

The ethics of confidentiality rest on the premise that clients have a right to expect what they discuss will be kept private except where legal statute dictates otherwise or where clients have given informed consent to the potential exceptions before entering therapy. Since confidentiality is not absolute, it is necessary that therapists be most familiar with those circumstances under which it can and cannot be maintained.

Malpractice

Unless therapists act in good faith and take due care, they are liable to a civil suit for failing to appropriately carry out their professional duties. When practitioners assume a professional role, they are expected to abide by legal standards and adhere to the ethical codes of their profession in providing services to clients. Malpractice may be viewed as the opposite of acting in good faith; civil liability means that therapists can be sued for not doing right or doing wrong to clients. Malpractice is therefore an act or omission by a therapist that is inconsistent with reasonable care and skill used by other reputable therapists of the same system and that results in injury to the client (Knapp, 1980).

Three conditions must be present for malpractice to have occurred (Burgum & Anderson, 1975): (1) the defendent must have had a duty to the plaintiff, (2) damages must have resulted through negligence or improper action, and (3) a causal relationship between the damages and negligence must have existed. Knapp (1980) points out that courts do not assume malpractice exists if a therapist has made a mistake in judgment, for it is possible to make mistakes and exercise reasonable care at the same time. Knapp also comments that the courts generally accept any treatment as legitimate if a substantial minority of therapists practice it. Further, therapists are typically evaluated in accordance with their theoretical orientation. For example, a behaviorally-oriented therapist would be evaluated according to acceptable standards within this theoretical approach and not within the framework of practices typical of Gestalt theory.

Some of the more frequent issues raised in malpractice action against therapists have included (Knapp, 1980):

☐ physical injuries sustained during encounter group therapy
☐ sexual relations with clients
☐ failure to exercise reasonable care in cases of suicide
☐ failure to warn and protect victims in cases involving violent clients

While beginning therapists may view the specter of malpractice with anxiety, knowledge of malpractice rules can help protect clients from harm as well as protect therapists from potential court actions. Even a malpractice claim settled out of court or later determined to be unfounded can be costly, time-consuming, and embarrassing. Corey et al. (1984) summarizes some of the safeguards that have been offered in this regard:

☐ Therapists can protect themselves and their clients by making use of informed consent procedures and by using written contracts to clarify the therapeutic relationship.
☐ Therapists should be concretely aware of local and state laws that limit their practice in addition to the policies of the agency that em-

ploys them. This rule particularly applies to statutes on privileged communication.

☐ Therapists should seek to engender positive feelings between themselves and their clients, since good relationships with clients not only facilitate therapeutic progress but also substantially reduce the likelihood of a malpractice action (Knapp, 1980).

☐ It is good practice for therapists to consult with supervisors or colleagues in situations involving difficult ethical and legal issues. It is foolish for therapists to think that they should not need to occasionally seek advice from other professionals.

☐ Having a theoretical orientation to guide one's practice, including a clear rationale for specific strategies, significantly contributes to assuring responsible practice.

☐ It is good practice to carefully document a client's treatment plan. Records can include references to symptomatology, diagnosis, and treatment strategies, documents verifying informed consent, relevant consultations and their outcomes, and a copy of the therapeutic contract (Knapp, 1980).

RESEARCH EFFORTS AND EFFECTIVE THERAPEUTIC PRACTICE

Research in counseling and psychotherapy serves several important purposes. In a broad sense, research is one of the three legs supporting the profession, the other two being theory and practice. Ideally, the three constantly interact. The theorist tries to formulate the most comprehensive and advanced explanation of the phenomena therapists deal with—persons' feelings, thoughts, and behaviors. The theorist builds on the experiences of therapists and their clients and the accumulated research. In doing so, the theorist offers a blueprint for potential practices and thus hypotheses for future research.

The researcher simultaneously looks to theorists for concepts to critically consider and to practitioners for sources of actual study. The practitioners' role in all this is twofold. First, they let the theorist and researcher know what problems they face, what lessons they are learning, what insights they are obtaining, and what methods seem to be producing specific results in practice. Second, practitioners look to published research for answers, insights, and suggestions that feed into their daily applied activities (Goldman, 1978).

Practicing therapists are, at times, theorists and researchers as well. Remer (1981) emphasizes the critical interplay between research and practice. He states that therapists need research relevant to the effectiveness of their practice because they "have an ethical, if not legal and moral, responsibility to both their clients and the public to know the effects and limits of the tools and techniques they use" (p. 569). Therapists obviously believe that their practice is effective. Research evidence is often called for to support therapists' positive suppositions.

Lewis and Hutson (1983) propose that the relationship between research and practice in counseling and psychotherapy is of special concern in the 1980s. Congress and agencies of the federal government have begun to show considerable interest in the efficacy of counseling and psychotherapy. For example, the 1980 Senate Bill 3029 included a section to create a 13-member national professional mental health commission to study the safety and efficacy of various mental health approaches. A similar bill, S. 647, was introduced in 1981. The ability to demonstrate the effectiveness of the therapeutic process will continue to be of the utmost concern to the future of the profession. Therapists must by necessity, therefore, be both consumers and creators of clinical research.

Types of Research

There are a number of ways to classify research, but perhaps the simplest manner is to identify research as either basic or applied. Basic research is mainly concerned with developing new knowledge and tends to be theoretical in orientation. The topic of applied research is assessing applications of existing knowledge. For example, after basic research determined the major factors required for therapists to communicate core conditions, applied research sought to develop ways whereby therapists would communicate these conditions more clearly, concisely, and efficiently.

Research is also classified by whether it is conducted in a laboratory or field setting. Laboratory settings lend themselves well to theoretical research and are therefore usually sites of basic research. In a laboratory setting, the factors thought to be most relevant to a particular problem under study can be controlled. Laboratory settings are not natural; instead, subjects are brought into some new situation (the laboratory) to participate in the research. Field settings, by contrast, are real, ongoing life situations. Research findings from laboratory settings are normally later tested in the field. For example, if laboratory research found that clients of certain backgrounds achieved greater therapeutic progress in a shorter time, field research might follow and consider whether assigning cases on the basis of client/therapist background has a significant effect on clients' progress in actual practice.

Research is also classified by the type of methodology or design used. Since any study can incorporate several methodologies, such classifications are not mutually exclusive. Some major methodological research classifications are survey, developmental, correlational, experimental, and case study.

Survey studies usually gather relatively limited data from many persons, typically through the use of questionnaires or interviews. A survey that covers the entire population being studied is called a census. A more typical study that involves only a portion of the population is the sample survey. From a sample survey inferences can be made about the entire population based on the sample population studied. For example, a frequent survey research topic has been identifying the needs of clients who are likely to seek therapy.

Developmental research is either longitudinal or cross-sectional, depending on the survey technique employed. In the longitudinal method, the same sample of subjects is studied over time, enabling intensive studies of subjects at various stages in their lives. However, longitudinal research has some inherent practical difficulties. Primarily, longitudinal research demands an extended commitment over time from researchers and their supporting agencies or institutions. Also, the subjects selected and variables chosen at the beginning of the study must remain constant even though subjects mature and concepts may be reconsidered. Finally, keeping track of the location of subjects and maintaining their cooperation for extended periods can be difficult.

Many of the practical difficulties of the longitudinal method are absent in the cross-sectional method. In cross-sectional research, a group having different characteristics is studied at one point in time. For example, to study the privacy needs of parents during varying periods of time after the birth of their first child, a cross-sectional study would analyze data on parents with children less than a year old, one to three years old, and so forth. Usually, a much larger sample population can be used in cross-sectional studies as opposed to longitudinal because cross-sectional studies allow for all data to be collected at one time. A major disadvantage of the cross-sectional approach is the possibility that extraneous variables can cause results to be invalid; that is, not reflect what is ostensibly being studied. For instance, in the aforementioned research on the privacy needs of parents, one important variable could significantly skew results: Parents who have considerable unmet privacy needs experience greater marital conflict resulting in divorce and separation, causing them to be exluded from the sample. Therefore, with the study designed as described, parents with possibly the greatest privacy needs would be left out.

Correlational research determines the extent of a relationship between two variables. For instance, on the basis of clinical experience, a therapist may believe that there is a relationship between clients' age and desire to learn to be more assertive in social situations. To test this belief or hypothesis, the therapist/researcher would have to select a sample from the population and gather data. The age of the subjects and their desire to acquire greater assertiveness in social situations would be measured, possibly by a test or self-report measure. The therapist/researcher then determines the degree of relationship between the two variables assessed.

Correlational research is particularly useful in making predictions. If there is a correlation between two variables, then a prediction can be made about some aspect of one based on the other. For example, the core conditions of empathic understanding, concreteness, genuineness, and respect have been shown to be highly correlated with a helpful therapeutic climate. Therapists should be cautioned, however, that correlation research does not suggest causation, which is in the domain of experimental research.

Experimental research begins with a population of subjects that can be randomly assigned to two or more treatment groups. Randomization enables the researcher to conclude that the only significant difference between the groups is the treatment they received. For instance, a sample of clients experiencing severe depression is randomly assigned to two different therapy groups, each designed to intervene in a specific manner. If the clients in one group progress more in alleviating their depression, it can be assumed that the different interventions determined the different degrees of progress. It is also assumed that if the groups were reversed the group receiving the less effective intervention would progress less. Thus, one of the specific interventions identified for study *caused* significantly greater client progress to occur. Further, the random assignment of subjects in this method assures that every client has as much chance of being assigned to one treatment group as to another. As a result, the characteristics of the clients assigned to each treatment group should be typical of the sample as a whole; this is critical to the validity of the study for general therapeutic application.

Case-study research is intensive investigation of one individual client. Most case studies arise from efforts to solve problems. Freud is well known for his case studies in which he tried to help clients resolve the problems with which they came to him. He felt that the relationship he observed between his individual clients and their environments, both external and intrapsychic or internal, were characteristic of other individuals with similar problems. Freud published detailed accounts of his therapy sessions with clients on the assumption that generalizations could be made from these case studies.

The greatest advantage of the case study method is its attempt to understand the client's whole being and situation in great detail. However, case studies have been criticized because of the possible skew of researcher bias and questionable generalization of findings. Still, it is a highly useful research method valued by many therapists.

The Therapist as Research Consumer

Harmon (1978) posits several reasons why therapists should be research consumers: (1) reading research contributes to professional development and effectiveness with clients; (2) given that practicing therapists should and do conduct research in their settings, therapists' own research will be influenced by their knowledge or lack thereof regarding previous research; (3) only therapists themselves can take ultimate responsibility for the quality of services they provide, and knowledge of recent research heavily affects therapists' ability to maintain the highest standard of quality.

The abundance of research articles in many professional journals makes a framework for evaluating worthwhile reading most valuable. Harmon (1978) presents such a framework in the following guidelines for reading research articles in the field of counseling and psychotherapy:

1. Read the abstract of the article if available and decide whether the article is of interest. If not, select another article and again evaluate by reading the abstract before proceeding.

2. The introduction of the article should describe the purpose of the research. It should have some theoretical or practical import. In experimental studies, formal hypotheses should be given in addition to a general statement of purpose.

3. In the introduction or in the methods sections, important terms and concepts should be operationally defined. These definitions should be consistent throughout the article.

4. If either the second or third step has been omitted, the article likely will be difficult to follow and therefore of limited benefit. It may be better to stop reading and select another article.

5. The methods section should include information sufficient to allow the reader to determine whether:
   a. the reliability and validity of the measures used are satisfactory.
   b. the subjects are appropriate for the study and the results can be generalized to other therapy situations.
   c. the research design tests the hypothesis or adequately explores the question or questions under consideration.
   d. the statistical analysis is appropriate for the problem.
   e. the overall logic of the methods employed is sound.

6. The discussion, conclusions, and recommendations should be consistent with the data; conclusions or recommendations that exceed the scope of the data probably are not valid.

7. Any concerns or ideas about the application of the findings to one's

own setting can be communicated to the author and/or extended by conducting another study oneself.

Many research studies published in professional journals do not adequately meet these guidelines. Of course, very few research studies, if any, are perfect. Because reading research articles is extremely important for staying current with developments in the profession, therapists should be aware that imperfect research is published and be prepared to read critically.

The Therapist/Researcher

More therapists are viewing themselves as researchers as well as service providers. They are realizing the increasing importance of evaluating the effectiveness of the approaches and interventions they employ. A great deal of creative thought and logical analysis is required to answer questions about therapeutic effectiveness. A more consistent and meaningful evaluation is possible when practitioners can demonstrate clearly defined therapeutic effects, clients' experiences of the effects, and meaningful outcomes. The therapist/researcher has a great responsibility as the professional in the position to generate research as well as benefit from it. Beginning therapists especially should understand how relevant research can be conducted in their setting. Since most of the research in counseling and psychotherapy is of a clinical, applied nature, therapists must learn the basic steps this kind of research requires. Ary, Jacobs, and Razavich (1979) offer the following guidelines for clinical research:

1. *Statement of the Problem.* The researcher must start with a clear statement of the problem. This definition concisely identifies the variables being studied and whether the study's purpose is to determine the status of these variables or to investigate relationships between them.

2. *Identification of Information Needed to Solve the Problem.* The information to be collected is listed, its nature is discussed, and the form the information is to take (such as test scores or responses to questionnaires) is specified.

3. *Selection or Development of Measures for Gathering Data.* The most frequently used measures are questionnaires, tests, sclaes, and interviews. If no suitable measure exists, the researcher must develop one.

4. *Identification of the Target Population and Determination of Any Necessary Sampling Procedure.* The researcher must determine the group about which the information is sought. If the entire target population is too large to study, the researcher should select a smaller sample that will adequately represent the larger population.

5. *Design of the Procedure for Data Collection.* The researcher develops a schedule for obtaining the sample of subjects and collecting the information.

6. *Collection of Data.* The procedure to collect data is implemented.

7. *Analysis of Data.* The data is examined to determine the answer to the problem stated in step one.

8. *Preparation of the Report.* The findings of the study are prepared so that they can be shared with others through a journal article, presentation at a professional meeting, or some other vehicle.

Applying Research to Practice

The most significant use of research findings is their day-to-day application in therapy. Many therapists, however, find it difficult to apply research findings they read in their professional journals. Burr, Mead, and Rollins (1973) propose three ways technical research findings might better be translated for more pragmatic use by practitioners: the popularization, empirical, and theoretical methods.

The popularization method involves changing research findings into a popularized form to be used by therapists. This method, although sometimes helpful, usually results in lost precision and therefore may not be of significant value to the practitioner. The empirical method involves the practitioner reading research reports and, when encountering a client with a problem similar to what has been reported, applying the findings to that client. Another way for therapists to employ the empirical method is to search the research literature for cases similar to ones with which they are currently working. After locating similar case descriptions, the practitioner can try to use the findings to develop a strategy for the case at hand.

The theoretical method is the process of going from technical research literature to theory and then from theory to practice. The therapist analyzes the research findings through appropriate theory rather than, as in the empirical method, trying to apply findings directly to a specific case. In other words, the practitioner who encounters a difficult case might find it advantageous to translate the present circumstances into theoretical terms to assess potential strategies, rather than attempting to garner strategies directly from specific case comparisons.

The following case study is offered to illustrate how these three methods can be applied. Schaefer (1976), a behaviorally-oriented therapist, describes a treatment case study of J, a thirty-eight-year-old married construction worker referred for treatment as part of a suspended sentence for repeatedly exhibiting himself on a construction site to two small school girls on their way to and from school. Schaefer's treatment plan was based on his hypothesis about exhibitionistic behavior:

If it were possible to elicit the behavior in the presence of stimuli other than highly specific ones in the presence of which it is normally emitted, then these new stimuli should weaken the exclusive control of the old. Among these new stimuli would be strong feelings of inappropriateness, shame, awareness of the situation, self-ridicule, and common sense, none of which is normally present during exhibitions, according to accounts by nearly all exhibitionists. These feelings, it should be pointed out, are well known to the exhibitionist, but they are invariably experienced after, never during, an exhibition. It is the presence of these stimuli, along with "vague" sexual urges, that probably prevents normal adults from exhibiting themselves in public. (p. 228)

The primary intervention strategy employed by Schaefer with J was to have him practice exhibitions once every hour, starting immediately after awakening in the morning and ending just before going to bed at night. He was asked to use discretion and to arrange for the exhibitions not to occur in crowded places (exhibitions it was hoped, without exhibitees). Using exhibition on cue (to the clock—once every hour—instead of to urges and fantasies) method, J was helped to gain control over his compulsive behavior.

Schaefer reported that by the end of the second week, J noted feeling silly and stupid when having to engage in the practice assignments. He stated that he had faithfully executed the exhibitions but asked that his "practices" be discontinued. It was pointed out to J that his urges to exhibit (which he had been recording daily since beginning therapy) had remained at zero every day between days 8 and 14.

Using the popularization method in applying Schaefer's findings could result in indiscriminately advising clients to regularly exhibit themselves, potentially without sufficient consideration of the necessary self-control/"urge" control therapeutic differential. Should a therapist use the empirical method in applying Schaefer's findings, he or she would have to wait until an exhibitionistic client sought therapeutic assistance. The theoretical method, by contrast, allows the therapist to use Schaefer's findings almost immediately. To do this, the therapist seeks to directly apply the findings by first considering the theoretical principles Schaefer used. One such principle, behavior on cue, enables the findings to be tested with a wide range of compulsive "urge"-controlled client actions, theoretically related but by appearance quite different from exhibitionism; for example, over-eating, excessive smoking, and compulsive gambling.

In conclusion, in applying research to practice, the theoretical method is of significant importance to therapists. In this method, the therapist does not try to apply findings from research studies directly to the clinical setting without first "going through" a theory. Research is viewed as support for or against the validity of theoretical concepts. The strategies therapists directly use in their practice should emanate from theoretical concepts supported by proven research outcomes.

To readers with fine long-term memory, this final point brings us back to where we began in chapter 1: theory and developing a pragmatic therapeutic position is of vital importance in working with clients.

SUMMARY

Therapists must not only be well-versed in theory and techniques for implementing it, but they must also respond daily to complex professional and ethical issues that directly affect both effective delivery of therapeutic services and public acceptance of these services. The profession as represented by its major associations must insist that its practitioners maintain recognized standards of competence and respected credentials and a high level of ethical practice. Further, research must be an extremely important and necessary part of therapists' professional responsibilities, with the roles of therapist/researcher and consumer of research carrying equal weight in clinical practice.

This chapter offers only a brief overview of these significant professional issues. A greater familiarity with their finer points will surely be called for as beginning therapists evolve into experienced practitioners. The suggested readings that follow can help you explore these issues in greater detail.

SUGGESTED READINGS

Professional Competence

Fretz, B. R., & Mills, D. H. (1980). *Licensing and certification of psychologists and counselors.* San Francisco: Jossey-Bass. Fretz and Mills offer a fine introduction to the organizations, regulations, and laws that govern professional licensing in the field of counseling and psychotherapy. The authors summarize various licensing laws, analyze court cases in which these laws have been challenged, and describe the actions of professional organizations that have affected licensing and certification regulations.

Hart, G. M. (1982). *The process of clinical supervision.* Baltimore: University Press. This book compares and contrasts supervisory models taken from psychology, psychiatry, social work, and education. In doing so it suggests specific conceptual frameworks, procedures for conducting supervision, and guidelines for formulating an applicable approach to one's own setting.

Professional Psychology: Research and practice. Washington, D.C. This journal, published by the American Psychological Association, addresses itself to issues relating to the professional practice and delivery of psychological services in a variety of contexts.

Ethical Issues

Goldberg, C. (1977). *Therapeutic partnership: Ethical concerns in psychotherapy.* New York: Springer. Goldberg offers an ethically enlightened examination of the practice of counseling and psychotherapy based on the importance of a concerted effort between therapist and client in creating a collaborative therapeutic climate.

Rosenbaum, M. (Ed.). (1982). *Ethics and values in psychotherapy: A guidebook.* New York: Free Press. This book provides an in-depth discussion of a wide range of ethical issues that are relevant to the professional practice of counseling and psychotherapy.

Van Hoose, W., & Kottler, J. (1977). *Ethical and legal issues in counseling and psychotherapy.* San Francisco: Jossey-Bass. Van Hoose and Kottler address a variety of ethical, legal, and values issues for the practicing therapist to consider in working with clients.

Research

Annual Review of Psychology. Palo Alto, CA: Annual Reviews. Each year, under varying editorship, this publication summarizes recent research findings in psychology including issues relevant to counseling and psychotherapy, behavior change, personality, and more.

Garfield, S., & Bergmin, A. (Eds.). (1978). *Handbook of psychotherapy and behavior change* (2nd ed). New York: Wiley. This book provides a discussion of a multitude of studies that address human change from individual, group, and community perspectives.

Goldman, L. (Ed.). (1978). *Research methods for counselors.* New York: Wiley. This is a superb resource for the therapist seeking a more practical position with relation to research. Goldman, for his part, frequently takes on an almost "anti" research stance and in doing so suggests a balance for the practitioner between traditional and more pragmatic points of view.

Appendices

APPENDIX A: Code of Ethics of the American Association for Counseling and Development

Section A: General

1. The member influences the development of the profession by continuous efforts to improve professional practices, teaching, services, and research. Professional growth is continuous throughout the member's career and is exemplified by the development of a philosophy that explains why and how a member functions in the helping relationship. Members must gather data on their effectiveness and be guided by the findings.

2. The member has a responsibility both to the individual who is served and to the institution within which the service is performed to maintain high standards of professional conduct. The member strives to maintain the highest levels of professional services offered to the individuals to be served. The member also strives to assist the agency, organization, or institution in providing the highest caliber of professional services. The acceptance of employment in an institution implies that the member is in agreement with the general policies and principles of the institution. Therefore the professional activities of the member are also in accord with the objectives of the institution. If, despite concerted efforts, the member cannot reach agreement with the employer as to acceptable standards of conduct that allow for changes in institutional policy conducive to the positive growth and development of clients, then terminating the affiliation should be seriously considered.

3. Ethical behavior among professional associates, both members and nonmembers, must be expected at all times. When information is possessed that raises doubt as to the ethical behavior of professional colleagues, whether Asso-ciation members or not, the member must take action to attempt to rectify such a condition. Such action shall use the institution's channels first and then use procedures established by the state Branch, Division, or Association.

4. The member neither claims nor implies professional qualifications exceeding those possessed and is responsible for correcting any misrepresentations of these qualifications by others.

5. In establishing fees for professional counseling services, members must consider the financial status of clients and locality. In the event that the established fee structure is inappropriate for a client, assistance must be provided in finding comparable services of acceptable cost.

6. When members provide information to the public or to subordinates, peers or supervisors, they have a responsibility to ensure that the content is general, unidentified client information that is accurate, unbiased, and consists of objective, factual data.

7. With regard to the delivery of professional services, members should accept only those positions for which they are professionally qualified.

8. In the counseling relationship the counselor is aware of the intimacy of the relationship and maintains respect for the client and avoids engaging in activities that seek to meet the counselor's personal needs at the expense of that client. Through awareness of the negative impact of both racial and sexual stereotyping and discrimination, the counselor guards the individual rights and personal dignity of the client in the counseling relationship.

351

Section B: Counseling Relationship

This section refers to practices and procedures of individual and/or group counseling relationships.

The member must recognize the need for client freedom of choice. Under those circumstances where this is not possible, the member must apprise clients of restrictions that may limit their freedom of choice.

1. The member's *primary* obligation is to respect the integrity and promote the welfare of the client(s), whether the client(s) is (are) assisted individually or in a group relationship. In a group setting, the member is also responsible for taking reasonable precautions to protect individuals from physical and/or psychological trauma resulting from interaction within the group.

2. The counseling relationship and information resulting therefrom should be kept confidential, consistent with the obligations of the member as a professional person. In a group counseling setting, the counselor must set a norm of confidentiality regarding all group participants' disclosures.

3. If an individual is already in a counseling relationship with another professional person, the member does not enter into a counseling relationship without first contacting and receiving the approval of that other professional. If the member discovers that the client is in another counseling relationship after the counseling relationship begins, the member must gain the consent of the other professional or terminate the relationship, unless the client elects to terminate the other relationship.

4. When the client's condition indicates that there is clear and imminent danger to the client or others, the member must take reasonable personal action or inform responsible authorities. Consultation with other professionals must be used where possible. The assumption of responsibility for the client(s)' behavior must be taken only after careful deliberation. The client must be involved in the resumption of responsibility as quickly as possible.

5. Records of the counseling relationship, including interview notes, test data, correspondence, tape recordings, and other documents, are to be considered professional information for use in counseling and they should not be considered a part of the records of the institution or agency in which the counselor is employed unless specified by state statute or regulation. Revelation to others of counseling material must occur only upon the expressed consent of the client.

6. Use of data derived from a counseling relationship for purposes of counselor training or research shall be confined to content that can be disguised to ensure full protection of the identity of the subject client.

7. The member must inform the client of the purposes, goals, techniques, rules of procedure and limitations that may affect the relationship at or before the time that the counseling relationship is entered.

8. The member must screen prospective group participants, especially when the emphasis is on self-understanding and growth through self-disclosure. The member must maintain an awareness of the group participants' compatibility throughout the life of the group.

9. The member may choose to consult with any other professionally competent person about a client. In choosing a consultant, the member must avoid placing the consultant in a conflict of interest situation that would preclude the consultant's being a proper party to the member's efforts to help the client.

10. If the member determines an inability to be of professional assistance to the client, the member must either avoid initiating the counseling relationship or immediately terminate that relationship. In either event, the member must suggest appropriate alternatives. (The member must be knowledgeable about referral resources so that a satisfactory referral can be initiated). In the event the client declines the suggested referral, the member is not obligated to continue the relationship.

11. When the member has other relationships, particularly of an administrative, supervisory and/or evaluative nature with an individual seeking counseling services, the member must not serve as the counselor but should refer the individual to another professional. Only in instances where such an alternative is unavailable and where the individual's situation warrants counseling intervention should the member enter into and/or maintain a counseling relationship. Dual relationships with clients that might impair the member's objectivity and professional judgment (e.g., as with close friends or relatives, sexual intimacies with any client) must be avoided and/or the counseling relationship terminated through referral to another competent professional.

12. All experimental methods of treatment must be clearly indicated to prospective recipients and safety precautions are to be adhered to by the member.

13. When the member is engaged in short-term group treatment/training programs (e.g., marathons and other encounter-type or growth groups), the member ensures that there is professional assistance available during and following the group experience.

14. Should the member be engaged in a work setting that calls for any variation from the above statements, the member is obligated to consult with other professionals whenever possible to consider justifiable alternatives.

Section C: Measurement and Evaluation

The primary purpose of educational and psychological testing is to provide descriptive measures that are objective and interpretable in either comparative or absolute terms. The member must recognize the need to interpret the statements that follow as applying to the whole range of appraisal techniques including test and nontest data. Test results constitute only one of a variety of pertinent sources of information for personnel, guidance, and counseling decisions.

1. The member must provide specific orientation or information to the examinee(s) prior to and following the

test administration so that the results of testing may be placed in proper perspective with other relevant factors. In so doing, the member must recognize the effects of socio-economic, ethnic and cultural factors on test scores. It is the member's professional responsibility to use additional unvalidated information carefully in modifying interpretation of the test results.

2. In selecting tests for use in a given situation or with a particular client, the member must consider carefully the specific validity, reliability, and appropriateness of the test(s). *General* validity, reliability and the like may be questioned legally as well as ethically when tests are used for vocational and educational selection, placement, or counseling.

3. When making any statements to the public about tests and testing, the member must give accurate information and avoid false claims or misconceptions. Special efforts are often required to avoid unwarranted connotations of such terms as *IQ* and *grade equivalent scores.*

4. Different tests demand different levels of competence for administration, scoring, and interpretation. Members must recognize the limits of their competence and perform only those functions for which they are prepared.

5. Tests must be administered under the same conditions that were established in their standardization. When tests are not administered under standard conditions or when unusual behavior or irregularities occur during the testing session, those conditions must be noted and the results designated as invalid or of questionable validity. Unsupervised or inadequately supervised test-taking, such as the use of tests through the mails, is considered unethical. On the other hand, the use of instruments that are so designed or standardized to be self-administered and self-scored, such as interest inventories, is to be encouraged.

6. The meaningfulness of test results used in personnel, guidance, and counseling functions generally depends on the examinee's unfamiliarity with the specific items on the test. Any prior coaching or dissemination of the test materials can invalidate test results. Therefore, test security is one of the professional obligations of the member. Conditions that produce most favorable test results must be made known to the examinee.

7. The purpose of testing and the explicit use of the results must be made known to the examinee prior to testing. The counselor must ensure that instrument limitations are not exceeded and that periodic review and/or retesting are made to prevent client stereotyping.

8. The examinee's welfare and explicit prior understanding must be the criteria for determining the recipients of the test results. The member must see that specific interpretation accompanies any release of individual or group test data. The interpretation of test data must be related to the examinee's particular concerns.

9. The member must be cautious when interpreting the results of research instruments possessing insufficient technical data. The specific purposes for the use of such instruments must be stated explicitly to examinees.

10. The member must proceed with caution when attempting to evaluate and interpret the performance of minority group members or other persons who are not represented in the norm group on which the instrument was standardized.

11. The member must guard against the appropriation, reproduction, or modifications of published tests or parts thereof without acknowledgment and permission from the previous publisher.

12. Regarding the preparation, publication and distribution of tests, reference should be made to:

a. *Standards for Educational and Psychological Tests and Manuals,* revised edition, 1974, published by the American Psychological Association on behalf of itself, the American Educational Research Association and the National Council on Measurement in Education.

b. The responsible use of tests: A position paper of AMEG, APGA, and NCME. *Measurement and Evaluation in Guidance,* 1972, 5, 385–388.

c. "Responsibilities of Users of Standardized Tests," APGA, *Guidepost,* October 5, 1978, pp. 5–8.

Section D: Research and Publication

1. Guidelines on research with human subjects shall be adhered to, such as:

a. *Ethical Principles in the Conduct of Research with Human Participants,* Washington, D.C.: American Psychological Association, Inc., 1973.

b. Code of Federal Regulations, Title 45, Subtitle A, Part 46, as currently issued.

2. In planning any research activity dealing with human subjects, the member must be aware of and responsive to all pertinent ethical principles and ensure that the research problem, design, and execution are in full compliance with them.

3. Responsibility for ethical research practice lies with the principal researcher, while others involved in the research activities share ethical obligation and full responsibility for their own actions.

4. In research with human subjects, researchers are responsible for the subjects' welfare throughout the experiment and they must take all reasonable precautions to avoid causing injurious psychological, physical, or social effects on their subjects.

5. All research subjects must be informed of the purpose of the study except when withholding information or providing misinformation to them is essential to the investigation. In such research the member must be responsible for corrective action as soon as possible following completion of the research.

6. Participation in research must be voluntary. Involuntary participation is appropriate only when it can be demonstrated that participation will have no harmful effects on subjects and is essential to the investigation.

7. When reporting research results, explicit mention must be made of all variables and conditions known to the

investigator that might affect the outcome of the investigation or the interpretation of the data.

8. The member must be responsible for conducting and reporting investigations in a manner that minimizes the possibility that results will be misleading.

9. The member has an obligation to make available sufficient original research data to qualified others who may wish to replicate the study.

10. When supplying data, aiding in the research of another person, reporting research results, or in making original data available, due care must be taken to disguise the identity of the subjects in the absence of specific authorization from such subjects to do otherwise.

11. When conducting and reporting research, the member must be familiar with, and give recognition to, previous work on the topic, as well as to observe all copyright laws and follow the principles of giving full credit to all to whom credit is due.

12. The member must give due credit through joint authorship, acknowledgment, footnote statements, or other appropriate means to those who have contributed significantly to the research and/or publication, in accordance with such contributions.

13. The member must communicate to other members the results of any research judged to be of professional or scientific value. Results reflecting unfavorably on institutions, programs, services, or vested interests must not be withheld for such reasons.

14. If members agree to cooperate with another individual in research and/or publications, they incur an obligation to cooperate as promised in terms of punctuality of performance and with full regard to the completeness and accuracy of the information required.

15. Ethical practice requires that authors not submit the same manuscript or one essentially similar in content, for simultaneous publication consideration by two or more journals. In addition, manuscripts published in whole or in substantial part, in another journal or published work should not be submitted for publication without acknowledgment and permission from the previous publication.

Section E: Consulting

Consultation refers to a voluntary relationship between a professional helper and help-needing individual, group or social unit in which the consultant is providing help to the client(s) in defining and solving a work-related problem or potential problem with a client or client system. (This definition is adapted from Kurpius, DeWayne. Consultation theory and process: An integrated model. *Personnel and Guidance Journal,* 1978, 56.

1. The member acting as consultant must have a high degree of self-awareness of his-her own values, knowledge, skills, limitations, and needs in entering a helping relationship that involves human and-or organizational change and that the focus of the relationship be on the issues to be resolved and not on the person(s) presenting the problem.

2. There must be understanding and agreement between member and client for the problem definition, change goals, and predicated consequences of interventions selected.

3. The member must be reasonably certain that she/he or the organization represented has the necessary competencies and resources for giving the kind of help that is needed now or may develop later and that appropriate referral resources are available to the consultant.

4. The consulting relationship must be one in which client adaptability and growth toward self-direction are encouraged and cultivated. The member must maintain this role consistently and not become a decision maker for the client or create a future dependency on the consultant.

5. When announcing consultant availability for services, the member conscientiously adheres to the Association's *Ethical Standards*.

6. The member must refuse a private fee or other remuneration for consultation with persons who are entitled to these services through the member's employing institution or agency. The policies of a particular agency may make explicit provisions for private practice with agency clients by members of its staff. In such instances, the clients must be apprised of other options open to them should they seek private counseling services.

Section F: Private Practice

1. The member should assist the profession by facilitating the availability of counseling services in private as well as public settings.

2. In advertising services as a private practitioner, the member must advertise the services in such a manner so as to accurately inform the public as to services, expertise, profession, and techniques of counseling in a professional manner. A member who assumes an executive leadership role in the organization shall not permit his/her name to be used in professional notices during periods when not actively engaged in the private practice of counseling.

The member may list the following: highest relevant degree, type and level of certification or license, type and/or description of services, and other relevant information. Such information must not contain false, inaccurate, misleading, partial, out-of-context, or deceptive material or statements.

3. Members may join in partnership/corporation with other members and-or other professionals provided that each member of the partnership or corporation makes clear the separate specialties by name in compliance with the regulations of the locality.

4. A member has an obligation to withdraw from a counseling relationship if it is believed that employment will result in violation of the *Ethical Standards*. If the mental or physical condition of the member renders it difficult to carry out an effective professional relationship or if the

member is discharged by the client because the counseling relationship is no longer productive for the client, then the member is obligated to terminate the counseling relationship.

5. A member must adhere to the regulations for private practice of the locality where the services are offered.

6. It is unethical to use one's institutional affiliation to recruit clients for one's private practice.

Section G: Personnel Administration

It is recognized that most members are employed in public or quasi-public institutions. The functioning of a member within an institution must contribute to the goals of the institution and vice versa if either is to accomplish their respective goals or objectives. It is therefore essential that the member and the institution function in ways to (a) make the institution's goals explicit and public; (b) make the member's contribution to institutional goals specific; and (c) foster mutual accountability for goal achievement.

To accomplish these objectives, it is recognized that the member and the employer must share responsibilities in the formulation and implementation of personnel policies.

1. Members must define and describe the parameters and levels of their professional competency.

2. Members must establish interpersonal relations and working agreements with supervisors and subordinates regarding counseling or clinical relationships, confidentiality, distinction between public and private material, maintenance, and dissemination of recorded information, work load and accountability. Working agreements in each instance must be specified and made known to those concerned.

3. Members must alert their employers to conditions that may be potentially disruptive or damaging.

4. Members must inform employers of conditions that may limit their effectiveness.

5. Members must submit regularly to professional review and evaluation.

6. Members must be responsible for inservice development of self and-or staff.

7. Members must inform their staff of goals and programs.

8. Members must provide personnel practices that guarantee and enhance the rights and welfare of each recipient of their service.

9. Members must select competent persons and assign responsibilities compatible with their skills and experiences.

Section H: Preparation Standards

Members who are responsible for training others must be guided by the preparation standards of the Association and relevant Division(s). The member who functions in the capacity of trainer assumes unique ethical responsibilities that frequently go beyond that of the member who does not function in a training capacity. These ethical responsibilities are outlined as follows:

1. Members must orient students to program expectations, basic skills development, and employment prospects prior to admission to the program.

2. Members in charge of learning experiences must establish programs that integrate academic study and supervised practice.

3. Members must establish a program directed toward developing students' skills, knowledge, and self-understanding, stated whenever possible in competency or performance terms.

4. Members must identify the levels of competencies of their students in compliance with relevant Division standards. These competencies must accommodate the para-professional as well as the professional.

5. Members, through continual student evaluation and appraisal, must be aware of the personal limitations of the learner that might impede future performance. The instructor must not only assist the learner in securing remedial assistance but also screen from the program those individuals who are unable to provide competent services.

6. Members must provide a program that includes training in research commensurate with levels of role functioning. Para-professional and technician-level personnel must be trained as consumers of research. In addition, these personnel must learn how to evaluate their own and their program's effectiveness. Graduate training, especially at the doctoral level, would include preparation for original research by the member.

7. Members must make students aware of the ethical responsibilities and standards of the profession.

8. Preparatory programs must encourage students to value the ideals of service to individuals and to society. In this regard, direct financial remuneration or lack thereof must not influence the quality of service rendered. Monetary considerations must not be allowed to overshadow professional and humanitarian needs.

9. Members responsible for educational programs must be skilled as teachers and practitioners.

10. Members must present thoroughly varied theoretical positions so that students may make comparisons and have the opportunity to select a position.

11. Members must develop clear policies within their educational institutions regarding field placement and the roles of the student and the instructor in such placements.

12. Members must ensure that forms of learning focusing on self-understanding or growth are voluntary, or if required as part of the education program, are made known to prospective students prior to entering the program. When the education program offers a growth experience with an emphasis on self-disclosure or other relatively intimate or personal involvement, the member must have no administrative, supervisory, or evaluating authority regarding the participant.

13. Members must conduct an educational program in keeping with the current relevant guidelines of the Association and its Divisions.

APPENDIX B: Code of Ethics of the American Psychological Association

Principle 1: Responsibility

In providing services, psychologists maintain the highest standards of their profession. They accept responsibility for the consequences of their acts and make every effort to ensure that their services are used appropriately.

a. As scientists, psychologists accept responsibility for the selection of their research topics and the methods used in investigation, analysis, and reporting. They plan their research in ways to minimize the possibility that their findings will be misleading. They provide thorough discussion of the limitations of their data, especially where their work touches on social policy or might be construed to the detriment of persons in specific age, sex, ethnic, socioeconomic, or other social groups. In publishing reports of their work, they never suppress disconfirming data, and they acknowledge the existence of alternative hypotheses and explanations of their findings. Psychologists take credit only for work they have actually done.

b. Psychologists clarify in advance with all appropriate persons and agencies the expectations for sharing and utilizing research data. They avoid relationships that may limit their objectivity or create a conflict of interest. Interference with the milieu in which data are collected is kept to a minimum.

c. Psychologists have the responsibility to attempt to prevent distortion, misuse, or suppression of psychological findings by the institution or agency of which they are employees.

d. As members of governmental or other organizational bodies, psychologists remain accountable as individuals to the highest standards of their profession.

e. As teachers, psychologists recognize their primary obligation to help others acquire knowledge and skill. They maintain high standards of scholarship by presenting psychological information objectively, fully, and accurately.

f. As practitioners, psychologists know that they bear a heavy social responsibility because their recommendations and professional actions may alter the lives of others. They are alert to personal, social, organizational, financial, or political situations and pressures that might lead to misuse of their influence.

Principle 2: Competence

The maintenance of high standards of competence is a responsibility shared by all psychologists in the interest of the public and the profession as a whole. Psychologists recognize the boundaries of their competence and the limitations of their techniques. They only provide services and only use techniques for which they are qualified by training and experience. In those areas in which recognized standards do not yet exist, psychologists take whatever precautions are necessary to protect the welfare of their clients.

They maintain knowledge of current scientific and professional information related to the services they render.

a. Psychologists accurately represent their competence, education, training, and experience. They claim as evidence of educational qualifications only those degrees obtained from institutions acceptable under the Bylaws and Rules of Council of the American Psychological Association.

b. As teachers, psychologists perform their duties on the basis of careful preparation so that their instruction is accurate, current, and scholarly.

c. Psychologists recognize the need for continuing education and are open to new procedures and changes in expectations and values over time.

d. Psychologists recognize differences among people, such as those that may be associated with age, sex, socioeconomic, and ethnic backgrounds. When necessary, they obtain training, experience, or counsel to assure competent service or research relating to such persons.

e. Psychologists responsible for decisions involving individuals or policies based on test results have an understanding of psychological or educational measurement, validation problems, and test research.

f. Psychologists recognize that personal problems and conflicts may interfere with professional effectiveness. Accordingly, they refrain from undertaking any activity in which their personal problems are likely to lead to inadequate performance or harm to a client, colleague, student, or research participant. If engaged in such activity when they become aware of their personal problems they seek competent professional assistance to determine whether they should suspend, terminate, or limit the scope of their professional and/or scientific activities.

Principle 3: Moral and Legal Standards

Psychologists' moral and ethical standards of behavior are a personal matter to the same degree as they are for any other citizen, except as these may compromise the fulfillment of their professional responsibilities or reduce the public trust in psychology and psychologists. Regarding their own behavior, psychologists are sensitive to prevailing community standards and to the possible impact that conformity to or deviation from these standards may have upon the quality of their performance as psychologists. Psychologists are also aware of the possible impact of their public behavior upon the ability of colleagues to perform their professional duties.

a. As teachers, psychologists are aware of the fact that their personal values may affect the selection and presentation of instructional materials. When dealing with topics that may give offense, they recognize and respect the diverse attitudes that students may have toward such materials.

b. As employees or employers, psychologists do not engage in or condone practices that are inhumane or that result in illegal or unjustifiable actions. Such practices include, but are not limited to, those based on considerations of race, handicap, age, gender, sexual preference, religion, or national origin in hiring, promotion, or training.

c. In their professional roles, psychologists avoid any action that will violate or diminish the legal and civil rights of clients or of others who may be affected by their actions.

d. As practitioners and researchers, psychologists act in accord with Association standards and guidelines related to practice and to the conduct of research with human beings and animals. In the ordinary course of events, psychologists adhere to relevant governmental laws and institutional regulations. When federal, state, provincial, organizational, or institutional laws, regulations, or practices are in conflict with Association standards and guidelines, psychologists make known their commitment to Association standards and guidelines and, wherever possible, work toward a resolution of the conflict. Both practitioners and researchers are concerned with the development of such legal and quasi-legal regulations as best serve the public interest, and they work toward changing existing regulations that are not beneficial to the public interest.

Principle 4: Public Statements

Public statements, announcements of services, advertising, and promotional activities of psychologists serve the purpose of helping the public make informed judgments and choices. Psychologists represent accurately and objectively their professional qualifications, affiliations, and functions, as well as those of the institutions or organizations with which they or the statements may be associated. In public statements providing psychological information or professional opinions or providing information about the availability of psychological products, publications, and services, psychologists base their statements on scientifically acceptable psychological findings and techniques with full recognition of the limits and uncertainties of such evidence.

a. When announcing or advertising professional services, psychologists may list the following information to describe the provider and services provided: name, highest relevant academic degree earned from a regionally accredited institution, date, type, and level of certification or licensure, diplomate status, APA membership status, address, telephone number, office hours, a brief listing of the type of psychological services offered, an appropriate presentation of fee information, foreign languages spoken, and policy with regard to third-party payments. Additional relevant or important consumer information may be included if not prohibited by other sections of these Ethical Principles.

b. In announcing or advertising the availability of psychological products, publications, or services, psychologists do not present their affiliation with any organization in a manner that falsely implies sponsorship or certification by that organization. In particular and for example, psychologists do not state APA membership or fellow status in a way to suggest that such status implies specialized professional competence or qualifications. Public statements include, but are not limited to, communication by means of

periodical, book, list, directory, television, radio, or motion picture. They do not contain (i) a false, fraudulent, misleading, deceptive, or unfair statement; (ii) a misinterpretation of fact or a statement likely to mislead or deceive because in context it makes only a partial disclosure of relevant facts; (iii) a testimonial from a patient regarding the quality of a psychologist's services or products; (iv) a statement intended or likely to create false or unjustified expectations of favorable results; (v) a statement implying unusual, unique, or one-of-a-kind abilities; (vi) a statement intended or likely to appeal to a client's fears, anxieties, or emotions concerning the possible results of failure to obtain the offered services; (vii) a statement concerning the comparative desirability of offered services; (viii) a statement of direct solicitation of individual clients.

c. Psychologists do not compensate or give anything of value to a representative of the press, radio, television, or other communication medium in anticipation of or in return for professional publicity in a news item. A paid advertisement must be identified as such, unless it is apparent from the context that it is a paid advertisement. If communicated to the public by use of radio or television, an advertisement is prerecorded and approved for broadcast by the psychologist, and a recording of the actual transmission is retained by the psychologist.

d. Announcements or advertisements of "personal growth groups," clinics, and agencies give a clear statement of purpose and a clear description of the experiences to be provided. The education, training, and experience of the staff members are appropriately specified.

e. Psychologists associated with the development or promotion of psychological devices, books, or other products offered for commercial sale make reasonable efforts to ensure that announcements and advertisements are presented in a professional, scientifically acceptable, and factually informative manner.

f. Psychologists do not participate for personal gain in commercial announcements or advertisements recommending to the public the purchase or use of proprietary or single-source products or services when that participation is based solely upon their identification as psychologists.

g. Psychologists present the science of psychology and offer their services, products, and publications fairly and accurately, avoiding misrepresentation through sensationalism, exaggeration, or superficiality. Psychologists are guided by the primary obligation to aid the public in developing informed judgments, opinions, and choices.

h. As teachers, psychologists ensure that statements in catalogs and course outlines are accurate and not misleading, particularly in terms of subject matter to be covered, bases for evaluating progress, and the nature of course experiences. Announcements, brochures, or advertisements describing workshops, seminars, or other educational programs accurately describe the audience for which the program is intended as well as eligibility requirements, educational objectives, and nature of the materials to be covered. These announcements also accurately represent the education, training, and experience of the psychologists presenting the programs and any fees involved.

i. Public announcements or advertisements soliciting research participants in which clinical services or other professional services are offered as an inducement make clear the nature of the services as well as the costs and other obligations to be accepted by participants in the research.

j. A psychologist accepts the obligation to correct others who represent the psychologist's professional qualifications, or associations with products or services, in a manner incompatible with these guidelines.

k. Individual diagnostic and therapeutic services are provided only in the context of a professional psychological relationship. When personal advice is given by means of public lectures or demonstrations, newspaper or magazine articles, radio or television programs, mail, or similar media, the psychologist utilizes the most current relevant data and exercises the highest level of professional judgment.

l. Products that are described or presented by means of public lectures or demonstrations, newspaper or magazine articles, radio or television programs, or similar media meet the same recognized standards as exist for products used in the context of a professional relationship.

Principle 5: Confidentiality

Psychologists have a primary obligation to respect the confidentiality of information obtained from persons in the course of their work as psychologists. They reveal such information to others only with the consent of the person or the person's legal representative, except in those unusual circumstances in which not to do so would result in clear danger to the person or to others. Where appropriate, psychologists inform their clients of the legal limits of confidentiality.

a. Information obtained in clinical or consulting relationships, or evaluative data concerning children, students, employees, and others, is discussed only for professional purposes and only with persons clearly concerned with the case. Written and oral reports present only data germane to the purposes of the evaluation, and every effort is made to avoid undue invasion of privacy.

b. Psychologists who present personal information obtained during the course of professional work in writings, lectures, or other public forums either obtain adequate prior consent to do so or adequately disguise all identifying information.

c. Psychologists make provisions for maintaining confidentiality in the storage and disposal of records.

d. When working with minors or other persons who are unable to give voluntary, informed consent, psychologists take special care to protect these persons' best interests.

Principle 6: Welfare of the Consumer

Psychologists respect the integrity and protect the welfare of the people and groups with whom they work. When

conflicts of interest arise between clients and psychologists' employing institutions, psychologists clarify the nature and direction of their loyalties and responsibilities and keep all parties informed of their commitments. Psychologists fully inform consumers as to the purpose and nature of an evaluative, treatment, educational, or training procedure, and they freely acknowledge that clients, students, or participants in research have freedom of choice with regard to participation.

a. Psychologists are continually cognizant of their own needs and of their potentially influential position vis-à-vis persons such as clients, students, and subordinates. They avoid exploiting the trust and dependency of such persons. Psychologists make every effort to avoid dual relationships that could impair their professional judgment or increase the risk of exploitation. Examples of such dual relationships include, but are not limited to, research with and treatment of employees, students, supervisees, close friends, or relatives. Sexual intimacies with clients are unethical.

b. When a psychologist agrees to provide services to a client at the request of a third party, the psychologist assumes the responsibility of clarifying the nature of the relationships to all parties concerned.

c. Where the demands of an organization require psychologists to violate these Ethical Principles, psychologists clarify the nature of the conflict between the demands and these principles. They inform all parties of psychologists' ethical responsibilities and take appropriate action.

d. Psychologists make advance financial arrangements that safeguard the best interests of and are clearly understood by their clients. They neither give nor receive any remuneration for referring clients for professional services. They contribute a portion of their services to work for which they receive little or no financial return.

e. Psychologists terminate a clinical or consulting relationship when it is reasonably clear that the consumer is not benefiting from it. They offer to help the consumer locate alternative sources of assistance.

Principle 7: Professional Relationships

Psychologists act with due regard for the needs, special competencies, and obligations of their colleagues in psychology and other professions. They respect the prerogatives and obligations of the institutions or organizations with which these other colleagues are associated.

a. Psychologists understand the areas of competence of related professions. They make full use of all the professional, technical, and administrative resources that serve the best interests of consumers. The absence of formal relationships with other professional workers does not relieve psychologists of the responsibility of securing for their clients the best possible professional service, nor does it relieve them of the obligation to exercise foresight, diligence, and tact in obtaining the complementary or alternative assistance needed by clients.

b. Psychologists know and take into account the traditions and practices of other professional groups with whom they work and cooperate fully with such groups. If a person is receiving similar services from another professional, psychologists do not offer their own services directly to such a person. If a psychologist is contacted by a person who is already receiving similar services from another professional, the psychologist carefully considers that professional relationship and proceeds with caution and sensitivity to the therapeutic issues as well as the client's welfare. The psychologist discusses these issues with the client so as to minimize the risk of confusion and conflict.

c. Psychologists who employ or supervise other professionals or professionals in training accept the obligation to facilitate the further professional development of these individuals. They provide appropriate working conditions, timely evaluations, constructive consultation, and experience opportunities.

d. Psychologists do not exploit their professional relationships with clients, supervisees, students, employees, or research participants sexually or otherwise. Psychologists do not condone or engage in sexual harassment. Sexual harassment is defined as deliberate or repeated comments, gestures, or physical contacts of a sexual nature that are unwanted by the recipient.

e. In conducting research in institutions or organizations, psychologists secure appropriate authorization to conduct such research. They are aware of their obligations to future research workers and ensure that host institutions receive adequate information about the research and proper acknowledgment of their contributions.

f. Publication credit is assigned to those who have contributed to a publication in proportion to their professional contributions. Major contributions of a professional character made by several persons to a common project are recognized by joint authorship, with the individual who made the principal contribution listed first. Minor contributions of a professional character and extensive clerical or similar nonprofessional assistance may be acknowledged in footnotes or in an introductory statement. Acknowledgment through specific citations is made for unpublished as well as published material that has directly influenced the research or writing. Psychologists who compile and edit material of others for publication publish the material in the name of the originating group, if appropriate, with their own name appearing as chairperson or editor. All contributors are to be acknowledged and named.

g. When psychologists know of an ethical violation by another psychologist, and it seems appropriate, they informally attempt to resolve the issue by bringing the behavior to the attention of the psychologist. If the misconduct is of a minor nature and/or appears to be due to lack of sensitivity, knowledge, or experience, such an informal solution is usually appropriate. Such informal corrective efforts are made with sensitivity to any rights to confidentiality involved. If the violation does not seem amenable to an informal solution, or is of a more serious nature, psychologists bring it to the attention of the appropriate local, state, and/or national committee on professional ethics and conduct.

Principle 8: Assessment Techniques

In the development, publication, and utilization of psychological assessment techniques, psychologists make every effort to promote the welfare and best interests of the client. They guard against the misuse of assessment results. They respect the client's right to know the results, the interpretations made, and the bases for their conclusions and recommendations. Psychologists make every effort to maintain the security of tests and other assessment techniques within limits of legal mandates. They strive to ensure the appropriate use of assessment techniques by others.

a. In using assessment techniques, psychologists respect the right of clients to have full explanations of the nature and purpose of the techniques in language the clients can understand, unless an explicit exception to this right has been agreed upon in advance. When the explanations are to be provided by others, psychologists establish procedures for ensuring the adequacy of these explanations.

b. Psychologists responsible for the development and standardization of psychological tests and other assessment techniques utilize established scientific procedures and observe the relevant APA standards.

c. In reporting assessment results, psychologists indicate any reservations that exist regarding validity or reliability because of the circumstances of the assessment or the inappropriateness of the norms for the person tested. Psychologists strive to ensure that the results of assessments and their interpretations are not misused by others.

d. Psychologists recognize that assessment results may become obsolete. They make every effort to avoid and prevent the misuse of obsolete measures.

e. Psychologists offering scoring and interpretation services are able to produce appropriate evidence for the validity of the programs and procedures used in arriving at interpretations. The public offering of an automated interpretation service is considered a professional-to-professional consultation. Psychologists make every effort to avoid misuse of assessment reports.

f. Psychologists do not encourage or promote the use of psychological assessment techniques by inappropriately trained or otherwise unqualified persons through teaching, sponsorship, or supervision.

Principle 9: Research with Human Participants

The decision to undertake research rests upon a considered judgment by the individual psychologist about how best to contribute to psychological science and human welfare. Having made the decision to conduct research, the psychologist considers alternative directions in which research energies and resources might be invested. On the basis of this consideration, the psychologist carries out the investigation with respect and concern for the dignity and welfare of the people who participate and with cognizance of federal and state regulations and professional standards governing the conduct of research with human participants.

a. In planning a study, the investigator has the responsibility to make a careful evaluation of its ethical acceptability. To the extent that the weighing of scientific and human values suggests a compromise of any principle, the investigator incurs a correspondingly serious obligation to seek ethical advice and to observe stringent safeguards to protect the rights of human participants.

b. Considering whether a participant in a planned study will be a "subject at risk" or a "subject at minimal risk," according to recognized standards, is of primary ethical concern to the investigator.

c. The investigator always retains the responsibility for ensuring ethical practice in research. The investigator is also responsible for the ethical treatment of research participants by collaborators, assistants, students, and employees, all of whom, however, incur similar obligations.

d. Except in minimal-risk research, the investigator establishes a clear and fair agreement with research participants, prior to their participation, that clarifies the obligations and responsibilities of each. The investigator has the obligation to honor all promises and commitments included in that agreement. The investigator informs the participants of all aspects of the research that might reasonably be expected to influence willingness to participate and explains all other aspects of the research about which the participants inquire. Failure to make full disclosure prior to obtaining informed consent requires additional safeguards to protect the welfare and dignity of the research participants. Research with children or with participants who have impairments that would limit understanding and/or communication requires special safeguarding procedures.

e. Methodological requirements of a study may make the use of concealment or deception necessary. Before conducting such a study, the investigator has a special responsibility to (i) determine whether the use of such techniques is justified by the study's prospective scientific, educational, or applied value; (ii) determine whether alternative procedures are available that do not use concealment or deception; and (iii) ensure that the participants are provided with sufficient explanation as soon as possible.

f. The investigator respects the individual's freedom to decline to participate in or to withdraw from the research at any time. The obligation to protect this freedom requires careful thought and consideration when the investigator is in a position of authority or influence over the participant. Such positions of authority include, but are not limited to, situations in which research participation is required as part of employment or in which the participant is a student, client, or employee of the investigator.

g. The investigator protects the participant from physical and mental discomfort, harm, and danger that may arise from research procedures. If risks of such consequences exist, the investigator informs the participant of that fact. Research procedures likely to cause serious or lasting harm to a participant are not used unless the failure to use these procedures might expose the participant to risk of greater harm, or unless the research has great potential benefit and fully informed and voluntary consent is obtained from each participant. The participant should be informed of procedures for contacting the investigator within a reasonable time period following participation should stress, potential harm, or related questions or concerns arise.

h. After the data are collected, the investigator provides the participant with information about the nature of the study and attempts to remove any misconceptions that may have arisen. Where scientific or humane values justify delaying or withholding this information, the investigator incurs a special responsibility to monitor the research and to ensure that there are no damaging consequences for the participant.

i. Where research procedures result in undesirable consequences for the individual participant, the investigator has the responsibility to detect and remove or correct these consequences, including long-term effects.

j. Information obtained about a research participant during the course of an investigation is confidential unless otherwise agreed upon in advance. When the possibility exists that others may obtain access to such information, this possibility, together with the plans for protecting confidentiality, is explained to the participant as part of the procedure for obtaining informed consent.

Principle 10: Care and Use of Animals

An investigator of animal behavior strives to advance understanding of basic behavioral principles and/or to contribute to the improvement of human health and welfare. In seeking these ends, the investigator ensures the welfare of animals and treats them humanely. Laws and regulations notwithstanding, an animal's immediate protection depends upon the scientist's own conscience.

a. The acquisition, care, use, and disposal of all animals are in compliance with current federal, state or provincial, and local laws and regulations.

b. A psychologist trained in research methods and experienced in the care of laboratory animals closely supervises all procedures involving animals and is responsible for ensuring appropriate consideration of their comfort, health, and humane treatment.

c. Psychologists ensure that all individuals using animals under their supervision have received explicit instruction in experimental methods and in the care, maintenance, and handling of the species being used. Responsibilities and activities of individuals participating in a research project are consistent with their respective competencies.

d. Psychologists make every effort to minimize discomfort, illness, and pain of animals. A procedure subjecting animals to pain, stress, or privation is used only when an alternative procedure is unavailable and the goal is justified by its prospective scientific, educational, or applied value. Surgical procedures are performed under appropriate anesthesia; techniques to avoid infection and minimize pain are followed during and after surgery.

e. When it is appropriate that the animal's life be terminated, it is done rapidly and painlessly.

APPENDIX C: Code of Ethics of the National Association of Social Workers

I. The Social Worker's Conduct and Comportment as a Social Worker

A. Propriety—The social worker should maintain high standards of personal conduct in the capacity or identity as social worker.

1. The private conduct of the social worker is a personal matter to the same degree as is any other person's, except when such conduct compromises the fulfillment of professional responsibilities.

2. The social worker should not participate in, condone, or be associated with dishonesty, fraud, deceit, or misrepresentation.

3. The social worker should distinguish clearly between statements and actions made as a private individual and as a representative of the social work profession or an organization or group.

B. Competence and Professional Development—The social worker should strive to become and remain proficient in professional practice and the performance of professional functions.

1. The social worker should accept responsibility or employment only on the basis of existing competence or the intention to acquire the necessary competence.

2. The social worker should not misrepresent professional qualifications, education, experience, or affiliations.

C. Service—The social worker should regard as primary the service obligation of the social work profession.

1. The social worker should retain ultimate responsibility for the quality and extent of the service that individual assumes, assigns, or performs.

2. The social worker should act to prevent practices that are inhumane or discriminatory against any person or group of persons.

D. Integrity—The social worker should act in accordance with the highest standards of professional integrity and impartiality.

1. The social worker should be alert to and resist the influences and pressures that interfere with the exercise of professional discretion and impartial judgment required for the performance of professional functions.

2. The social worker should not exploit professional relationships for personal gain.

E. Scholarship and Research—The social worker engaged in study and research should be guided by the conventions of scholarly inquiry.

1. The social worker engaged in research should consider carefully its possible consequences for human beings.

2. The social worker engaged in research should ascertain that the consent of participants in the research is voluntary and informed, without any implied deprivation or penalty for refusal to participate, and with due regard for participants' privacy and dignity.

3. The social worker engaged in research should protect participants from unwarranted physical or mental discomfort, distress, harm, danger, or deprivation.

4. The social worker who engages in the evaluation of services or cases should discuss them only for the professional purposes and only with persons directly and professionally concerned with them.

5. Information obtained about participants in research should be treated as confidential.

6. The social worker should take credit only for work actually done in connection with scholarly and research endeavors and credit contributions made by others.

II. The Social Worker's Ethical Responsibility to Clients

F. Primacy of Clients' Interests—The social worker's primary responsibility is to clients.

1. The social worker should serve clients with devotion, loyalty, determination, and the maximum application of professional skill and competence.

2. The social worker should not exploit relationships with clients for personal advantage, or solicit the clients of one's agency for private practice.

3. The social worker should not practice, condone, facilitate or collaborate with any form of discrimination on the basis of race, color, sex, sexual orientation, age, religion, national origin, marital status, political belief, mental or physical handicap, or any other preference or personal characteristic, condition or status.

4. The social worker should avoid relationships or commitments that conflict with the interests of clients.

5. The social worker should under no circumstances engage in sexual activities with clients.

6. The social worker should provide clients with accurate and complete information regarding the extent and nature of the services available to them.

7. The social worker should apprise clients of their risks, rights, opportunities, and obligations associated with social service to them.

8. The social worker should seek advice and counsel of colleagues and supervisors whenever such consultation is in the best interest of clients.

9. The social worker should terminate service to clients, and professional relationships with them, when such service and relationships are no longer required or no longer serve the clients' needs or interests.

10. The social worker should withdraw services precipitously only under unusual circumstances, giving careful consideration to all factors in the situation and taking care, to minimize possible adverse effects.

11. The social worker who anticipates the termination or interruption of service to clients should notify clients promptly and seek the transfer, referral, or continuation of service in relation to the clients' needs and preferences.

G. Rights and Prerogatives of Clients—The social worker should make every effort to foster maximum self-determination on the part of clients.

1. When the social worker must act on behalf of a client who has been adjudged legally incompetent, the social worker should safeguard the interests and rights of that client.

2. When another individual has been legally authorized to act in behalf of a client, the social worker should deal with that person always with the client's best interest in mind.

3. The social worker should not engage in any action that violates or diminishes the civil or legal rights of clients.

H. Confidentiality and Privacy—The social worker should respect the privacy of clients and hold in confidence all information obtained in the course of professional service.

1. The social worker should share with others confidences revealed by clients, without their consent, only for compelling professional reasons.

2. The social worker should inform clients fully about the limits of confidentiality in a given situation, the purposes for which information is obtained, and how it may be used.

3. The social worker should afford clients reasonable access to any official social work records concerning them.

4. When providing clients with access to records, the social worker should take due care to protect the confidences of others contained in those records.

5. The social worker should obtain informed consent of clients before taping, recording, or permitting third party observation of their activities.

I. Fees—When setting fees, the social worker should ensure that they are fair, reasonable, considerate, and commensurate with the service performed and with due regard for the clients' ability to pay.

1. The social worker should not divide a fee or accept or give anything of value for receiving or making a referral.

ation for the interest, character, and reputation of that colleague.

6. The social worker should not exploit a dispute between a colleague and employers to obtain a position or otherwise advance the social worker's interest.

7. The social worker should seek arbitration or mediation when conflicts with colleagues require resolution for compelling professional reasons.

8. The social worker should extend to colleagues of other professions the same respect and cooperation that is extended to social work colleagues.

9. The social worker who serves as an employer, supervisor, or mentor to colleagues should make orderly and explicit arrangements regarding the conditions of their continuing professional relationship.

10. The social worker who has the responsibility for employing and evaluating the performance of other staff members, should fulfill such responsibility in a fair, considerate, and equitable manner, on the basis of clearly enunciated criteria.

11. The social worker who has the responsibility for evaluating the performance of employees, supervisees, or students should share evaluations with them.

K. Dealing with Colleagues' Clients—The social worker has the responsibility to relate to the clients of colleagues with full professional consideration.

1. The social worker should not solicit the clients of colleagues.

2. The social worker should not assume professional responsibility for the clients of another agency or a colleague without appropriate communication with that agency or colleague.

3. The social worker who serves the clients of colleagues, during a temporary absence or emergency, should serve those clients with the same consideration as that afforded any client.

III. The Social Worker's Ethical Responsibility to Colleagues

J. Respect, Fairness, and Courtesy– The social worker should treat colleagues with respect courtesy, fairness, and good faith.

1. The social worker should cooperate with colleagues to promote professional interests and concerns.

2. The social worker should respect confidences shared by colleagues in the course of their professional relationships and transactions.

3. The social worker should create and maintain conditions of practice that facilitate ethical and competent professional performance by colleagues.

4. The social worker should treat with respect, and represent accurately and fairly, the qualifications, views, and findings of colleagues and use appropriate channels to express judgments on these matters.

5. The social worker who replaces or is replaced by a colleague in professional practice should act with consider-

IV. The Social Worker's Ethical Responsibility to Employers and Employing Organizations

L. Commitments to Employing Organization—The social worker should adhere to commitments made to the employing organization.

1. The social worker should work to improve the employing agency's policies and procedures, and the efficiency and effectiveness of its services.

2. The social worker should not accept employment or arrange student field placements in an organization which is currently under public sanction by NASW for violating personnel standards, or imposing limitations on or penalties for professional actions on behalf of clients.

3. The social worker should act to prevent and eliminate discrimination in the employing organization's work assignments and in its employment policies and practices.

4. The social worker should use with scrupulous regard, and only for the purpose for which they are intended, the resources of the employing organization.

V. The Social Worker's Ethical Responsibility to the Social Work Profession

M. Maintaining the Integrity of the Profession—The social worker should uphold and advance the values, ethics, knowledge, and mission of the profession.

1. The social worker should protect and enhance the dignity and integrity of the profession and should be responsible and vigorous in discussion and criticism of the profession.

2. The social worker should take action through appropriate channels against unethical conduct by any other member of the profession.

3. The social worker should act to prevent the unauthorized and unqualified practice of social work.

4. The social worker should make no misrepresentation in advertising as to qualifications, competence, service, or results to be achieved.

N. Community Service—The social worker should assist the profession in making social services available to the general public.

1. The social worker should contribute time and professional expertise to activities that promote respect for the utility, the integrity, and the competence of the social work profession.

2. The social worker should support the formulation, development, enactment and implementation of social policies of concern to the profession.

O. Development of Knowledge—The social worker should take responsibility for identifying, developing, and fully utilizing knowledge for professional practice.

1. The social worker should base practice upon recognized knowledge relevant to social work.

2. The social worker should critically examine, and keep current with emerging knowledge relevant to social work.

3. The social worker should contribute to the knowledge base of social work and share research knowledge and practice wisdom with colleagues.

VI. The Social Worker's Ethical Responsibility to Society

P. Promoting the General Welfare—The social worker should promote the general welfare of society.

1. The social worker should act to prevent and eliminate discrimination against any person or group on the basis of race, color, sex, sexual orientation, age, religion, national origin, marital status, political belief, mental or physical handicap, or any other preference or personal characteristic, condition, or status.

2. The social worker should act to ensure that all persons have access to the resources, services, and opportunities which they require.

3. The social worker should act to expand choice and opportunity for all persons, with special regard for disadvantaged or oppressed groups and persons.

4. The social worker should promote conditions that encourage respect for the diversity of cultures which constitute American society.

5. The social worker should provide appropriate professional services in public emergencies.

6. The social worker should advocate changes in policy and legislation to improve social conditions and to promote social justice.

7. The social worker should encourage informed participation by the public in shaping social policies and institutions.

References

American Association for Counseling and Development (formerly American Personnel and Guidance Association). (1981). *Ethical standards* (Rev. ed.). Alexandria, VA: Author.

American Psychological Association. (1981). *Ethical principles of psychologists* (Rev. ed.). Washington, D.C.: Author.

Arbuckle, D. (1975). *Counseling and psychotherapy: An existential-humanistic view* (3rd ed.). Boston: Houghton Mifflin.

Ary, D., Jacobs, L. C., & Razavich, A. (1979). *Introduction to research in education* (2nd ed.). New York: Holt, Rinehart and Winston.

Atkinson, D. R., & Carskadden, G. (1975). A prestigious introduction, psychological jargon, and perceived counselor credibility. *Journal of Counseling Psychology, 22,* 180–186.

Atkinson, D. R., Maruyama, M., & Matsui, S. (1978). Effects of counselor race and counseling approach on Asian Americans' perceptions of counselor credibility and utility. *Journal of Counseling Psychology, 25,* 76–83.

Aubrey, R. F. (1967). Misapplication of therapy models to school counseling. *Personnel and Guidance Journal, 48,* 273–278.

Bandura, A. (1969). *Principles of behavior modification.* New York: Holt, Rinehart and Winston.

Bandura, A. (1971). Psychotherapy based upon modeling principles. In A. E. Bergin & S. L. Garfield (Eds.), *Handbook of psychotherapy and behavior change.* New York: Wiley.

Bandura, A. (1976). Effecting change through participant modeling. In J. D. Krumboltz & C. E. Thoresen (Eds.), *Counseling Methods* (pp. 248–265). New York: Holt, Rinehart and Winston.

Bandura, A. (1977). *Social learning theory.* Englewood Cliffs, NJ: Prentice-Hall.

Bandura, A. & Adams, N. E. (1977). Analysis of self-efficacy theory of behavioral change. *Cognitive Therapy and Research, 1,* 287–310.

Bandura, A., Adams, N. E., & Beyer, J. (1977). Cognitive processes mediating behavioral change. *Journal of Personality and Social Psychology, 35,* 125–139.

Barak, A., & LaCrosse, M. B. (1975). Multidimensional perception of counselor behavior. *Journal of Counseling Psychology, 24,* 288–292.

Barnhart, C. (1950). *American college dictionary.* New York: Harper & Row.

Beck, A. T. (1963). Thinking and depression: I. Idiosyncratic content and cognitive distortions. *Archives of General Psychiatry, 9,* 324–333.

Beck, A. T. (1964). Thinking and depression: II. Theory and therapy. *Archives of General Psychiatry, 10,* 561–571.

Beck, A. T. (1967). Depression: Clinical, experimental, and theoretical aspects. New York: Harper & Row.

Beck, A. T. (1972). *Depression: Causes and treatment.* Philadelphia: University of Pennsylvania Press.

Beck, A. T. (1976). *Cognitive therapy and the emotional disorders.* New York: International Universities Press.

Beck, A. T., & Shaw, B. F. (1977). Cognitive approaches to depression. In A. Ellis & R. Grieger (Eds.), *Handbook of rational-emotive therapy* (pp. 119–134). New York: Springer.

Beier, G. W. (1966). *The silent language of psychotherapy.* Chicago: Adline.

Belkin, G. S. (1980). *An introduction to counseling.* Dubuque, IA: Wm. C. Brown.

Benjamin, A. (1974). *The helping interview* (2nd ed.). Boston: Houghton Mifflin.

Benoit, R. B., & Mayer, G. R. (1974). Extinction: Guidelines for its selection and use. *Personnel and Guidance Journal, 52,* 290–295.

Benoit, R. B., & Mayer, G. R. (1976). Extinction and timeout: Guidelines for their selection and use. In G. S. Belkin (Ed.), *Counseling: Directions in theory and practice* (pp. 179–189). Dubuque, IA: Kendall/Hunt.

Berenson, B. G., & Carkhuff, R. R. (1967). *Sources of gain in counseling and psychotherapy.* New York: Holt, Rinehart and Winston.

Berne, E. (1964). *Games people play.* New York: Grove Press.

Berne, E. (1966). *Principles of group treatment.* New York: Oxford University Press.

Berne, E. (1972). *What do you say after you say hello?* New York: Grove Press.

Bordin, E. S. (1968). *Psychological counseling.* New York: Appleton-Century-Crofts.

Boudin, H. M. (1972). Contingency contracting as a therapeutic tool in the deceleration of amphetamine use. *Journal of Applied Behavioral Analysis, 3,* 604–608.

Boy, A. V., & Pine, G. J. (1982). *Client-centered counseling: A renewal.* Boston: Allyn and Bacon.

Brammer, L. (1973). *The helping relationship: Process and skills.* Englewood Cliffs, NJ: Prentice-Hall.

Brammer, L. M., & Shostrom, E. L. (1982). *Therapeutic psychology: Fundamentals of counseling and psychotherapy* (4th ed.). Englewood Cliffs, NJ: Prentice-Hall.

Bryer, J. W., & Egan, G. (1979). *Training the skilled helper.* Monterey, CA: Brooks/Cole.

Bugental, J. F. T. (1965). *The search for authenticity: An existential-analytic approach to psychotherapy.* New York: Holt, Rinehart, and Winston.

Bugental, J. F. T. (1969). Someone needs to worry: The existential anxiety of responsibility and decision. *Journal of Contemporary Psychotherapy, 2,* 41–53.

Bugental, J. F. T. (1976). *The search for existential identity.* San Francisco: Jossey-Bass.

Bugg, C. A. (1972). Systematic desensitization: A technique worth trying. *Personnel and Guidance Journal, 50,* 823–828.

Burgum, T., & Anderson, S. (1975). *The counselor and the law.* Washington, D.C.: APGA Press.

Burns, D. D. (1980). *Feeling good: The new mood therapy.* New York: The New American Library.

Burr, W. R., Mead, D. E., & Rollins, B. C. (1973). A model for the application of research findings by the educator and counselor: Research to theory to practice. *Family Coordinator, 22,* 285–290.

Camus, A. (1942). *The stranger.* New York: Random House.

Camus, A. (1958). *The myth of Sisyphus.* New York: Knopf.

Cantrell, R. P., Cantrell, M. L., Huddleston, C. M., & Woolridge, R. L. (1969). Contingency contracting with school problems. *Journal of Applied Behavioral Analysis, 2,* 215–220.

Carkhuff, R. R. (1969). *Helping and human relations: Vol. 1. Selection and training.* New York: Holt, Rinehart and Winston. (a)

Carkhuff, R. R. (1969). *Helping and human relations:*

Vol. 2. Practice and research. New York: Holt, Rinehart and Winston. (b)

Carkhuff, R. R. (1971). *The development of human resources.* New York: Holt, Rinehart and Winston.

Carkhuff, R. R. (1972). *The art of helping.* Amherst, MA: Human Resource Development Press. (a)

Carkhuff, R. R. (1972). The development of a systematic human resource development model. *The Counseling Psychologist, 3,* 4–30. (b)

Carkhuff, R. R. (1973). *The art of problem-solving.* Amherst, MA: Human Resource Development Press.

Carkhuff, R. R., & Anthony, W. A. (1979). *The skills of helping: An introduction to counseling.* Amherst, MA: Human Resource Development Press.

Carkhuff, R. R., & Berenson, B. G. (1967). *Beyond counseling and therapy.* New York: Holt, Rinehart and Winston.

Carkhuff, R. R., & Berenson, B. G. (1976). *Teaching as treatment.* Amherst, MA: Human Resource Development Press.

Carkhuff, R. R., & Berenson, B. G. (1977). *Beyond counseling and therapy* (2nd ed.). New York: Holt, Rinehart and Winston.

Chambless, D. L., & Goldstein, A. J. (1979). In R. J. Corsini (Ed.), *Current psychotherapies* (2nd ed.) (pp. 230–272). Itasca, IL: Peacock.

Ciminero, A., Nelson, R., & Lipinski, D. (1977). Self-monitoring procedures. In A. Ciminero, H. Calhoun, & H. Adams (Eds.), *Handbook of behavioral assessment.* New York: Wiley.

Conyne, R. K. (1977). Ecological counselor education: Tonic for a lethargic profession. *Counselor Education and Supervision, 16,* 310–313.

Corey, G. (1977). *Theory and practice of counseling and psychotherapy.* Monterey, CA: Brooks/Cole.

Corey, G. (1982). *Theory and practice of counseling and psychotherapy* (2nd ed.). Monterey, CA: Brooks/Cole.

Corey, G., Corey, M. S., & Callanan, P. (1984). *Issues and ethics in the helping professions* (2nd ed.). Monterey, CA: Brooks/Cole.

Cormier, L. S., & Cormier, W. H. (1975). *Behavioral counseling: Operant procedures, self-management strategies, and recent innovations.* Boston: Houghton Mifflin.

Cormier, W. H., & Cormier, L. S. (1979). *Interviewing strategies for helpers: A guide to assessment, treatment, and evaluation.* Monterey, CA: Brooks/Cole.

Corrigan, J. D., Dell, D. M., Lewis, K. N., & Schmidt, L. D. (1980). Counseling as a social influence process: A review. *Journal of Counseling Psychology Monograph, 27,* 395–431.

Cozby, P. C. (1973). Self-disclosure: A literature review. *Psychological Bulletin, 79,* 73–91.

Cronbach, L. J. (1970). *Essentials of psychological testing* (3rd ed.). New York: Harper & Row.

Daher, D. M., & Banikiotes, P. G. (1976). Interpersonal attraction and rewarding aspects of disclosure content and level. *Journal of Personality and Social Psychology, 33,* 492-496.

Daubner, E. V., & Daubner, E. S. (1970). Ethics and counseling decisions. *Personnel and Guidance Journal, 48,* 433–436.

Davis, J. W. (1981). Counselor licensure: Overkill? *Personnel and Guidance Journal, 60,* 83–85.

Day, R. W., & Sparacio, R. T. (1980). Structuring the counseling process. *Personnel and Guidance Journal, 59,* 246–249.

DeKraai, M. B., & Sales, B. D. (1982). Privileged communications of psychologists. *Professional Psychology, 13,* 372–388.

Dell, D. M., & Schmidt, L. D. (1976). Behavioral cues to counselor expertness. *Journal of Counseling Psychology, 23,* 197–201.

Denkowski, K. M., & Denkowski, G. C. (1982). Client-counselor confidentiality: An update. *Personnel and Guidance Journal, 60,* 371–375.

Dimond, R. E., Havens, R. E., & Jones, A. C. (1978). A conceptual framework for the practice of prescriptive eclecticism in psychotherapy. *American Psychologist, 33,* 239–248.

Dinkmeyer, D. C., Pew, W. L., & Dinkmeyer, D. C., Jr. (1979). *Adlerian counseling and psychotherapy.* Monterey, CA: Brooks/Cole.

Doster, J. A., & Nesbitt, J. G. (1979). Psychotherapy and self-disclosure. In G. J. Chelune (Ed.), *Self-disclosure: Origins, patterns, and implications of openness in interpersonal relationships,* San Francisco: Jossey-Bass.

Dryfus, E. A. (1971). *An existential approach to counseling.* In E. Beck (Ed.), *Philosophical guidelines for counseling.* Dubuque, IA: Wm. C. Brown.

Dusay, J., & Dusay, K. M. (1979). Transactional analysis. In R. Corsini (Ed.), *Current psychotherapies* (2nd ed.) (pp. 374–427). Itasca, IL: Peacock.

Dworkin, S. (1984). Traditionally defined client, meet feminist therapist: Feminist therapy as attitude change. *Personnel and Guidance Journal, 62,* 301–305.

Dyer, W. W., & Vriend, J. (1977). A goal-setting checklist for counselors. *Personnel and Guidance Journal, 55,* 469–471.

Egan, G. (1975). *The skilled helper: A model for systematic helping and interpersonal relating.* Monterey, CA: Brooks/Cole.

Egan, G. (1976). *Interpersonal living: A skills/contract approach to human relations training in groups.* Monterey, CA: Brooks/Cole.

Egan, G. (1982). *The skilled helper: model, skills, and methods for effective helping* (2nd ed.). Monterey, CA: Brooks/Cole.

Eisenberg, S., & Delaney, D. J. (1977). *The counseling process* (2nd ed.). Chicago: Rand McNally.

Ellis, A. (1962). *Reason and emotion in psychotherapy.* New York: Lyle Stuart.

Ellis, A. (1965). Showing clients they are not worthless individuals. *Voices, 2,* 74–77.

Ellis, A. (1971). Emotional disturbance and its treatment in a nutshell. *Canadian Counselor, 5,* 168–171.

Ellis, A. (1973). *Humanistic psychotherapy.* New York: McGraw-Hill.

Ellis, A. (1977). The basic clinical theory of rational-emotive therapy. In A. Ellis & R. Grieger (Eds.), *Handbook of rational-emotive therapy* (pp. 3–34). New York: Springer.

Ellis, A. (1982). Major systems. *Personnel and Guidance Journal, 61,* 6–7.

Ellis, A., & Grieger, R. (Eds.). (1977). *Handbook of rational-emotive therapy.* New York: Springer.

Erikson, E. H. (1963). *Childhood and society.* New York: Norton.

Evans, D. R., Hearn, M. T., Uhlemann, M. R., & Ivey, A. E. (1979). *Essential interviewing: A programmed approach to effective communication.* Monterey, CA: Brooks/Cole.

Everstine, L., Everstine, D. S., Heymann, G. M., True, R. H., Frey, D. H., Johnson, H. G., & Seiden, R. H. (1980). Privacy and confidentiality in psychotherapy. *American Psychologist, 35,* 828-840.

Eysenck, H. J. (1970). A mish-mash of theories. *International Journal of Psychiatry, 9,* 140–146.

Fay, A. (1976). The drug modality. In A. A. Lazarus (Ed.), *Multimodal behavior therapy* (pp. 65–85). New York: Springer.

Festinger, L. (1957). *A theory of cognitive dissonance.* Evanston, IL: Row-Peterson.

Foxx, R. M., & Azrin, N. H. (1973). The elimination of autistic self-stimulatory behavior by overcorrection. *Journal of Applied Behavior Analysis, 6,* 1–14.

Frank, J. D. (1973). *Persuasion and healing* (2nd ed.). Baltimore: Johns Hopkins University Press.

Frankl, V. (1959). *Man's search for meaning.* New York: Washington Square Press.

Fretz, B. R., & Mills, D. H. (1980). *Licensing and certification of psychologists and counselors.* San Francisco: Jossey-Bass.

Gambrill, E. D., & Richey, C. A. (1975). An assertion inventory for use in assessment and research. *Behavior Therapy, 6,* 550–561.

Garfield, S. L., & Kurtz, R. (1974). A survey of clinical psychologists: Characteristics, activities, and orientations. *The Clinical Psychologist, 28,* 7–10.

Garfield, S. L., & Kurtz, R. (1977). A study of eclectic views. *Journal of Consulting and Clinical Psychology, 45,* 78–83.

Gartner, A., & Riessman, F. (1977). *Self-help in the human services.* San Francisco: Jossey-Bass.

Gazda, G. M., Asbury, F. R., Balzer, F. J., Childers, W. C., & Walters, R. (1977). *Human relations development: A manual for educators.* Boston: Allyn & Bacon.

Gazda, G. M., Walters, R., & Childers, W. C. (1975). *Human relations development: A manual for health sciences.* Boston: Allyn & Bacon.

Gelatt, H., Varenhorst, B., Carey, R., & Miller, G. (1973). *Decisions and outcomes: A leader's guide.* Princeton, NJ: College Entrance Examination Board.

George, R. L., & Christiani, T. S. (1981). *Theory, methods, and processes of counseling and psychotherapy.* Englewood Cliffs, NJ: Prentice-Hall.

Gilbert, T. F. (1978). *Human competence: Engineering worthy performance.* New York: McGraw-Hill.

Gill, S. J. (1982). Professional disclosure and consumer protection in counseling. *Personnel and Guidance Journal, 60,* 443–446.

Gillis, P. (1980). The new-girl network. *Parents, 55,* 34, 36, 38, 40.

Glasser, W. (1965). *Reality therapy: A new approach to psychiatry.* New York: Harper & Row.

Glasser, W. (1972). *The identity society.* New York: Harper & Row.

Glasser, W., & Zunin, L. M. (1979). In R. Corsini (Ed.), *Current psychotherapies* (2nd ed.) (pp. 302–338). Itasca, IL: Peacock.

Goldfried, M. R., & Davison, G. C. (1976). *Clinical behavior therapy.* New York: Holt, Rinehart and Winston.

Goldman, L. (1978). Introduction and a point of view. In L. Goldman (Ed.), *Research methods for counselors.* New York: Wiley.

Goldstein, A. (1971). *Psychotherapeutic attraction.* New York: Pergamon.

Goldstein, A. (1973). Behavior therapy. In R. Corsini (Ed.), *Current psychotherapies.* Itasca, IL: Peacock.

Gottman, J. M., & Leiblum, S. R. (1974). *How to do psychotherapy and how to evaluate it.* New York: Holt, Rinehart and Winston.

Gould, R. (1972). The phases of adult life: A study in developmental psychology. *American Journal of Psychiatry, 129,* 521–531.

Goulding, M., & Goulding, R. (1979). *Changing lives through redecision therapy.* New York: Brunner/Mazel.

Groden, G., & Cautela, J. R. (1981). Behavior therapy: A survey of procedures for counselors. *Personnel and Guidance Journal, 60,* 175–180.

Gross, S. (1977). Professional disclosure: An alternative to licensure. *Personnel and Guidance Journal, 55,* 586–588.

Hackett, G., Horan, J. J., Stone, C., Linberg, S., Nicholas, W., & Lukaski, H. (1976). *Further outcomes and tentative predictor variables from an evolving comprehensive program for the behavioral control of smoking.* Paper presented at the annual meeting of the American Educational Research Association, San Francisco.

Hackney, H. L., & Nye, S. (1973). *Counseling strategies and objectives.* Englewood Cliffs, NJ: Prentice-Hall.

Hackney, H. L., & Cormier, L. S. (1979). *Counseling strategies and objectives (2nd ed.).* Englewood Cliffs, NJ: Prentice-Hall.

Haley, J. (1977). *Problem-solving therapy.* San Francisco: Jossey-Bass.

Hansen, J. C., Stevic, R. R., & Warner, R. W. (1982). *Counseling: Theory and process* (3rd ed.). Boston: Allyn and Bacon.

Hare-Mustin, R. T., Marecek, J., Kaplan, A. G., & Liss-Levinson, N. (1979). Rights of clients, responsibilities of therapists. *American Psychologist, 34,* 3–16.

Harmon, L. W. (1978). The counselor as consumer of research. In L. Goldman (Ed.), *Research methods for counselors.* New York: Wiley.

Harper, F. D. (1978). Outcomes of jogging: Implications for counseling. *Personnel and Guidance Journal, 57,* 74–78.

Harper, F. D. (1981). Biological foundations of behavior: Implications for counseling. *Personnel and Guidance Journal, 60,* 25–30.

Harris, T. (1967). *I'm ok, you're ok.* New York: Harper & Row.

Hasse, R. F., & Tepper, D. T. (1972). Nonverbal components of emphatic communication. *Journal of Counseling Psychology, 19,* 417–424.

Heidegger, M. (1962). *Being and time* (J. Macquarrie & E. Robinson, Trans.). London: SCM Press.

Herink, R. (Ed.). (1980). *The psychotherapy handbook.* New York: New American Library.

Hilgard, E. R., & Bower, G. H. (1966). *Theories of learning.* New York: Appleton.

Hosford, R. E. (1969). Behavioral counseling—A contemporary overview. *Counseling Psychologist, 1,* 1–33.

Hoveland, C. T., Janis, I. L., & Kelly, H. H. (1953). *Communication and persuasion: Psychological studies of opinion change.* New Haven, CT: Yale University Press.

Huber, C. H. (1983). A social-ecological approach to the counseling process. *AMHCA Journal, 5,* 4–11.

Hutchens, D. E. (1979). Systematic counseling: The T-F-A model for counselor intervention. *Personnel and Guidance Journal, 57,* 529–531.

Hutchens, D. E. (1982). Ranking major counseling strategies with the TFA matrix. *Personnel and Guidance Journal, 60,* 427–431.

Ivey, A. E. (1971). *Microcounseling: Innovations in interviewing training.* Springfield, IL: Charles C. Thomas.

Ivey, A. E. (1983). *Intention interviewing and counseling.* Monterey, CA: Brooks/Cole.

Ivey, A. E., & Authier, J. (1978). *Microcounseling* (2nd ed). Springfield, IL: Charles C. Thomas.

Ivey, A. E., & Gluckstern, N. (1976). *Basic influencing skills participant manual.* North Amherst, MA: Microtraining.

Ivey, A. E., & Simek-Downing, L. (1980). *Counseling and psychotherapy: Skills, theories, and practice.* Englewood Cliffs, NJ: Prentice-Hall.

Jacobson, E. (1938). *Progressive relaxation.* Chicago: University of Chicago Press.

James, M., & Jongeward, D. (1971). *Born to win: Transactional analysis with gestalt experiments.* Reading, MA: Addison-Wesley.

Johnson, D. W. (1981). *Reaching out: Interpersonal effectiveness and self-actualization* (2nd ed.). Englewood Cliffs, NJ: Prentice-Hall.

Johnson, M. (1976). An approach to feminist therapy. *Psychotherapy: Theory, Research and Practice, 13,* 72–76.

Jones, R. T., Nelson, R. E., & Kazdin, A. E. (1977). The role of external variables in self-reinforcement: A review. *Behavior Modification, 1,* 147–178.

Jongeward, D., & James, M. (1973). *Winning with people:*

Group exercises in transactional analysis. Reading, MA: Addison-Wesley.

Jourard, S. (1971). *The transparent self* (Rev. ed.). New York: Van Nostrand Reinhold.

Kadushin, A. (1973). *Supervision in social work.* New York: Columbia University Press.

Kagan, N. (1973). Can technology help us toward reliability in influencing human interaction? *Educational Technology, 13,* 44–51.

Kanfer, F. H. (1975). Self-management methods. In F. H. Kanfer & A. P. Goldstein (Eds.), *Helping people change.* New York: Pergamon Press.

Kanfer, F. H., & Karoly, P. (1972). Self-control: A behavioristic excursion into the lion's den. *Behavior Therapy, 3,* 398–416.

Kazdin, A. (1973). Covert modeling and the reduction of avoidance behavior. *Journal of Abnormal Psychology, 81,* 89–95.

Kazdin, A. (1974). Comparative effects of some variations of covert modeling. *Journal of Behavior Therapy and Experimental Psychiatry, 5,* 225–231.

Kazdin, A. (1975). *Behavior modification in applied settings.* Homewood, IL: Dorsey Press.

Kazdin, A. (1977). Assessing the clinical or applied importance of behavior change through social validation. *Behavior Modification, 1,* 427–452.

Kazdin, A. (1978). *History of behavior modification: Experimental foundations of contemporary research.* Baltimore: University Park Press.

Keith, D. V., & Whitaker, C. A. (1980). Experiential/symbolic family therapy. In A. S. Gurman & D. P. Kniskern (Eds.), *Handbook for family therapy.* New York: Brunner/Mazel.

Kelly, G. (1955). *The psychology of personal constructs.* New York: Norton.

Kemp, C. G. (1971). Existential counseling. *The Counseling Psychologist, 2,* 2–30.

Kemp, C. G. (1976). Existential counseling. In G. S. Belkin (Ed.), *Counseling directions in theory and practice* (pp. 109–144). Dubuque, IA: Kendall/Hunt.

Kempe, C. H., & Helfer, R. E. (Eds.). (1980). *Child abuse and neglect: The family and the community* (2nd ed.). Cambridge, MA: Ballinger.

Kempler, W. (1973). Gestalt therapy. In R. Corsini (Ed.), *Current psychotherapies.* Itasca, IL: Peacock.

Kerr, B. A., & Dell, D. M. (1976). Perceived interviewer expertness and attractiveness: Effects of interviewer behavior and attire and interview setting. *Journal of Counseling Psychology, 23,* 553–556.

Kimmel, D. (1974). *Adulthood and aging.* New York: Wiley.

Kirman, W. J. (1977). *Modern psychoanalysis in the schools.* Dubuque, IA: Kendall/Hunt.

Klein, M. J. (1976). Feminist concepts of therapy outcome. *Psychotherapy: Theory, Research and Practice, 12,* 89–95.

Knapp, M. L. (1978). *Nonverbal communication in human interaction* (2nd ed.). New York: Holt, Rinehart and Winston.

Knapp, S. (1980). A primer on malpractice for psychologists. *Professional Psychology, 11,* 606–612.

Knapp, S., & Vandecreek, L. (1982). Tarasoff: Five years later. *Professional Psychology, 13,* 511–516.

Kronsky, B. J. (1971). Feminism and psychotherapy. *Journal of Contemporary Psychotherapy, 3,* 89–98.

Krumboltz, J. D. (1966). Promoting adaptive behavior. In J. D. Krumboltz (Ed.), *Revolution in counseling: Implications of behavioral science.* Boston: Houghton Mifflin.

Krumboltz, J. D. (1980). A second look at the revolution in counseling. *The Personnel and Guidance Journal, 58,* 463–466.

Krumboltz, J. D., & Thoresen, C. E. (1976). *Counseling methods.* New York: Holt, Rinehart and Winston.

Kurpius, D., & Robinson, S. E. (1978). An overview of consultation. *Personnel and Guidance Journal, 56,* 321–323.

L'Abate, L. (1981). Classification of counseling therapy theorists, methods, processes, and goals: The E-R-A model. *Personnel and Guidance Journal, 59,* 263–265.

LaCrosse, M. B. (1975). Nonverbal behavior and perceived counselor attractiveness and persuasiveness. *Journal of Counseling Psychology, 22,* 563–566.

Latner, J. (1973). *The gestalt therapy book.* New York: Julian Press.

Lazarus, A. A. (1977). Has behavior therapy outlived its usefulness? *American Psychologist, 32,* 550–554.

Lazarus, A. A. (1981). *The practice of multimodal therapy.* New York: McGraw-Hill.

Leaman, D. (1973). The counselor's use of existential sharing in a synergistic relationship. *Counseling and Values, 18,* 40–44.

Levitsky, A., & Perls, F. S. (1970). The rules and games of gestalt therapy. In J. Fagan & I. L. Shepherd (Eds.), *Gestalt therapy now* (pp. 140–149). Palo Alto, CA: Science and Behavior Books.

Lewis, E. C. (1970). *The psychology of counseling.* New York: Holt, Rinehart and Winston.

Lewis, J., & Lewis, M. (1977). *Community counseling: A human services approach.* New York: Wiley.

Lewis, W. A., & Hutson, S. P. (1983). The gap between research and practice on the question of counseling effectiveness. *Personnel and Guidance Journal, 61,* 532–535.

Lieberman, R. P., Wheeler, E. G., deVisser, L., Kuehnel, J., & Kuehnel, T. (1980). *Handbook of marital therapy.* New York: Plenum.

Luft, J. (1970). *Group processes: An introduction to group dynamics.* Palo Alto, CA: National Press Books.

Mahoney, M. J. (1974). *Cognition and behavior modification.* Cambridge, MA: Ballinger.

Mahoney, M. J. (1977). Some applied issues in self-monitoring. In J. D. Cone & R. P. Hawkins (Eds.), *Behavioral assessment: New directions in clinical psychology.* New York: Brunner/Mazel.

Mahoney, M. J., & Thoresen, C. E. (Eds.). (1974). *Self-control: Power to the person.* Monterey, CA: Brooks/Cole.

Mann, R. A. (1972). The behavior-therapeutic use of contingency contracting to control an adult behavior problem: Weight control. *Journal of Applied Behavior Analysis, 5,* 99–109.

Mann, B., & Murphy, K. C. (1975). Timing of self-disclosure, reciprocity of self-disclosure, and reactions as to initial interview. *Journal of Counseling Psychology, 22,* 304–308.

Marlett, G. A., & Perry, M. A. (1980). Modeling methods. In F. H. Kanfer & A. P. Goldstein (Eds.), *Helping people change.* New York: Pergamon Press.

Maultsby, M. C. (1975). *Help yourself to happiness.* New York: Institute for Rational Living.

May, R. (1953). *Man's search for himself.* New York: Dell (Delta).

May, R. (1958). The origins and significance of the existential movement in psychology. In R. May, E. Angel, & H. Ellenberger (Eds.), *Existence* (pp. 3-36). New York: Basic Books

May, R. (Ed.). (1961). *Existential psychology.* New York: Random House.

May, R. (1969). *Love and will.* New York: Norton.

May, R. (1967). *Psychology and the human dilemma.* Princeton, NJ: Van Nostrand.

Meador, B. D., & Rogers, C. (1979). Person-centered therapy. In R. Corsini (Ed.), *Current psychotherapies* (2nd ed.) (pp. 131–184). Itasca, IL: F. E. Peacock.

Mehrabian, A. (1971). *Silent messages.* Belmont, CA: Wadsworth.

Meichenbaum, D. (1977). *Cognitive behavior modification.* New York: Plenum.

Merluzzi, T., Banikiotes, P. G., & Missbach, J. W. (1978). Perceptions of counselor characteristics: Contributions of counselor sex, experience, and disclosure level. *Journal of Counseling Psychology, 25,* 479–482.

Merluzzi, T., Merluzzi, B. H., & Kaul, T. J. (1977). Counselor race and power base: Effects on attitudes and behavior. *Journal of Counseling Psychology, 24,* 430–436.

Moos, R. (1973). Conceptualization of human environments. *American Psychologist, 28,* 652–665.

Moos, R. (1974). *Evaluating treatment environments: A social ecological approach.* New York: Wiley.

Morse, S. J., Watson, R. I. (Eds.). (1977). *Psychotherapies: A comparative casebook.* New York: Holt, Rinehart and Winston.

Murphy, K. C., & Strong, S. R. (1972). Some effects of similarity self-disclosure. *Journal of Counseling Psychology, 19,* 121–124.

National Association of Social Workers. (1979). *Code of ethics.* Washington, D.C.: Author.

Nay, W. R. (1977). Analogue measures. In A. Ciminero, K. Calhoun, & H. Adams (Eds.), *Handbook of behavioral assessment.* New York: Wiley.

Neugarten, B. L. (1977). Adaptation and the life cycle. In N. K. Schlossberg & A. D. Entine (Eds.), *Counseling adults* (pp. 34–46). Monterey, CA: Brooks/Cole.

Nye, L. S. (1973). Obtaining results through modeling. *Personnel and Guidance Journal, 51,* 380–384.

Okun, B. F. (1976). *Effective helping: Interviewing and counseling techniques.* North Scituate, MA: Duxbury Press.

Okun, B. F. (1982). *Effective helping: Interviewing and counseling techniques* (2nd ed). Monterey, CA: Brooks/Cole.

Passons, W. R. (1975). *Gestalt approaches in counseling.* New York: Holt, Rinehart and Winston.

Patterson, C. H. (1969). A current view of client-centered or relationship therapy. *The Counseling Psychologist, 1,* 2–24.

Patterson, C. H. (1973). *Theories of counseling and psychotherapy* (2nd ed.). New York: Harper & Row.

Patterson, L. E., & Eisenberg, S. (1983). *The counseling process* (3rd ed.). Boston: Houghton Mifflin.

Perls, F. S. (1969). *Gestalt therapy verbatim.* Moab, Utah: Real People Press.

Phillips-Jones, L. (1982). *Mentors and proteges.* New York: Arbor House.

Pietrofesa, J. J., Hoffman, A., Splete, H. H., & Pinto, D. V. (1978). *Counseling: Theory, research and practice.* Chicago: Rand McNally.

Polster, E., & Polster, M. (1973). *Gestalt therapy integrated: Contours of theory and practice.* New York: Brunner/Mazel.

Ponzo, Z. (1976). Integrating techniques from five counseling theories. *Personnel and Guidance Journal, 54,* 415–419.

Premack, D. (1965). Reinforcement theory. In D. Levine (Ed.), *Nebraska symposium on motivation.* Lincoln: University of Nebraska Press.

Rachin, R. L. (1974). Reality therapy: Helping people help themselves. *Crime and Delinquency, 20,* 45–53.

Rachlin, H. (1970). *Introduction to modern behaviorism.* San Francisco: W. H. Freeman.

Radov, C. G., Masnick, B. R., & Hauser, B. R. (1977). Issues in feminist therapy: The work of a women's study group. *Social Work, 22,* 507–509.

Raimy, V. (1975). *Misunderstandings of the self: Cognitive psychotherapy and the misconception hypothesis.* San Francisco: Jossey-Bass.

Rawlins, M. E., & Rawlins, L. (1983). Mentoring and networking for helping professionals. *Personnel and Guidance Journal, 62,* 116–118.

Remer, R. (1981). The counselor and research: Introduction. *Personnel and Guidance Journal, 59,* 567–571.

Repp, A. C., & Dietz, S. M. (1974). Reducing aggressive and self-injurious behavior of institutionalized retarded children through reinforcement of other behaviors. *Journal of Applied Behavior Analysis, 7,* 313–325.

Rimm, D. C., & Masters, J. C. (1979). *Behavior therapy: Techniques and empirical findings* (2nd ed.). New York: Academic Press.

Rogers, C. (1942). *Counseling and psychotherapy.* Boston: Houghton Mifflin.

Rogers, C. (1951). *Client-centered therapy.* Boston: Houghton Mifflin.

Rogers, C. (1957). The necessary and sufficient conditions of therapeutic personality change. *Journal of Consulting Psychology, 21,* 95–103. (a)

Rogers, C. (1957). A note on "the nature of man." *Journal of Counseling Psychology, 4,* 199–203. (b)

Rogers, C. (1959). A theory of therapy, personality, and interpersonal relationships as developed in the client-centered framework. In S. Koch (Ed.), *Psychology: A study of a science: Vol. III. Formulations of the person and the social context.* New York: McGraw-Hill.

Rogers, C. (1961). *On becoming a person.* Boston: Houghton Mifflin.

Rogers, C. (1967). The conditions of change from a client-centered viewpoint. In B. Berenson & R. Carkhuff (Eds.), *Sources of gain in counseling and psychotherapy.* New York: Holt, Rinehart and Winston.

Rogers, C. (1970). *Carl Rogers on encounter groups.* New York: Harper & Row.

Rogers, C. (1972). *Becoming partners: Marriage and its alternatives.* New York: Delacorte.

Rogers, C. (1975). Empathic: An unappreciated way of being. *The Counseling Psychologist, 5,* 2–10.

Rogers, C. (1976). The interpersonal relationship: The core of guidance. In G. S. Belkin (Ed.), *Counseling directions in theory and practice* (pp. 96–108). Dubuque, IA: Kendall/Hunt.

Rogers, C. (1977). *Carl Rogers on personal power: Inner strength and its revolutionary impact.* New York: Delacorte.

Rogers, C., Gendlin, E. T., Kiessler, D., & Truax, C. B. (1967). *The therapeutic relationship and its impact.* Madison: University of Wisconsin Press.

Rose, S. D. (1973). *Treating children in groups: A behavioral approach.* San Francisco: Jossey-Bass.

Rosen, G. M. (1976). Subjects' initial therapeutic expectancies and subjects' awareness of therapeutic goals in systematic desensitization: A review. *Behavior Therapy, 7,* 14–27.

Rosen, S. (1972). Recent experiences with gestalt, encounter, and hypnotic techniques. *American Journal of Psychoanalysis, 32,* 90–102.

Rosenthal, T. (1976). Modeling therapies. In M. Hersen, R. Eisler, & P. Miller (Eds.), *Progress in behavior modification* (Vol. 2). New York: Academic Press.

Russell, R. K., & Sipich, J. F. (1973). Cue-controlled relaxation in the treatment of test anxiety. *Journal of Behavior Therapy and Experimental Psychiatry, 4,* 47–49.

Saral, T. B. (1972). Cross-cultural generality of communication via facial expressions. *Comparative Group Studies, 3,* 473–486.

Sartre, J. (1946). *No exit.* New York: Knopf.

Sartre, J. (1956). *Being and nothingness.* London: Methuen.

Schaefer, H. H. (1976). Treatment for exhibitionism. In J. D. Krumboltz & C. E. Thoresen (Eds.), *Counseling methods* (pp. 226–234). New York: Holt, Rinehart and Winston.

Scheid, A. B. (1976). Clients' perception of the counselor: The influence of counselor introduction and behavior. *Journal of Counseling Psychology, 23,* 503–508.

Schmidt, J. A., & Wolfe, J. S. (1980). The mentor partnership: Discovery of professionalism. *NASPA Journal, 17,* 45–51.

Schmidt, L. D., & Strong, S. R. (1971). Attractiveness and influence in counseling. *Journal of Counseling Psychology, 18,* 348–351.

Schultz, B. (1982). *Legal liability in psychotherapy.* San Francisco: Jossey-Bass.

Shaefer, A. B. (1981). Clinical supervision. In E. E. Walker (Ed.), *Clinical practice of psychology: A guide for mental health professionals* (pp. 50–61). New York: Pergamon Press.

Shaffer, B. P. (1978). *Humanistic psychology.* Englewood Cliffs, NJ: Prentice-Hall.

Shah, S. (1969). Privileged communications, confidentiality, and privacy: Privileged communications. *Professional Psychology, 1,* 56–69.

Shah, S. (1970). Privileged communications, confidentiality, and privacy: Confidentiality. *Professional Psychology, 1,* 159–164.

Shapiro, M. B. (1966). The single case in clinical psychological research. *Journal of General Psychology, 74,* 3–23.

Shaw, B. F., & Beck, A. T. (1977). The treatment of depression with cognitive therapy. In A. Ellis & R. Grieger (Eds.), *Handbook of rational-emotive therapy* (pp. 309–326). New York: Springer.

Shepherd, I. E. (1970). Limitations and cautions in the gestalt approach. In J. Fagan & I. L. Shepherd (Eds.), *Gestalt therapy now* (pp. 234–238). Palo Alto, CA: Science and Behavior Books.

Shertzer, B., & Stone, S. C. (1974). *Fundamentals of counseling.* Boston: Houghton Mifflin.

Shimberg, B. (1981). Testing for licensure and certification. *American Psychologist, 36,* 1138–1146.

Skinner, B. F. (1953). *Science and human behavior.* New York: Macmillan.

Slovenko, R. (1973). *Psychiatry and the law.* Boston: Little, Brown.

Sprafkin, R. P. (1970). Communicator expertness and changes in word meaning in psychological treatment. *Journal of Counseling Psychology, 17,* 191–196.

Sprinthall, N. (1971). *Guidance for human growth.* New York: Van Nostrand Reinhold.

Stedman, J. M. (1976). Family counseling with a school-phobic child. In J. D. Krumboltz & C. E. Thoresen (Eds.), *Counseling methods* (pp. 280–288). New York: Holt, Rinehart and Winston.

Steinman, A. (1974). Cultural values, female role expectancies and therapeutic goals: Research and interpretation. In V. Granks & V. Burtle (Eds.), *Women in therapy* (pp. 51–82). New York: Brunner/Mazel.

Stewart, N. R., Winborn, B. B., Johnson, R. G., Burks, H. M., & Engelkes, J. R. (1978). *Systematic counseling.* Englewood Cliffs, NJ: Prentice-Hall.

Strickland, B. (1969). The philosophy-theory-practice continuum. *Counselor Education and Supervision, 8,* 165–175.

Strong, S. R. (1968). Counseling: An interpersonal influence process. *Journal of Counseling Psychology, 15,* 215–224.

Strong, S. R., & Matross, R. P. (1973). Change process in counseling and psychotherapy. *Journal of Counseling Psychology, 20,* 25-37.

Strong, S. R., & Schmidt, L. D. (1970). Expertness and influence in counseling. *Journal of Counseling Psychology, 17,* 81–87. (a)

Strong, S. R., & Schmidt, L. D. (1970). Trustworthiness and influence in counseling. *Journal of Counseling Psychology, 17,* 197–204. (b)

Stuart, R. B. (1971). Behavioral contracting within the families of delinquents. *Journal of Behavior Therapy and Experimental Psychiatry, 2,* 1–11.

Stuart, R. B. (1980). *Helping couples change.* New York: Guilford.

Stude, E. W., & McKelvey, J. (1979). Ethics and the law: Friend or foe? *Personnel and Guidance Journal, 57,* 453–456.

Swan, G. E. (1979). On the structure of eclecticism: Cluster analysis of eclectic behavior therapists. *Professional Psychology, 10,* 732–739.

Swanson, J. L. (1979). Counseling directory and consumer's guide: Implementing professional disclosure and consumer protection. *Personnel and Guidance Journal, 58,* 190–193.

Talbutt, L. C. (1981). Ethical standards: Assets and limitations. *Personnel and Guidance Journal, 60,* 110–112.

Tasto, D. L. (1977). Self-report schedules and inventories. In A. Ciminero, K. Calhoun, & H. Adams (Eds.), *Handbook of behavioral assessment.* New York: Wiley.

Thomas, S. A. (1977). Theory and practice in feminist therapy. *Social Work, 22,* 447–454.

Thoresen, C. E., & Coates, T. J. (1980). What does it mean to be a behavior therapist? In C. E. Thoresen (Ed.). *The behavior therapist.* Monterey, CA: Brooks/Cole.

Thorne, F. C. (1973). Eclectic psychotherapy. In R. Corsini (Ed.), *Current psychotherapies.* Itasca, IL: Peacock.

Toffler, A. (1970). *Future shock.* New York: Random House.

Toffler, A. (1980). *The Third wave.* New York: William Morrow.

Tricket, E. J., & Todd, D. M. (1973). High school culture: An ecological perspective. *Journal of Theory into Practice, 11,* 28–37.

Truax, C. B., & Carkhuff, R. R. (1967). *Toward effective counseling and psychotherapy: Training and practice.* Chicago: Aldine.

Truax, C. B., & Mitchell, K. M. (1971). Research on certain therapist interpersonal skills in relation to process and outcome. In A. E. Bergin & S. L. Garfield (Eds.), *Hand-book of psychotherapy and behavior change.* New York: Wiley.

Turock, A. (1980). Immediacy in counseling: Recognizing clients' unspoken messages. *Personnel and Guidance Journal, 59,* 168–172.

Vance, B. (1976). Using contracts to control weight and improve cardiovascular physical fitness. In J. D. Krumboltz & C. E. Thoresen (Eds.), *Counseling methods* (pp. 527–541). New York: Holt, Rinehart and Winston.

Van Hoose, W. H., & Kottler, J. (1978). *Ethical and legal issues in counseling and psychotherapy.* San Francisco: Jossey-Bass.

Walen, S. R., DiGiuseppe, R., & Wessler, R. L. (1980). *A practitioner's guide to rational-emotive therapy.* New York: Oxford University Press.

Ward, D. E. (1983). The trend toward eclecticism and the development of comprehensive models to guide counseling and psychotherapy. *Personnel and Guidance Journal, 62,* 154–157.

Watson, D., & Tharp, R. (1981). *Self-directed behavior* (3rd ed.). Monterey, CA: Brooks/Cole.

Watson, R. I., & Morse, S. J. (1977). An introduction to psychotherapy. In S. J. Morse & R. I. Watson (Eds.), *Psychotherapies: A comparative casebook* (pp. 1–14). New York: Holt, Rinehart and Winston.

Weathers, L., & Lieberman, R. P. (1975). The family contracting exercise. *Journal of Behavior Therapy and Experimental Psychiatry, 6,* 208–214.

Welch, M. S. (1980). *Networking: The great way for women to get ahead.* New York: Harcourt Brace Jovanovich.

Wessler, R. L. (1982). Varieties of cognitions in the cognitively-oriented psychotherapies. *Rational Living, 17,* 3-10.

Wessler, R. A., & Wessler, R. L. (1980). *The principles and practice of rational-emotive therapy.* San Francisco: Jossey-Bass.

Williams, R. L., Long, J. D., & Yoakley, R. W. (1972). The utility of behavior contracts and behavior proclamations with advanced senior high school students. *Journal of School Psychology, 10,* 329–338.

Williamson, E. G. (1962). The counselor as technique. *Personnel and Guidance Journal, 41,* 108–111.

Williamson, E. G. (1965). *Vocational counseling: Some historical, philosophical, and theoretical perspectives.* New York: McGraw-Hill.

Winborn, B. B. (1977). Honest labeling and other procedures for the protection of consumers of counseling. *Personnel and Guidance Journal, 56,* 206–209.

Wolpe, J. (1958). *Psychotherapy by reciprocal inhibition.* Stanford, CA: Stanford University Press.

Wolpe, J., & Lazarus, A. (1966). *Behavior therapy techniques.* New York: Pergamon Press.

Woolfolk, R. L. (1976). A multimodal perspective on emotion. In A. A. Lazarus (Ed.), *Multimodal behavior therapy* (pp. 48–64). New York: Springer.

Author Index

373

Subject Index